NANOPARTICULATE DRUG DELIVERY SYSTEMS FOR CANCER THERAPY

Sachin Naik

ACKNOWLEDGEMENTS

This thesis arose in part out of years of research that has been done since I came to Professor Ambikanandan Misra's group. By that time, I have worked with a great number of people whose contribution in assorted ways to the research and the making of the thesis deserved special mention. It is a pleasure to convey my gratitude to them all in my humble acknowledgment.

In the first place I owe my deepest gratitude to my mentor, Dr. Ambikanandan Misra, Professor in Pharmaceutics, Pharmacy Department, The Maharaja Sayajirao University of Baroda for his supervision, advice, and guidance from the very early stage of this research as well as giving me extraordinary experiences through out the work. Above all and the most needed, he provided me unflinching encouragement, requisite facilities, and support in various ways. His truly scientist intuition has made him as a constant oasis of ideas and passions in science, which exceptionally inspire and enrich my growth as a student, a researcher and a scientist want to be. I am indebted to him more than he knows.

I would like to record my gratitude to Professor Hamid Ghandehari, Departments of Pharmaceutics & Pharmaceutical Chemistry and Bioengineering, University of Utah, USA for providing supervision, financial support, lab facilities and guidance to complete my part of research work.

I shall like to thank Dr. R. Balaraman, Head and Professor, Pharmacy Department, The Maharaja Sayajirao University of Baroda for providing me the necessary facilities for the research work. Dr. M.R. Yadav, Professor in Pharmaceutical Chemistry, Dr. S.H. Mishra, Professor in Herbal Drug Technology, Dr. R.S.R. Murthy, Professor in Pharmaceutics, Dr. (Mrs.) Rajani Giridhar, Professor in Pharmaceutical Chemistry, Dr.

(Mrs.) K.K. Sawant, Professor in Pharmaceutics, Dr. (Mrs.) S.J. Rajput, Professor in Pharmaceutical Quality Assurance and Dr. R.C. Mashru, Reader of Pharmaceutical Quality Assurance, Pharmacy Department, The Maharaja Sayajirao University of Baroda for their invaluable support during the research work. My sincere thanks are due to the Dean, Faculty of Tech. and Engg. M.S. University of Baroda, for providing me necessary facilities.

I am extending my sincere thanks to Dr. Abhijit Ray, Research Assistant Professor, Dr. Alexander Malugin (Sasha) , Research Associate and Dr. Khaled Greish , Research Associte, Departments of Pharmaceutics & Pharmaceutical Chemistry and Bioengineering, University of Utah, for their advice, supervision, and crucial contribution, their involvement with their originality has triggered and nourished my intellectual maturity. I am grateful in every possible way and hope to keep up our collaboration in the future.

I am very thankful to University Grant Commission (UGC), New Delhi, India for awarding "Junior Research Fellowship" to me during research work.

I am extending my sincere thanks to American Association of Cancer Research for selecting my abstract and providing me financial support to attend the special conference at San Diego, California.

I also express my gratitude to Panacea Biotech Ltd, Lalru, and Torrent Research Center, Ahmedabad for providing me a partial financial support to complete my part of research work at University of Utah, USA.

I express my special thanks to my friend Mr. Mahavir Chougule, Post Doctoral research fellow, University of Florida, Mr. Bhagirath, Mr. Gaurang, and Mr. Umang shah and his family for their kind help and support.

I would to thank to my all colleagues, Dr. Pranav, Dr.Viral, Dr. Nazneen, Ms. Pinki, Mr. Hamsaraj, Mr. Yogesh, Mr. Kamal, Mr. Nirav, Mr. Bhavik, Mr. Divyen, Ms. Florence, Ms. Gitanjali, Mr. Prashant, Ms. Shraddha, Ms. Vijayalakshmi, Ms. Arnida, Ms. Tian, Mr. Phillip, Mr. Dan, Mr. Nat, Mr. Mak, Mr. Gagan, Mr. Hammad, Mr. Antony and Mr. Josh for their fruitful advice and constant co operation.

I take a special note of thanks to all office and Laboratory staff of the G. H. Patel Building and Pharmacy Department, Kalabhavan, M. S. University of Baroda, for their constant support during my studies. Thanks are also due to Office staff, Faculty of Tech. and Engg., and M. S. University of Baroda for there support and cooperation.

I am feeling out of word to code an appropriate thanks to parents. It was the love and indispensable support of my family who despite all inconvenience and typically perpetual insolence provided me with the best possible of every thing in my ascent to the present accomplishment. I take this opportunity to convey my special thank Ms. Deepa for her great support and help to fulfill the completion of my thesis work.

Last but not the least, I thank my spiritual Guru "Shri Asaramji Bapu" for empowering me with courage and strength to take up and accomplish the task.

Finally, my sincere apologies to all those; whose name could not be included in this section. No names have been intentionally missed out.

Sachin Naik

TABLE OF CONTENTS

LIST OF FIGURES

LIST OF TABLES

Chapter 1
Introduction

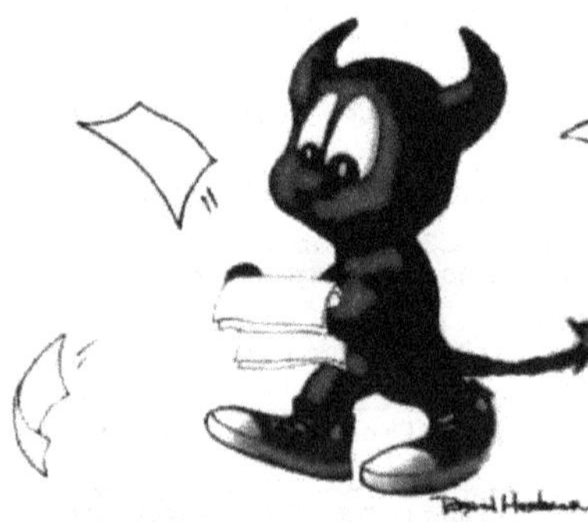

1.1. Introduction

Molecular medicine has discovered many new therapeutic modalities by using state-of-the-art techniques in molecular biology. High through-put, in-vitro assays that screen for pharmacological actions on the desired cell type are frequently used to design new drugs. Although such agents are certainly justified by their success in-vitro, they frequently perform much less effectively in-vivo where the agent must reach its target cells in a tissue in sufficient quantities to be potent while sparing bystander organs. Depending on the route of administration, the endothelium and/or epithelium form significant barriers that greatly limit the in-vivo accessibility of many drugs, antibodies, and gene vectors to their intended target sites of pharmacological action, namely, the cells inside the tissue (Jain, R. K. et al., 1998). Hence, the major challenge for formulation development scientist is to design drug delivery strategies that deliver the therapeutic agents to the desired intracellular targets based on ability to understand, utilize, modify and exploit membrane trafficking pathways (Miller, N. et al., 1995).

Intracellular drug delivery refers to the delivery of therapeutic agents to specific compartments or organelles within the cell. The therapeutic agent could be a low molecular weight drug or a macromolecule like protein or DNA. Thus targeted intracellular drug delivery results in higher bioavailability of a therapeutic agent at its site of action (i.e. distinct intracellular compartments or microenvironments), potentiates the pharmacologic effect of the drug, and at the same time, reduces the side effects. (Jayanth Panyam et al., 2004). There are a number of pathways through which a therapeutic agent or a carrier can enter a cell. Such as Endocytosis, Caveolar endocytosis, Pinocytosis, Phagocytosis, In receptor-mediated endocytosis, Folate Receptor-Mediated Endocytosis, Transferrin Receptor-Mediated Endocytosis, Biotin Receptor-Mediated Endocytosis, Wheat Germ Agglutinin-Mediated Endocytosis, ICAM-1-Mediated Endocytosis, Antibody-Mediated Endocytosis, Physical or mechanical methods use force to traverse the cell membrane, e.g. Particle bombardment accelerates ,Microinjection and Electroporation. The various Intracellular Targets are Endo-Lysosomal Targeting, Cytoplasmic Delivery, Nuclear Targeting, and Mitochondrial Targeting.

A number of different carriers have been used for targeting different organelles including viral vectors, cationic lipids, polymer conjugates, micelles, protein transduction domains, nanoparticles and liposomes.

Nanoparticles are defined as particulate dispersions or solid particles with a size in the range of 10-1000nm. The drug is dissolved, entrapped, encapsulated or attached to a nanoparticles matrix. Depending upon the method of preparation, nanoparticles, nanospheres or nanocapsules can be obtained. Nanocapsules are systems in which the drug is confined to a cavity surrounded by a unique polymer membrane, while nanospheres are matrix systems in which the drug is physically and uniformly dispersed. In recent years, biodegradable polymeric nanoparticles, particularly those coated with hydrophilic polymer such as poly(ethylene glycol) (PEG) known as long-circulating particles, have been used as potential drug delivery devices because of their ability to circulate for a prolonged period time target a particular organ, as carriers of DNA in gene therapy, and their ability to deliver proteins, peptides and genes. (Mohanraj, V.J. et al., 2006) Biodegradable nanoparticles for pharmaceutical use are prepared from a variety of synthetic and natural polymers. Synthetic polymers such as polyacrylates, polycaprolactones, polylactides and its copolymers with polyglycolides are widely used.

A wide spectrum of synthetic and natural polymers is available for nanoparticle formation, but their biocompatibility and biodegradability are the major limiting factors for their use in the drug delivery area. Natural polymers are more restricted due to variation in their purity. Also, some natural polymers require crosslinking, which can inactivate the entrapped drug (Hans, M.L. et al., 2002). Synthetic polymers, on the other hand, offer better reproducibility of the chemical characteristics of the synthesized nanoparticles as compared to the natural polymers. Synthetic polymers from the ester family, such as poly(lactic acid), poly(hydroxybutyrate), poly(caprolactone), poly(dioxanone), or other families such as poly(cyanoacrylates), poly(acrylic acid), poly(anhydrides), poly(amides), poly(ortho esters), poly(ethylene glycol), and poly(vinyl alcohol) are suitable for drug delivery due to their biodegradability, special release profiles and biocompatibility (Ghosh, S. et al., 2004). Poly(lactide-co-glycolide acid) (PLGA), from the ester family, has been widely used in the biomedical industry as a major components in biodegradable sutures, bone fixation nails and screw. It is a well-characterized polymer, its degradation sub products are non toxic, it provides controlled drug release profiles by changing the PLGA copolymer ratio which affects the crystallinity (low crystallinity, more amorphous polymer means more fast degradation) of PLGA (Moghimi, S.M. et al 2001). FDA approved biodegradable and biocompatible polymers, poly (D,L-lactide-*co*-glycolide) (PLGA) in the with a therapeutic agent encapsulated into the polymer is widely used for localized and sustained drug and macro-molecular delivery (Jayanth Panyama et al., 2003)

Two main procedures can be followed to form polymeric nanoparticles, namely top-down and bottom-up techniques. The top-down methods use size reduction to obtain controlled-size nanoparticles. This size reduction is based on the application of strong shear stress by wave sound emission (sonication), high pressure (microfluidization), and high speed agitation (homogenization). The bottom-up methods start from individual molecules to form nanoparticles, by polymerization. Liposomes are vesicles in which an aqueous volume is entirely enclosed by a membrane composed of lipid molecules, usually phospholipids. Spontaneously formed upon dispersion in aqueous media, the size of such vesicles can range from tens of nanometres to tens of microns in diameter. In pharmaceutical sciences, liposomes have been used traditionally as formulation ingredients to assist in formulation of poorly soluble therapeutic agents for oral or parenteral administration. Liposomes can be made of natural constituents. Their membrane is very similar to natural cell membranes and provides great convenience as models for membrane systems. Such naturally occurring constituents are cholesterol, phospholipids or fatty acids that make them a biocompatible and safe vehicle for medical *in vivo* applications. Those favourable properties can be adjusted by chemical modifications of the phospholipid-bilayer membrane of the liposome. Chemical modifications, such as saturation or pegylation of phospholipids are well established and numerous possibilities are described, which results in a vast versatility and flexibility of such phospholipid-bilayer membrane liposomes.

Conventional preparation of liposomes unfortunately involves evaporation of organic solvent, preparation of vesicles by sonication, and dialysis to provide Unilamellar vesicles. Use of SCF CO_2 to provide a "clean" and effective alternative to traditional methods of drug processing, related to micronization, encapsulation, and impregnation of molecules of interest to pharmaceutical industry; formation of micron sized particles with SCF CO2 by rapid expansion of supercritical solutions (RESS) or phase separation by gas saturated solutions (PGSS), gas antisolvent (GAS) techniques by solubilizing the drug in an organic solvent and introducing SCF to solubilize the solvent and allow the drug to precipitate and also incorporating drugs into controlled matrices; based on these techniques, nanoparticles of cyclosporine A in phospholipid and ibuprofen nanoparticles in aqueous solution were made. In the gas antisolvent (GAS) technique, in which the gas is used as an antisolvent to reduce the solvating power of the organic solvent, the ability of the SCFs to dissolve and expand the organic solvents for precipitation of solids from organic solution is exploited (Udaya Sankar Kadimi et al., 2007). Conventional drug particle precipitation uses organic solvents as antisolvents for precipitation or as emulsifiers for emulsion process. Traces of residual organic solvents, such as methylene chloride, that may still be in the drug particles have motivated researchers to find alternative methods for particle formation. Organic solvent use should be limited for pharmaceutical manufacturing operations, based on United States Pharmacopeia (USP) standards. An alternative to reduce this problem is to use supercritical carbon dioxide (CO_2) as an antisolvent to precipitate drug particles from solution since CO_2 is nonflammable, non-toxic, inexpensive, renewable, and environmentally benign (McHugh, M.A. et al., 1994).

Polymeric conjugates have been used for targeted delivery of drugs to tumor sites because the attachment of drugs to water soluble polymer increases their solubility, reduces the side effect, and overcomes multi-drug resistance; the large size of conjugates increases blood half life and significantly alters the drug properties and pharmacokinetics; the conjugates can be tailor-made (i.e., side-chain content, molecular weight, charge etc.) for specific targeting and delivery needs; they can be designed to passively (EPR) or actively target tumor sites; and site specific drug release can be achieved by designing biodegradable spacers that can be enzymatically cleaved or that are pH sensitive. The advantages have led to the development of a wide range of plolymer-anti-cancer drug conjugates, some of which are currently in clinical trials. One of the most promising systems is based on water soluble N-(2-hydroxypropyl) methacrylamide (HPMA). HPMA homopolymer was originally developed by Kopecek and colleagues as a plasma expander (Ruth Duncan et al., 2003) HPMA copolymers has been employed to modify the in vivo biodistribution of chemotherapeutics agents and enzymes. The advantage of HPMA copolymer over other water soluble polymers is that they can be tailor-made with simple chemical modification to regulate drug and targeting moiety content for biorecognization, internalization, or subcellular trafficking depending on specific therapeutics needs. The over all molecular weight of HPMA copolymers is determined by the polymerization conditions, particularly the concentration of initiator and chain transfer agents. Various side chain moieties (isotope chelator, targeting moieties and drug) may be directly linked to the polymer chain via a biodegradable or non-biodegradable spacer.

Polymeric based delivery systems have been used as carriers for passive and active targeting of drugs in the treatment of various diseases and as novel imagine agents. Without a specific targeting ligand moderate-size (> 30 kD) polymer can passively (*via* EPR) accumulate in tumor tissues. The EPR .effect has been used to deliver macromolecular bioactive agents to solid tumors including anti-angiogenic drugs. There are number of important differences between small molecular weight drugs and polymeric conjugates of these small molecules. The advantages of polymer-based delivery system stem decreased extravasation in normal tissues because of the large molecular weight of the conjugates. Low extravasation of polymer conjugates in normal tissues generally results in reduced systemic toxicity. In this regard, predominant liver and kidney uptake of small RGD peptides has been identified as a significant disadvantage of targeting tumor angiogenesis with small peptides.

Peptide-targeted delivery has a basis in nature as many peptides are used as attachment ligands by bacteria and viruses. A major objective in the design of functionalized polymer surfaces for tissue engineering applications has been the covalent attachment of peptides that regulate cell adhesion: specifically those that promote integrin-mediated cell attachment (Shakesheff, K.M. et al., 1998 and Rezania, A. et al., 1999). Since the vast majority of mammalian cells are anchorage-dependent, they must attach and spread on a substrate to proliferate and function normally (Madri, J.A. et al., 1988 and Baldwin, S.P. et al., 1998). By controlling the surface properties of the substrate, cell attachment and growth *in vitro* can be altered (Kim, B.S. et al., 1999). A great deal of work has focused on RGD containing peptides to regulate cell adhesion (Shakesheff, K.M. et al., 1998, Besselink, G.A.J, et al., 1998 and Chinn, J.A. et al., 1998). Peptides containing the RGD (R=arginine, G=glycine, D=aspartic acid) sequence are considered important small cell-adhesive ligands (Shakesheff, K.M. et al., 1998, Besselink, G.A.J, et al., 1998). This cell-binding sequence is present in adhesive proteins like fibrinogen, vitronectin, collagens, and fibronectin (Ruoslahti, E. et al., 1987). Membrane proteins of blood platelets, endothelial cells, and several other cell types can bind RGD-containing peptides whether the peptide is in solution or immobilized onto a solid surface (Hynes, R.O. et al., 1992 and Plow, E.F et al., 1986).

RGD-based therapeutics functions as agonists to promote the interaction of cells and tissues with artificial matrices, or as antagonists to control the nature of cell-cell and cell-ECM interactions (Craig, W. S. et al., 1995). At this state of the art many different

RGD peptides have been developed. Linear and cyclic RGD peptides, and chemically designed peptidomimeticsare currently being tested by researchers.

Breast cancers are potentially life-threatening malignancies that develop in one or both breasts. Breast cancer is either noninvasive (referred to as *in situ*, confined to the site of origin) or invasive (spreading).

Noninvasive breast cancers include

- Ductal carcinoma in situ (also called intraductal carcinoma or DCIS). DCIS consist of cancer cells in the lining of the duct. DCIS is a non-invasive, early cancer, but if left untreated, it may sometimes progress to an invasive, infiltrating ductal breast cancer. DCIS is the most common type of noninvasive breast cancer.
- Lobular carcinoma in situ, or LCIS. Although it is technically not a cancer, lobular carcinoma in situ is a marker for an increased risk of invasive cancer the same or both breasts.

A diagnosis of these early cancers (DCIS and LCIS) is made when there is no evidence of invasion.

Invasive Breast Cancer

Invasive cancer occurs when cancer cells spread beyond the basement membrane, which covers the underlying connective tissue in the breast. This tissue is rich in blood vessels and lymphatic channels that are capable of carrying cancer cells beyond the breast. Invasive breast cancers include the following:

- Invasive (also called infiltrating) ductal carcinoma. This is invasive breast cancer that penetrates the wall of a milk-passage duct. It comprises between 70 - 80% of all breast cancer cases.
- Invasive (also called infiltrating) lobular carcinoma. This invasive cancer has spread through the wall of a milk-producing lobule. It accounts for 10 ÷ 15% of all breast cancers. It may sometimes appear in both breasts, sometimes in several separate locations.

Docetaxel is a clinically well established anti-neoplastic medication used mainly for the treatment of breast, ovarian and non-small cell lung cancer. Docetaxel has an approved claim for treatment of patients who have locally advanced, or metastatic breast or non small-cell lung cancer who have undergone anthracycline-based chemotherapy and failed to stop cancer progression or relapsed. The cytotoxic activity of docetaxel is exerted by promoting and stabilising microtubule assembly, while preventing physiological microtubule depolymerisation/disassembly in the absence of guanosine triphosphate (GTP). This leads to a significant decrease in free tubulin, needed for microtubule formation and results in inhibition of mitotic cell division between metaphase and anaphase, preventing further cancer cell progeny.

The main mode of therapeutic action of docetaxel is the suppression of microtubule dynamic assembly and disassembly, rather than microtubule bundling leading to apoptosis, or the blocking of bcl-2. Intravenous administration of docetaxel results in 100% bioavailability and absorption is immediate. Oral bioavailability has been found to be 8% ± 6% on its own and when co-administered with cyclosporine, bioavailability increased to 90% ± 44%. In practice, docetaxel is administered intravenously only to increase dose precession. Docetaxel is used for the treatment of Breast cancer, Nonsmall cell lung cancer Prostate cancer Gastric adenocarcinoma Head and neck cancer.

It was hypothesized that RGD conjugated PLGA nanoparticles and liposomes loaded with docetaxel would result in higher cellular uptake and hence higher and sustained intracellular levels of drugs compared to unconjugated nanoparticles and liposomes or plain drugs by both passive and active targeting. Active targeting will be achieved by specific receptor binding of peptide and passive targeting will be achieved by EPR effect and hence present as a potential delivery system to treat breast cancer.

1.2. Research envisaged

The objectives of present investigation were development of three types nanoconstructs of docetaxel (PLGA nanoparticles, liposomes and HPMA copolymer drug conjugates), RGD-conjugation onto the nanoconstructs systems, characterization, and evaluation of these nanoconstructs on breast cancer cell lines to understand their role in breast cancer chemotherapy.

The proposed plan of work may be divided into following specific aims:

I. Literature reviews covering mechanisms, barriers and various approaches to intracellular drug delivery.

II. To prepare nanoconstructs systems of the drug docetaxel, to conjugate RGD onto the surface of these nanoconstructs and to characterize them for particle size, zeta potential, entrapment efficiency, surface morphology and *in-vitro* drug release.

III. To study the stability of unconjugated and conjugated systems with respect to appearance, particle size, zeta potential and drug content.

IV. To study the cellular uptake of unconjugated and conjugated of 6-coumarin loaded nanoconstructs using confocal microscopy.

V. To evaluate the unconjugated and conjugated nanoconstructs for their *in-vitro* antiproliferative activity using breast cell line.

VI. To study the effect of unconjugated and conjugated nanoconstructs on cell cycle and mode of cell death on breast cancer cells.

1.3. References

Baldwin, S.P. et al, 1998, Materials for protein delivery in tissue engineering, Advanced Drug Delivery Reviews, **33**, 71-86.

Besselink, G.A.J. et al, Affinity-binding of cells to sephadex derivatized with peptides and proteins, in Frontiers in biomedical polymer applications, Technomic: Lancaster, 201-213.

Chinn, J.A. et al, 1998, Blood and tissue compatibility of modified polyester: Thrombosis, inflammation, and healing, J. Biomed. Mater. Res., **39**, 130-140.

Craig, W. S. et al, 1995, Concept and progress in the development of RGD-containing peptide pharmaceuticals, Biopolymers, **37**, 157–175.

Ghosh, S. et al, 2004, Recent research and development in synthetic polymer-based drug delivery systems. Journal of Chemical Reaserach, 241-246.

Hans, M.L. et al, 2002, Biodegradable nanoparticles for drug delivery and targeting, Current Opinion Solid State Matter Science, **6**, 319-327.

Hynes, R.O. et al, Integrins: Versatility, modulation, and signaling in cell adhesion, Cell, **69, 53,** 11-25.

Jain, R. K. et al, 1998, Nat. Med., **4**, 655–657.

Jayanth Panyama et al, 2003, Biodegradable nanoparticles for drug and gene delivery to cells and tissue, Advanced Drug Delivery Reviews, **55**,329–347.

Kadimi, U.S. et al, 2007, In vitro studies on liposomal amphotericin B obtained by supercritical carbon dioxide–mediated process, Nanomedicine: Nanotechnology, Biology, and Medicine, **3**, 273–280.

Kim, B.S. et al, 1999, Engineered smooth muscle tissues: Regulating cell phenotype with the scaffold. Experimental Cell Research, **251**, 318-328.

Madri, J.A. et al, 1988, Endothelial cell-extracellular matrix interactions: Matrix as a modulator of cell functions, in Endothelial cell biology in health and disease, Plenum Press: New York, 167-188.

McHugh, M.A. et al, 1994, Supercritical Fluid Extraction, 2nd ed., Newton, MA: Butterworth-Heinemann.

Miller, N. et al, 1995, FASEB J., **9**, 190–199.

Moghimi, S.M. et al, 2001, Long-circulating and target-specific nanoparticles: Theory to practice. Pharmacological Reviews, **53**, 283-318.

Mohanraj, V.J. et al, 2006, Nanoparticles – A Review, Trop. J. Pharm. Res, **5 (1)**, 561-573.

Rezania, A. et al, 1999, Biomimetic peptide surfaces that regulate adhesion, spreading, cytoskeletal organization, and mineralization of the matrix deposited by osteoblast-like cells, Biotechnol. Prog., **15**, 19-32.

Ruoslahti, E. et al, 1987, New perspectives in cell adhesion: RGD and integrins, Science, **238**, 491-497.

Ruth Duncan et al, 2003, The Dawning Era of Polymer Therapeutics, Nature Reviews Drug Discovery, **2**, 347-360.

Shakesheff, K.M. et al, 1998, Creating biomimetic microenvironments with synthetic polymer-peptide hybrid molecules, in Polymers for tissue engineering, VSP: Utrecht., 113-124.

Chapter 2
Literature Review

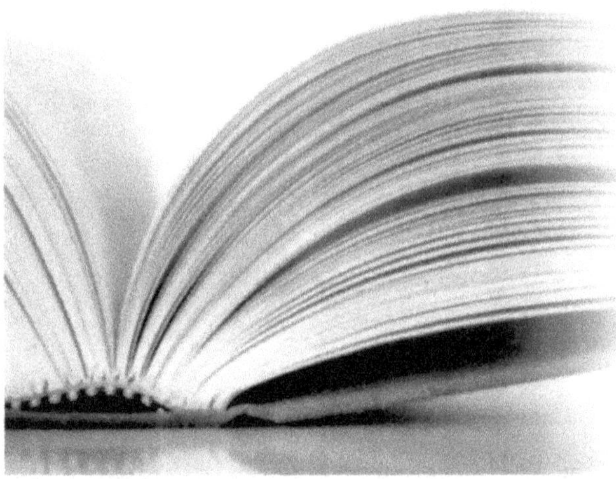

2.1. Intracellular Drug Delivery

The efficacy of drug therapy depends on identifying a target and designing a pharmaceutical agent that will be able to reach that target. The increased understanding of molecular pathology provides us with many targets relating to the primary cause of diseases. The information tells us that no intracellular compartment can claim to be free from being implicated in the cause or effect of at least one disease. Drugs may therefore need to be delivered not only to specific organs and cells but also to distinct intracellular compartments or microenvironments. Molecular medicine has discovered many new therapeutic modalities by using state-of-the-art techniques in molecular biology. High through-put, in-vitro assays that screen for pharmacological actions on the desired cell type are frequently used to design new drugs. Although such agents are certainly justified by their success in-vitro, they frequently perform much less effectively *in-vivo* where the agent must reach its target cells in a tissue in sufficient quantities to be potent while sparing bystander organs. Depending on the route of administration, the endothelium and/or epithelium form significant barriers that greatly limit the *in-vivo* accessibility of many drugs, antibodies, and gene vectors to their intended target sites of pharmacological action, namely, the cells inside the tissue (Jain, R. K. et al., 1998). Hence, the major challenge for formulation development scientist is to design drug delivery strategies that deliver the therapeutic agents to the desired intracellular targets based on ability to understand, utilize, modify and exploit membrane trafficking pathways (Miller, N. et al., 1995).

Intracellular drug delivery refers to the delivery of therapeutic agents to specific compartments or organelles within the cell. The therapeutic agent could be a low molecular weight drug or a macromolecule like protein or DNA. Thus targeted intracellular drug delivery results in higher bioavailability of a therapeutic agent at its site of action (i.e. distinct intracellular compartments or microenvironments), potentiates the pharmacologic effect of the drug, and at the same time, reduces the side effects. (Jayanth Panyam et al., 2004).

Factors that limit the intracellular delivery of drugs include poor permeability of the drug through the cell membrane, low accessibility of the drug to its site of action within the cell, degradation of the drug in specific cell compartments and toxicity due to the exposure of the drug and/or the delivery system to different cellular organelles

2.1.1. Mechanisms of Intracellular Delivery

There are a number of pathways through which a therapeutic agent or a carrier can enter a cell. The simplest mechanism is diffusion across cell membrane. Low molecular weight lipophilic compounds cross the cell membrane by simple diffusion method. Water soluble substrates need a means of facilitating their passage into the cell. They can enter the cell when membrane protein form channels allowing substances to diffuse across the cell membrane. E.g. ligand-gated channels, voltage gated channels. Simple and facilitated diffusion allow the transport of molecules from an area of high concentration to that of lower concentration. Active transport utilizes ATP-derived energy to pump substances against a concentration gradient.

- Endocytosis
- Caveolar endocytosis
- Pinocytosis
- Phagocytosis
- In receptor-mediated endocytosis,
- Folate Receptor-Mediated Endocytosis
- Transferrin Receptor-Mediated Endocytosis
- Biotin Receptor-Mediated Endocytosis
- Wheat Germ Agglutinin-Mediated Endocytosis
- ICAM-1-Mediated Endocytosis
- Antibody-Mediated Endocytosis
- Physical or mechanical methods use force to traverse the cell membrane
  -Particle bombardment accelerates
  -Microinjection
  -Electroporation

2.1.2. Barriers to Intracellular Delivery of Therapeutic Agents

There are a number of barriers to the intracellular delivery of therapeutic agents. Low molecular lipophilic drugs can diffuse across the cell, but once the concentration gradient is removed, they diffuse back out or efflux out of the cell rapidly. Presences of transporters such as MRP of P-gp are responsible for drug efflux e.g. anti-tumor agents. For high molecular drugs, which are transported by endocytosis- pH is lowered in the pathway (Extracellular fluid 7.4, endosomes 5.5-6.5, lysosomes 3.0-5.5). Unless there are special mechanisms of escape from the endosomes to the cytoplasm, these macromolecules are delivered to lysosomes where they are degraded. Endosomes and lysosomes contain proteases (e.g. cathepsins), lipases, glycolases, and phophatases. Thus, most macromolecules have very poor availability inside the cell. Two major strategies for delivery of bio-active molecules to the cytoplasm are destabilization of endosomal/lysosomal membrane and direct penetration through the plasma membrane.

Extracellular barriers

The mononuclear phagocyte system is a system of phagocytic components which recognize, capture and remove foreign material from the body. Circulatory monocytes and fixed tissue macrophages (e.g. Kupffer cells) remove drug delivery systems from the bloodstream before degradation within macrophage-rich organs such as the liver, spleen and bone marrow. A reduction in phagocytic cell interaction increases the circulation time of the delivery system which is a prerequisite for site specific drug accumulation.

2.1.3. Intracellular Targets

- Endo-Lysosomal Targeting
- Cytoplasmic Delivery
- Nuclear Targeting
- Mitochondrial Targeting

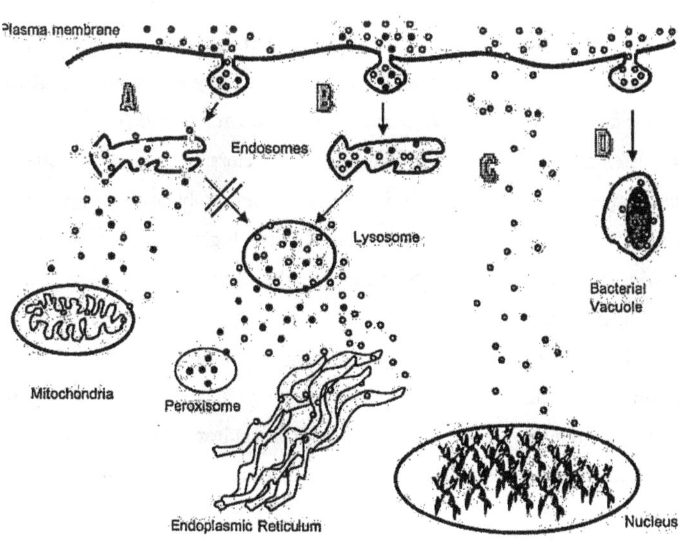

Figure: 2.1. Examples of targets, barriers and strategies for intracellular drug delivery. (A, B) Internalisation of the drug or drug complex into the endocytic pathway precedes drug release into the cytosol. This may be mediated by cleavage of a labile drug-complex linker or physical membrane destabilisation by, for example, a virus or a liposome. In A, the drug complex (red) is endosomotropic, and the drug needs to be released prior to encountering the degrading proteases and nucleases of the lysosome. (B) The ER (yellow)- and peroxisome (black)-targeted drugs are lysosomotropic; there is a requirement for them to be ®rst delivered to the lysosomes. (C) The nuclear-targeted drug (blue) permeates through biological membranes or alternatively is attached to a membrane-permeable carrier. (D) The drug (green) is targeted via the endocytic pathway to a bacterium (purple) inside the vacuole. (Arwyn, T. Jones et al., 2001)

2.2. Intracellular Drug Delivery Approaches

Once administered, a drug may have to traverse several biological membranes or organelles before intracellular targeting is complete. In order to achieve this, it may be necessary to develop carriers, with specific properties, that would enable them to localize in those compartments. A number of different carriers have been used for targeting different organelles including viral vectors, cationic lipids, polymer conjugates, micelles, protein transduction domains, nanoparticles and liposomes.

2.2.1 Viral Vectors

These are by far the most efficient means of delivering DNA (gene therapy), usually achieving success rates of higher than 90% for both delivery and expression. Adenovirus, adeno-associated virus and lenti virus are some of the viral vectors (replication-deficient) that have been studied. Limitations of using viral vectors are immunogenicity, toxicity, restricted targeting of specific cell types, costs and problems with production and packaging. Viral peptide transporters typically use highly stable hydrophobic helix peptide which is structural similarity to transmembrane protein tails, which help them to cross the plasma membrane.

Viral peptides evolved for endosomal escape are (1) HIV-tat peptide (Mudit Tyagi et al., 2001). Current mechanism hypothesis is that positively-charged residues bind polyanionic proteoglycans, triggering rapid internalization. It is unclear how escape from endosome occurs. (2) Influenza hemagluttinin peptide: Undergoes conformational change at reduced pH. Inserts in membrane, reduced pH causes a membrane-destabilizing change in conformation.

2.2.2. Cationic Lipids and Polymers (Lipoplexes/polyplexes)

Cationic lipids and cationic polymers have been used as non-viral transfection vectors for efficient intracellular delivery of DNA. Lipoplexes are complexes between cationic lipids and DNA and polyplexes are complexes are complexes between DNA and cationic polymers. Complexes between cationic lipids [such as Lipofectin®, an equimolar mixture of N-[1-(2, 3-dioleyloxy)propyl]-N,N,N-trimethylammonium chloride (DOTMA) and dioleoyl phosphatidylethanolamine (DOPE)] and DNA and complexes between cationic polymers, such as polyethyleneimine (PEI), and DNA are formed because of strong electrostatic interactions between the positively charged carrier and negatively charged DNA (Kunath, K. et al., 2003)

2.2.3. Micelles

Micelles are colloidal dispersions and have the particle size within the 5 to 50–100 nm range. An important property of micelles is their ability to increase the solubility and bioavailability of poorly soluble pharmaceuticals. The use of certain special amphiphilic molecules as micelle building blocks can also introduce the property of micelle extended blood half-life upon intravenous administration. Because of their small size (5–50 nm), micelles demonstrate a spontaneous penetration into the interstitium in the body compartments with the leaky vasculature (tumors and infarcts) by the enhanced permeability and retention (EPR) effect, a form of selective delivery termed as "passive targeting"(Maeda, H. et al., 2000). Specific ligands (such as antibodies and/or certain sugar moieties) can be attached to the water exposed termini of hydrophilic blocks (Torchilin, V.P. et al., 2001). In the case of targeted micelles, a local release of a free drug from micelles in the target organ should lead to the increased efficacy of the drug, whereas the stability of the micelles en route to the target organ or tissue should contribute better drug solubility and toxicity reduction owing to less interaction with non-target organs.

Micelles (polymeric micelles) can also demonstrate pH-sensitivity and ability to escape from endosomes. Thus, micelles prepared from PEG-poly(aspartate hydrazone adriamycin) easily release an active drug at lowered pH values typical for endosomes and facilitate its cytoplasmic delivery and toxicity against cancer cells (Bae, Y. et al., 2005).

Alternatively, micelles for intracellular delivery of antisense oligonucleotides (ODN) were prepared from ODN-PEG conjugates complexes with a cationic fusogenic peptide, KALA, and provided much higher intracellular delivery of the ODN than could be achieved with free ODN (Jeong, J.H. et al., 2003).

Vladimir P et al prepared tumor-specific 2C5 immunomicelles loaded with a sparingly soluble anticancer agent, taxol. Immunomicelles with attached antitumor mAb 2C5 effectively recognized and bound various cancer cells *in vitro* and showed an increased accumulation in experimental tumors in mice when compared with nontargeted micelles (Torchilin, V.P. et al., 2003).

2.2.4. Protein Transduction Domains

It was observed that certain proteins entered cells when added to the surrounding media. From these proteins, short basic peptide sequences (Protein Transduction Domains, PTDs) were identified that could cross the plasma membrane and in doing so take the rest of the protein with them. Most of the currently recognized CPP are of cationic nature and derived from viral, insect or mammalian proteins endowed with membrane translocation properties. The exact mechanisms underlying the translocation of CPP across the cellular membrane are still poorly understood. However, several similarities in translocation can be found. Early studies on CPP translocation mechanisms tended to suggest that the internalization of these peptides was neither significantly inhibited by low temperature, depletion of the cellular adenosine triphosphate (ATP) pool, nor by inhibitors of endocytosis. Moreover, chemical modification of the peptide sequence, such as the synthesis of retro-, enantio- or retroenantio-analogs, appeared not to affect the internalization properties. Therefore, translocation was concluded to result from direct, physical transfer through the lipid bilayer of the cell membrane. Later studies, however, showed convincing evidence for the involvement of endocytosis as the dominating mechanism for cellular internalization. Cellular delivery using PTDs has several advantages over conventional techniques because it is efficient for a range of cell types and has a potential therapeutic application

There is no DNA, no risk of genome modification or transgene dissemination, an efficient passage through the blood-brain barrier, the capacity to bypass the multidrug resistance system, and the direct incorporation inside the cytoplasm, avoiding the problem of endosome efflux. PTD carriers suffer from certain limitations such as cell toxicity, possible immunogenicity, and negative interference with the activity of the transported molecules. They also require cross-linking to the therapeutic peptide or protein. Also, some of these systems such as PTDs derived from HIV-1 TAT protein require denaturation of the protein before delivery to increase the accessibility of the PTD domains. More recently, a short synthetic amphipathic carrier, Pep-1, was developed to deliver functionally active proteins and peptides intracellularly without the need for cross-linking or denaturation. *Torchilin V.P et al* *and Levchenk T. S et al* attached TAT peptide to the surface of plain and PEGylated liposomes. TAT peptide-liposomes were made slightly cationic by adding up to 10 mol % of a cationic lipid (DOTAP). These slightly cationic liposomes were non-toxic towards cells, formed firm complexes with DNA (plasmid encoding for the formation of the Green Fluorescent Protein), and efficiently transfected a variety of cells. (Torchilin, V.P. et al., 2003).

2.2.5. Nanoparticles

Nanoparticles are defined as particulate dispersions or solid particles with a size in the range of 10-1000nm. The drug is dissolved, entrapped, encapsulated or attached to a nanoparticles matrix. Depending upon the method of preparation, nanoparticles, nanospheres or nanocapsules can be obtained. Nanocapsules are systems in which the drug is confined to a cavity surrounded by a unique polymer membrane, while nanospheres are matrix systems in which the drug is physically and uniformly dispersed. In recent years, biodegradable polymeric nanoparticles, particularly those coated with hydrophilic polymer such as poly(ethylene glycol) (PEG) known as long-circulating particles, have been used as potential drug delivery devices because of their ability to circulate for a prolonged period time target a particular organ, as carriers of DNA in gene therapy, and their ability to deliver proteins, peptides and genes. (Mohanraj, V.J. et al., 2006)

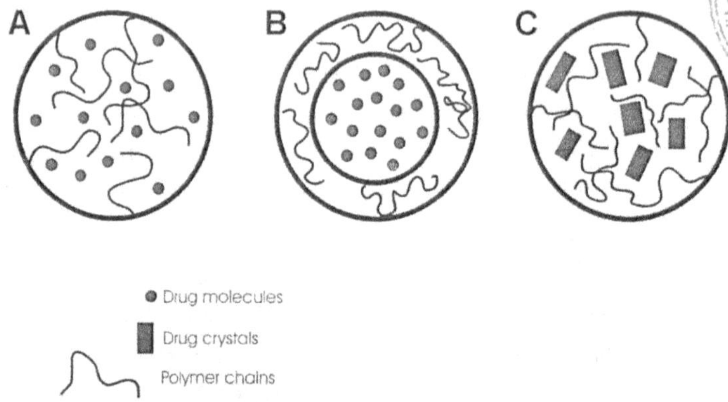

Figure: 2.2. Schematics of exemplary types of drug nanoparticles. A. Matrix type nanosphere, drug molecules are evenly dispersed in the polymer matrix. B. Core shell nanocapsule, drug molecule is presented in a core covered with a polymer shell. C. Matrix type nanosphere where drug crystals are embedded in a polymer matrix (Vauthier-Holtzscherer, C. et al., 1991).

The advantages of using nanoparticles as a drug delivery system include the following:

1. Particle size and surface characteristics of nanoparticles can be easily manipulated to achieve both passive and active drug targeting after paranteral parenteral administration.
2. They control and sustain release of the drug during the transportation and at the site of localization, altering organ distribution of the drug and subsequent clearance of the drug so as to achieve increase in drug therapeutic efficacy and reduction in side effects.
3. Controlled release and particle degradation characteristics can be readily modulated by the choice of matrix constituents. Drug loading is relatively high and drugs can be incorporated into the systems without any chemical reaction; this is an important factor for preserving the drug activity.
4. Site-specific targeting can be achieved by attaching targeting ligands to surface of particles or use of magnetic guidance.
5. The system can be used for various routes of administration including oral, nasal, parenteral, intra-ocular etc.

In spite of these advantages, nanoparticles do have limitations. For example, their small size and large surface area can lead to particle-particle aggregation, making physical handling of nanoparticles difficult in liquid and dry forms. In addition, small particles size and large surface area readily result in limited drug loading and burst release. These practical problems have to be overcome before nanoparticles can be used clinically or made commercially available.

Nanoparticle components:

Organic materials

- Polymers: natural (chitosan, sodium alginate, agarose)

  Synthetic (PLGA, PBCA, PVP)
- Proteins: gelatin, albumin
- Lipids: triglycerides, fatty acids, sterols
- Calcium phosphate
- Silica
- Iron oxide

Inorganic materials

- Calcium phosphate
- Silica
- Iron oxide

Biodegradable nanoparticles for pharmaceutical use are prepared from a variety of synthetic and natural polymers. Synthetic polymers such as polyacrylates, polycaprolactones, polylactides and its copolymers with polyglycolides are widely used.

Polymer (PLGA)

A wide spectrum of synthetic and natural polymers is available for nanoparticles formation, but their biocompatibility and biodegradability are the major limiting factors for their use in the drug delivery area. Natural polymers are more restricted due to variation in their purity. Also, some natural polymers require crosslinking, which can inactivate the entrapped drug (Hans, M.L. et al., 2002). Synthetic polymers, on the other hand, offer better reproducibility of the chemical characteristics of the synthesized nanoparticles as compared to the natural polymers. Synthetic polymers from the ester family, such as poly(lactic acid), poly(-hydroxybutyrate), poly(caprolactone), poly(dioxanone), or other families such as poly(cyanoacrylates), poly(acrylic acid), poly(anhydrides), poly(amides), poly(ortho esters), poly(ethylene glycol), and poly(vinyl alcohol) are suitable for drug delivery due to their biodegradability, special release profiles and biocompatibility (Ghosh, S. et al., 2004). Poly(lactide-co-glycolide acid) (PLGA), from the ester family, has been widely used in the biomedical industry as a major components in biodegradable sutures, bone fixation nails and screw. It is a well-characterized polymer, its degradation sub products are non toxic, it provides controlled drug release profiles by changing the PLGA copolymer ratio which affects the crystallinity (low crystallinity, more amorphous polymer means more fast degradation) of PLGA (Moghimi, S.M. et al 2001). For these reasons, PLGA has been selected as the polymer of choice in the present research. PLGA of different molecular weights (from 10 kDa to over 100 kDa) and different copolymer molar ratios (50:50, 75:25, and 85:15) is available on the market. Molecular weight and copolymer molar ratio influence the degradation process and release profile of the drug 4 entrapped. In general, low molecular weight PLGA with higher amounts of glycolic acid offer faster degradations rates (Alexis, F. et al., 2005).

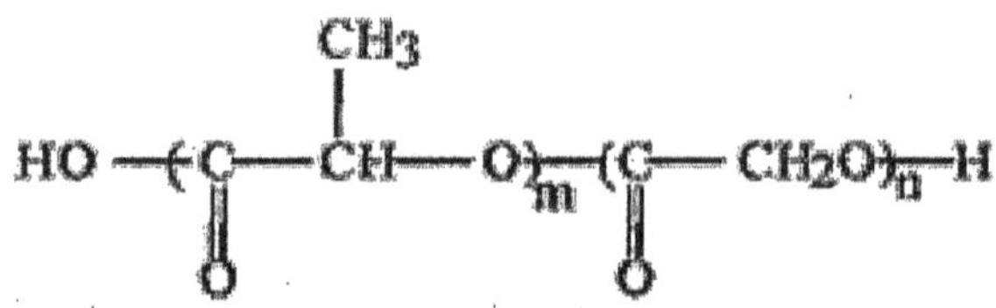

Chemical structure of PLGA polymer. The "m" component represents lactic acid and "n" component represents glycolic acid.

Figure: 2.3. Chemical Structure of PLGA

FDA approved biodegradable and biocompatible polymers, poly (D, L-lactide-co-glycolide) (PLGA) in the with a therapeutic agent encapsulated into the polymer is widely used for localized and sustained drug and macro-molecular delivery (Jayanth Panyama et al., 2003)

Pharmaceutical nanoparticles are submicron-sized, colloidal vehicles that carry drugs to the target or release drugs in a controlled way in the body. After preparation, nanoparticles are usually dispersed in liquid. Such a system can be administered to humans for example by injection, by the oral route, or used in ointments and ocular products. Alternatively, nanoparticles can be dried to a powder, which allows pulmonary delivery or further processing to tablets or capsules. In drug delivery, nanoparticles should readily be biocompatible (not harmful for humans) and biodegradable (deteriorate and expulse in the body conditions). These properties, as well as targeting and controlled release, can be affected by nanoparticles material selection and by surface modification.

Materials such as synthetic polymers, proteins or other natural macromolecules are used in the preparation of nanoparticles. To process these materials into nanoparticles, a variety of preparation techniques exist ranging from polymerization of monomers to different polymer deposition methods (Kreuter, J. et al., 1994 and Pinto Reis et al., 2006).

Nanoparticles in pharmaceutical applications have gained plenty of research attention during recent decades (Couvreur, P. et al., 2006). Although the research concerning formulation of nanoparticles into drug delivery devices has been extensive, only a few polymeric nanoparticulate products have reached the market. One known product, Abraxane™, consist of intravenously administered 130nm nanoparticles prepared from the protein albumin bound with paclitaxel, a drug used in cancer therapy (Rios, M. et al., 2006). Another cancer drug, Doxorubicin Transdrug®, consisting of doxorubicin-loaded poly(isohexylcyanoacrylate) nanoparticles is currently at the Phase II/III clinical trials (Bio-Alliance Pharma., 2006). Among the drugs used in nanoparticles formulations, particularly cancer therapeutics are widely studied because the formulation might reduce toxicity of the drug while improving efficacy of the treatment. In addition to drug molecules, other candidates to be encapsulated in or coupled with nanoparticles include macromolecules like proteins, peptides and genes (nucleic acids) (Morishita, M. et al.,2006 and Cohen, H. et al., 2000). These kinds of molecules tend to be inactivated in the body by enzymatic degradation. In terms of controlled release, nanoparticles provide protection against the body conditions resulting in sustained release maintenance of bioactivity before the drug reaches the target. After intravenous administration, nano sized particles are mainly taken up by the macrophages of the mononuclear phagocyte system (MPS) (Grislain, L. et al., 1983, Illum, L. Davis et al., 1982) and, thus, can be localized in the liver, spleen and lungs (Couvreur, P. et al., 1980). By modifying particle surface, e.g., by coating, defense mechanisms of the body can be avoided to some extent leading to longer circulation times of nanoparticles in the blood (Storm, G. et al., 1995). Tailored coating also enables another promising application of nanoparticles: drug delivery across the blood-brain barrier (BBB) (Garcia-Garcia et al., 2005). From the intestine, after oral administration, intracellular uptake may occur and prior to that, the nanoparticles can adhere to the mucosa (bioadhesion) and thus improve pharmacokinetics of the drug (Florence, A.T. et al., 1997). As a summary of the above mentioned facts, the benefits of nanoparticles include protection of the encapsulated pharmaceutical substance, improved efficacy, fewer adverse effects, controlled release and drug targeting.

Correspondingly, potential active substances in nanoparticles formulations could be expensive molecules applicable in small amounts.

At the present time, several successful laboratory-scale nanoparticulate drug targeting systems are available (Pinto Reis, C et al., 2006), and some processes have been scaled up (Galindo-Rodriguez et al., 2005) the time approaches when an increasing number of nanoparticulate drug delivery systems reach the market and the systems are transferred from animal tests to human use, concerns about the safety of the products are emerging. More attention will be paid to stability and toxicology of nanoparticles and their constituents. According to recent opinion, proper physicochemical characterization of nanoparticles should be included in risk assessment and toxicology considerations of nanoparticulate systems, in addition to pharmaceutical in vitro and in vivo testing (Oberdörster, G. et al., 2005).

Preparation of nanoparticles

Two main procedures can be followed to form polymeric nanoparticles, namely top-down and bottom-up techniques. The top-down methods use size reduction to obtain controlled-size nanoparticles. This size reduction is based on the application of strong shear stress by wave sound emission (sonication), high pressure (microfluidization), and high speed agitation (homogenization). The bottom-up methods start from individual molecules to form nanoparticles, by polymerization. The polymerization methods commonly used are emulsion polymerization (water in oil, oil in water, and polymerization in bicontinuous structures), dispersion polymerization, and interfacial polymerization (Nakache, E. et al., 2000). Monomers, initiators, additives, and solvent are the basic chemical components used in the polymerization methods. The main drawbacks of the bottom-up methods are the presence of residual sub-products in the final nanoparticles that can impart toxicity to the nanoparticles, the difficulty in the prediction of polymer molecular weight, affecting the biodistribution and release behavior of the drug from the nanoparticle; and the possibility for drug inhibitions due to interactions, or cross reactions of the drug with activated monomers and H+ ions present during polymerization (De Jaeghere, F. et al., 1999). To overcome these limitations, top-down methods were developed using naturals and synthetic polymers. The emulsion evaporation, salting out, nanoprecipitation, and emulsion diffusion are the main top-down methods used to form polymeric nanoparticles. modifications of these methods have been developed in an attempt to avoid the use of toxic solvents and surfactants, to improve drug entrapment efficiency and nanoparticles stability, and to more efficiently use energy in droplet size reduction. All these methods involve two liquid phases, the organic phase which can dissolve the polymer and the other hydrophobic components, and the continuous aqueous phase.

1. Dispersion of preformed polymers (Kumaresh, S. et al., 2001 and Mohanraj, V.J. et al., 2006)

Several methods have been suggested to prepare biodegradable NPs from PLA, PLG, PLGA and poly(e-caprolactone) by dispersing the preformed polymers.

1.1. Solvent evaporation method

In this method, the polymer is dissolved in an organic solvent like dichloromethane, chloroform or ethyl acetate. The drug is dissolved or dispersed into the preformed polymer solution, and this mixture is then emulsified into an aqueous solution to make an oil (O) in water (W) i.e., O/W emulsion by using a surfactant/emulsifying agent like gelatin, poly(vinyl alcohol), polysorbate-80, poloxamer-188, etc. After the formation of a stable emulsion, the organic solvent is evaporated by increasing the temperature/under pressure or by continuous stirring. The W/O/W method has also been used to prepare the water-soluble drug-loaded NPs. Both the above methods use a high-speed homogenization or sonication. However, these procedures are good for a laboratory-scale operation, but for a large-scale pilot production, alternative methods using low-energy emulsification are required. In this pursuit, following approaches have been attempted.

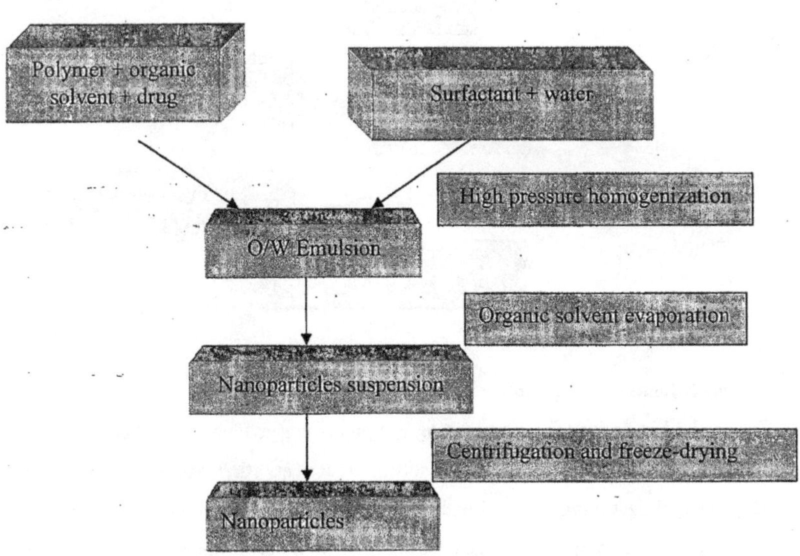

1.2. Spontaneous emulsification /solvent diffusion method

In a modified version of the solvent evaporation method the water-soluble solvent like acetone or methanol along with the water insoluble organic solvent like dichloromethane or chloroform were used as an oil phase. Due to the spontaneous diffusion of water-soluble solvent (acetone or methanol), an interfacial turbulence is created between two phases leading to the formation of smaller particles. As the concentration of water-soluble solvent (acetone) increases, a considerable decrease in particle size can be achieved.

1.3. Salting out

This technique involves the addition of polymer and drug solution in a slightly water-miscible solvent such as acetone to an aqueous solution containing the salting out agent and a colloidal stabilizer under vigorous mechanical stirring. When this O/W emulsion is diluted with a sufficient volume of water, it induces the formation of nanoparticles by enhancing the diffusion of acetone into the aqueous phase.

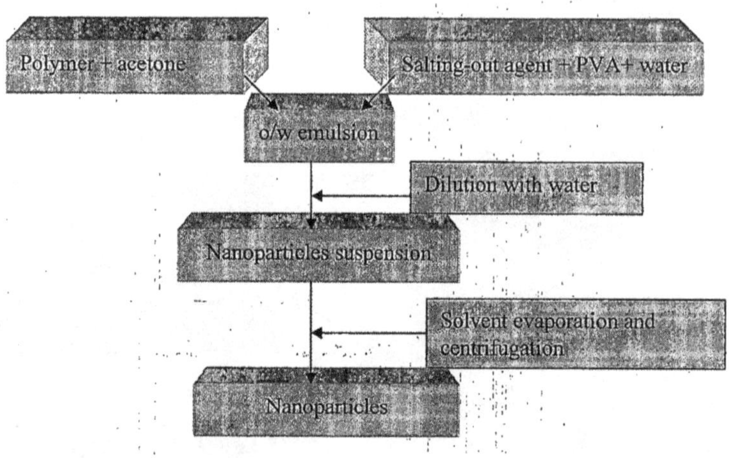

1.4. Emulsification-diffusion

This method is derived from the salting-out procedure. It involves adding of a polymer solution, in partially water miscible solvent (such as ethyl acetate, benzyl alcohol, propylene carbonate) presaturated with water, to an aqueous solution containing stabilizer under vigorous stirring. The subsequent addition of water to the system destabilizes the equilibrium between the two phases and causes the solvent to diffuse into the external phase, resulting in reduction of the interfacial tension and in nanoparticles formation.

1.5. Solvent displacement/Nanoprecipitation

This method is usually employed to incorporate lipophilic drugs into the carriers based on the interfacial deposition of a polymer following displacement of a semi-polar solvent miscible with water from a lipophilic solution. The particle formation is based on precipitation and subsequent solidification of the polymer at the interface of a solvent and a non-solvent. Thus, the process is often called solvent displacement or interfacial deposition. The polymer is dissolved in a water miscible organic solvent (or solvent mixture) and added to an aqueous solution, in which the organic solvent diffuses. Particle formation is spontaneous, because the polymer precipitates in the aqueous environment. According to the current opinion, the Marangoni effect is considered to explain the process solvent flow, diffusion and surface tensions at the interface of the organic solvent and the aqueous phase cause turbulences, which form small droplets containing the polymer. Subsequently, as the solvent diffuses out from the droplets, the polymer precipitates. Finally, the organic solvent is typically evaporated with the help of a vacuum. No emulsification step (which is usually part of a nanoparticles preparation process), laborious processing conditions or special laboratory ware is needed. The size of the nanoparticles prepared by nanoprecipitation varies typically from 100 to 500 nm (Schwendeman, S. et al., 1997).

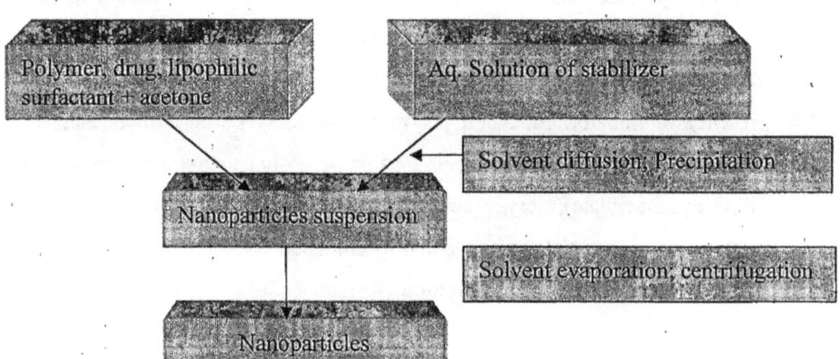

2. Polymerization method (Kumaresh, S. et al., 2001 and Mohanraj, V.J. et al., 2006)

In this method, monomers are polymerized to form nanoparticles in an aqueous solution. Drug is incorporated either by being dissolved in the polymerization medium or by adsorption onto the nanoparticles after polymerization completed. The nanoparticles suspension is then purified to remove various stabilizers and surfactants employed for polymerization by ultracentrifugation and re-suspending the particles in an isotonic surfactant-free medium. This technique has been reported for making polybutylcyanoacrylate or poly (alkylcyanoacrylate) nanoparticles. Nanocapsule formation and their particle size depend on the concentration of the surfactants and stabilizers used.

Two types of polymerization processes have been adopted to prepare polymeric nanoparticles

1. Dispersion polymerization: Dispersion polymerization starts with monomer, an initiator, solvent in which the formed polymer is insoluble, and a polymeric stabilizer. Polymer forms in the continuous phase and precipitates into a new particle phase stabilized by the polymeric stabilizer. Small particles are formed by aggregation of growing polymer chains precipitating from the continuous phase as these chins exceed a critical chain length. Coalescence of these precursor particles with themselves and with their aggregates results in the formation of stable colloidal particles, which occurs when sufficient stabilizer covers the particles.
2. Emulsion polymerization: In this technique the monomer is emulsified in non-solvent containing surfactant, which leads to the formation of monomer swollen micelles and stabilized monomer droplets. The polymerization is performed in the presence of initiator. Emulsion polymerization may be performed using either organic or aqueous media as continuous phase. Poly (methyl methacrylate), poly (alkyl cyanoacrylate), acrylic copolymer, polystyrene, poly(vinyl pyridine) and polyacrolen nanoparticles are prepared by emulsion polymerization technique.

3. Coacervation or ionic gelation method (Kumaresh, S. et al., 2001 and Mohanraj, V.J. et al., 2006)

Much research has been focused on the preparation of nanoparticles using biodegradable hydrophilic polymers such as chitosan, gelatin and sodium alginate. *Calvo et al 1997* developed a method for preparing hydrophilic chitosan nanoparticles by ionic gelation. The method involves a mixture of two aqueous phases, of which one is the polymer chitosan, a di-block co-polymer ethylene oxide or propylene oxide (PEO-PPO) and the other is a polyanion sodium tripolyphosphate. In this method, positively charged amino group of chitosan interacts with negative charged tripolyphosphate to form coacervates with a size in the range of nanometer. Coacervates are formed as a result of electrostatic interaction between two aqueous phases, whereas, ionic gelation involves the material undergoing transition from liquid to gel due to ionic interaction conditions at room temperature.

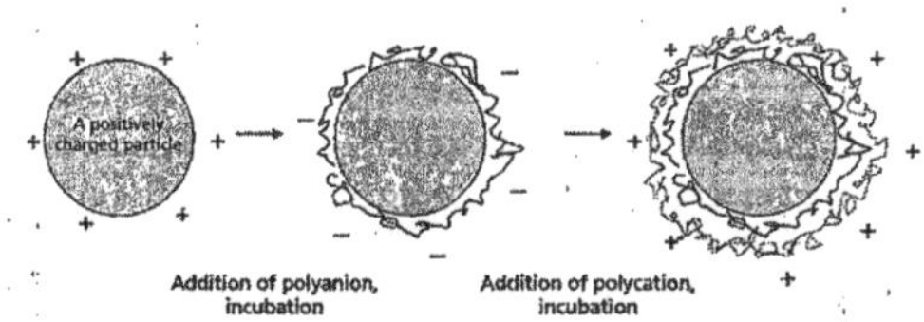

Figure: 2.4. Sequential adsorption of polyelectrolytes on a charged particle. (Sukhorukov, G.B. et al., 1998 and Decher, G. et al., 1997)

4. Production of Nanoparticles (NPs) using supercritical fluid technology (Kumaresh, S. et al., 2001)

Production of NPs with the desired physicochemical properties to facilitate the targeted drug delivery has been a topic of renewed interest in pharmaceutical industries. Conventional methods like solvent evaporation, coacervation and in situ polymerization often require the use of toxic solvents and/or surfactants. Therefore, research efforts have been directed to develop the environmentally safer encapsulation methods to produce the drug-loaded micron and submicron size particles. If solvent impurities remain in the drug-loaded NPs, then these become toxic and may degrade the pharmaceuticals within the polymer matrix. Supercritical fluids have now became the attractive alternatives because these are environmentally friendly solvents and the method can be profitably used to process particles in high purity and without any trace amount of the organic solvent.

In the rapid expansion of supercritical solution (RESS) method the solute of interest is solubilized in a supercritical fluid and the solution is expanded through a nozzle. Thus, the solvent power of super- critical fluid dramatically decreases and the solute eventually precipitates. This technique is clean because the precipitated solute is completely solvent-free. Unfortunately, most polymers exhibit little or no solubility in supercritical fluids, thus making the technique less of practical interest. RESS was very popular in the late 80s and early 90s for particle production of bioerodible drug-loaded polymers like PLA. A uniform distribution of drug inside the polymer matrix can be achieved by this method for low molecular mass (10 000) polymers. However, the RESS method cannot be used for high molecular mass polymers due to their limited solubility in supercritical fluids. For these reasons, much less information is found in the literature over the past 6–7 years on this technique.

In the supercritical anti-solvent (SAS) method the solution is charged with the supercritical fluid in the precipitation vessel containing solute of interest in an organic solvent. At high pressures, enough anti-solvent will enter into the liquid phase so that the solvent power will be lowered and the solute precipitates. After precipitation, when the final operating pressure is reached, the anti-solvent flows through the vessel so as to strip the residual solvent. When the solvent content has been reduced to the desired level, the vessel is depressurized and the solid product is collected. A schematic of the SAS method is shown in **Figure: 2.5.**

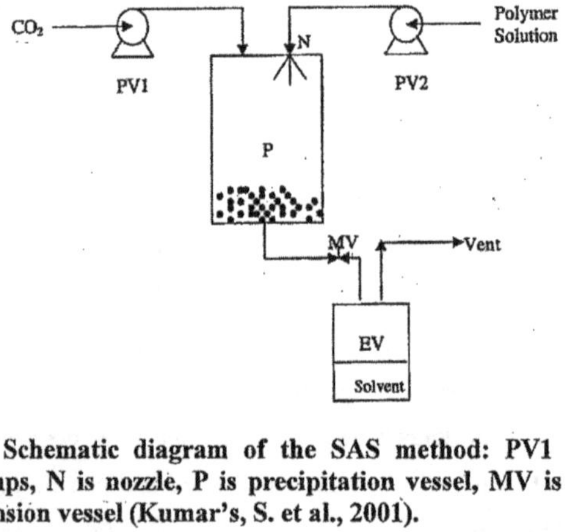

Figure: 2.5. Schematic diagram of the SAS method: PV1 and PV2 are two volumetric pumps, N is nozzle, P is precipitation vessel, MV is micrometric valve and EV is expansion vessel (Kumar's, S. et al., 2001).

Stability of Nanoparticles

Freeze-drying is one of the well established methods for the preservation of unstable molecules over long periods of time. (Corveleyn, S. et al., 1996; Diminsky, D. et al., 1999; Li B. et al., 2000). Most studies have shown a good preservation of the physicochemical properties of the particles when the lyoprotectant was employed in a sufficient concentration.

Characterization methods of Nanoparticles

Characterization of the nanoparticles carrier systems to thoroughly understand the properties is essential before putting them to pharmaceutical application. After preparation, nanoparticles are characterized at two levels. The physicochemical characterization consists of the evaluation of the particle size, size distribution, and surface properties (composition, charge, hydrophobicity) of the nanoparticles. The biopharmaceutical characterization includes measurements of drug encapsulation, in vitro drug release rates, and *in vivo* studies revealing biodistribution, bioavailability, and efficacy of the drug.

There are many sensitive techniques for characterizing nanoparticles, depending upon the parameter being looked at; laser light scattering (LLS) or photon correlation spectroscopy (PCS) for particle size and size distribution; scanning electron microscopy (SEM), transmission electron microscopy (TEM), and atomic force microscopy (AFM) for morphological properties; X-ray photoelectron spectroscopy (XPS), Fourier transform infrared spectroscopy (FTIR),a and nuclear magnetic resonance spectroscopy (NMR) for surface chemistry; and differential scanning calorimetry (DSC) for thermal properties (Figure below). Parameters such as density, molecular weight, and crystallinity affect release and degradation properties, where as surface charge, hydrophilicity, and hydrophobicity significantly influence interaction with the biological environment.

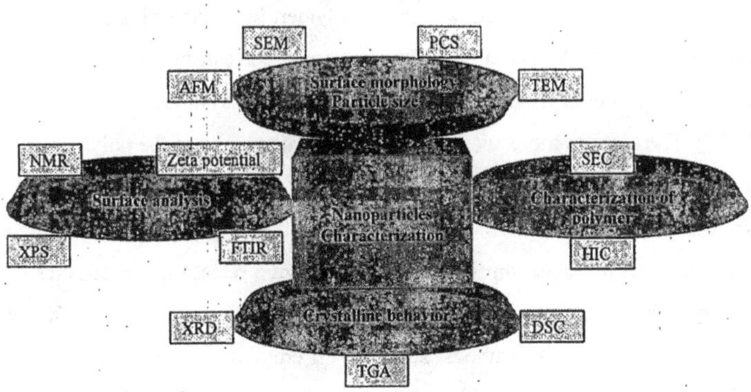

Figure: 2.6.Various techniques to characterize nanoparticles.

Particle size and Morphology:

Particle size and size distribution are the most important characteristics of nanoparticles systems. They determine the *in vivo* distribution, biological fate, toxicity and the targeting ability of nanoparticles systems. In addition, they can also influence the drug loading, drug release and stability of nanoparticles. Generally nanoparticles have relatively higher intracellular uptake compared to microparticles and available to a wider range of biological targets due to their small size and relative mobility. Drug release is affected by particle size. Smaller particles have larger surface area, therefore, most of the drug associated would be at or near the particle surface, leading to fast drug release. Whereas, larger particles have large cores which allow more drug to be encapsulated and slowly diffuse out 30. Smaller particles also have greater risk of aggregation of particles during storage and transportation of nanoparticles dispersion. It is always a challenge to formulate nanoparticles with the smallest size possible but maximum stability. (Mohanrajs, V.J. et al., 2006). Nan particles size is critical not only in determining its release and degradation behaviour (Dunne, M. et al, 2000) but also in determining the efficacy of the therapeutic agent by affecting tissue penetration or even intracellular uptake. Particle size can be determined by Photon correlation spectroscopy, Scanning electron microscopy (SEM), Transmission electron microscopy (TEM), Atomic force microscopy.

Surface chemistry analysis: X-ray photon spectroscopy, Fourier transform infrared spectroscopy, nuclear magnetic spectroscopy are the techniques employed to analyze the surface chemistry.

Molecular weight: Polymer molecular weight influences the nanoparticles size, encapsulation efficiency and degradation rate of the polymer, hence affecting the release rate of the therapeutic agent. A low molecular weight polymer can be used to prepare small-sized nanoparticles but at the expense of reduced encapsulation efficiency. (Hans, M. L. et al., 2002). The average molecular weights and polydispersity of the polymers are found by size exclusion chromatography.

Crystallinity: The physical state of both the drug and the polymer are determined because this will have an influence on the in vitro and in vivo release characteristics of the drug. The crystalline behavior of polymeric nanoparticles is studied using X-ray diffraction and thermo-analytical methods such as differential scanning calorimetry (Ubrich, N. et al., 2004) (DSC) and differential thermal analysis (DTA) (Oh, I. et al., 1999) DSC and X-ray diffraction techniques are often combined to get useful information on the structural characteristics of both drugs and polymers.

Surface charge: The zeta potential of a Nanoparticle is commonly used to characterize the surface charge property of nanoparticles. It reflects the electrical potential of particles and is influenced by the composition of the particle and the medium in which it is dispersed. Nanoparticles with a zeta potential above (+/-) 30 mV have been shown to be stable in suspension, as the surface charge prevents aggregation of the particles (Mohanraj, V.J. et al., 2006). The zeta potential can also be used to determine whether a charged active material is encapsulated within the centre of the nanocapsule or adsorbed onto the surface. Zeta potential is measure of the surface charge of the nanoparticles. The zeta potential value can influence particle stability and mucoadhesive as well as intracellular trafficking of nanoparticles as a function of pH. High zeta potential values, either positive or negative, should be achieved in order ensures stability and avoids aggregation of the particles. The extent of surface hydrophilicity can then be predicted from the values of zeta potential (Soppimath et al., 2001). Surface charge is generally determined by well-known electrophoresis method with the help of zetasizer (Panagi, Z. et al, 2001).

Encapsulation efficiency and drug release studies:

The encapsulation efficiency depends on the preparation method, nanoparticles size, molecular weight and nature of the polymer and drug. It is mostly measured by HPLC. HPLC assay analyses, size exclusion chromatography, and spectroscopic measurements are used to monitor drug release from nanoparticles. All of these techniques require separation of liberated drug from nanoparticles dispersion. To develop a successful nanoparticulate system, both drug release and polymer biodegradation are important consideration factors. In general, drug release rate depends on: (1) solubility of drug; (2) desorption of the surface bound/ adsorbed drug; (3) drug diffusion through the nanoparticles matrix; (4) nanoparticles matrix erosion/degradation; and (5) combination of erosion/diffusion process. Thus solubility, diffusion and biodegradation of the matrix materials govern the release process. Various methods which can be used to study the *in vitro* release of the drug are: (1) side-by-side diffusion cells with artificial or biological membranes; (2) dialysis bag diffusion technique; (3) reverse dialysis bag technique; (4) agitation followed by ultracentrifugation/centrifugation; (5) Ultra-filtration or centrifugal ultra-filtration techniques. Usually the release study is carried out by controlled agitation followed by centrifugation. Due to the time-consuming nature and technical difficulties encountered in the separation of nanoparticles from release media, the dialysis technique is generally preferred (Mohanraj, V.J. et al., 2006).

Drug-polymer interactions

Drug loading can be performed during the preparation of nanoparticles or by adsorbing/absorbing in preformed particles. Within the particle-forming polymer, drug can be present as a solid solution (individual drug molecules) or as a solid dispersion (amorphous/crystalline drug). It can be adsorbed on the particle surface [150] or bound chemically within the nanoparticles (Page-Clisson et al., 1998). The preparation process can also modify the crystal structure of the drug. The polymer is usually amorphous or semi-crystalline. Differential scanning calorimetry (DSC), (powder) x-ray diffractometry (XRPD) and FTIR are commonly used techniques to reveal the physicochemical state and possible interactions of the drug and the polymer in pharmaceutical micro- and nanoparticles. Polymer MW is determined e.g. by size exclusion chromatography (SEC) [58, 70] (the term gel permeation chromatography (GPC) is interchangeably used (Panyam, J. et al., 2003). DSC detects phase transitions such as glass transition, (exothermic) crystallization and (endothermic) melting: the nanoparticle sample is heated and changes in heat flow, compared to reference, are registered (Dubernet, C. et al., 1995). Crystallinity/amorphicity properties are obtained from XRPD analysis when diffraction pattern of the x-ray from the sample is determined as a function of scattering angle (Suryanarayanan, R., et al., 1995). In FTIR, a vibrational spectrum, characteristics for a given crystal structure, is obtained (Brittain, H.G, et al., 1991).

2.2.6. Liposomes

Liposomes are vesicles in which an aqueous volume is entirely enclosed by a membrane composed of lipid molecules, usually phospholipids (Figure: 2.7). Spontaneously formed upon dispersion in aqueous media, the size of such vesicles can range from tens of nanometers to tens of microns in diameter. In pharmaceutical sciences, liposomes have been used traditionally as formulation ingredients to assist in formulation of poorly soluble therapeutic agents for oral or parenteral administration. The antibiotic amphotericin B is an example of a marketed drug that makes use of this formulation principle for intravenous infusion (Gulati et al., 1998).

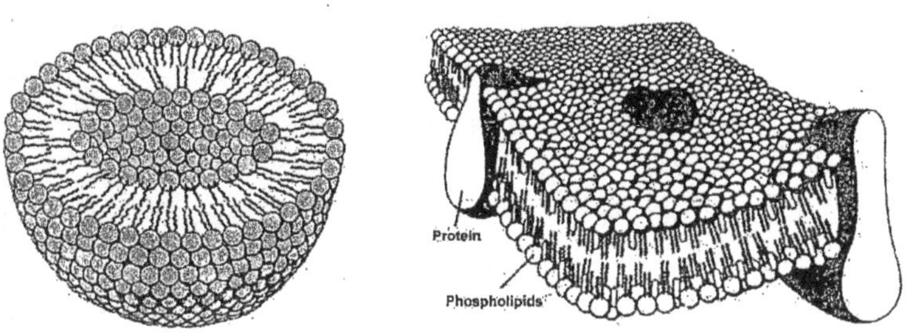

Figure: 2.7. Schematic representation of membranes: Liposome structure (left panel) and human cell membrane (right panel).

Both of them are formed by phospholipid molecules that have arranged themselves to form a membrane. Under certain physical conditions they will spontaneously form liposomes (left panel) whose walls are very similar in construction to the actual cell membrane shown on the right side.

Liposomes can contain large amounts of small molecules either within their aqueous interior or dissolved in the lipophilic region of their membrane bilayers. Enzymes have no longer access to the encapsulated substance which is hence protected from degradation and metabolism. This is one of the reasons why such liposomal delivery systems acquired much attention during the last years. Liposomes can be made of natural constituents. Their membrane is very similar to natural cell membranes (Figure: 2.7) and provides great convenience as models for membrane systems. Such naturally occurring constituents are cholesterol, phospholipids or fatty acids that make them a biocompatible and safe vehicle for medical *in vivo* applications. Those favourable properties can be adjusted by chemical modifications of the phospholipid-bilayer membrane of the liposome. Chemical modifications, such as saturation or pegylation of phospholipids are well established and numerous possibilities are described, which results in a vast versatility and flexibility of such phospholipid-bilayer membrane liposomes.

Pegylation of liposomes

Pharmacokinetics of conventional liposomes, i.e. liposomes that consist of naturally occurring phospholipids and cholesterol, are characterized by a very high systemic plasma clearance. After intravenous administration, such vesicles are rapidly removed from the circulation by macrophages of the reticuloendothelial system, namely the liver, the spleen, and the bone marrow. The liposome half-life in the circulation can considerably be prolonged by incorporation of gangliosides (such as monosialoganglioside GM1 derived from bovine brain or polyethylene glycol (PEG) derivatized lipids within the phospholipid bilayer of conventional liposomes. Conventional liposomes coated with the inert and biocompatible polymer PEG are often referred to as 'sterically stabilized' liposomes. The PEG coating is believed to prevent binding of opsonins from physiological fluids such as plasma, which in turn avoids the recognition by phagocytotic cells PEG phospholipids are safe and can be prepared synthetically at high purity and in large quantities, which has led to their acceptance for clinical applications. Animal and human studies have demonstrated pronounced differences with respect to pharmacokinetic parameters between conventional and sterically stabilized PEG-liposomes: in humans, pegylation of liposomes resulted in a 50-fold decrease in plasma volume of distribution to a value similar to the plasma volume (from 200 to 4.5 liters), a 200-fold decrease in systemic plasma clearance (from 22 to 0.1 l/hour) and a nearly 100-fold increase in area under the time-concentration curve. The apparent terminal half-life of PEG-liposomes reached up to 90 h in humans. The extended circulation half-life of sterically stabilized liposomes in combination with an increased permeability of tumor vasculature results in passive accumulation of PEG-liposomes in solid end-stage tumors. This principle of passive targeting to tumor tissue has been applied to commercial formulations of doxorubicin used for the chemotherapy of malignant Kaposi's sarcoma or breast cancer.

Aside from the effects described above, pegylation of liposomes offers an additional advantage. As it has been shown several times, incorporation of PEG derivatized lipids within the phospholipid bilayer provides liposomes with an enhanced stability. The underlying mechanism is in particular inhibition of membrane fusion, whereat PEG acts on three independent levels: First, inhibition of phospholipase C-induced liposome fusion, second, prevention of membrane apposition and third, stabilization of the lamellar phase. These effects may act together and lead, along with formerly discussed items, to a remarkably enhanced lifetime of liposomal carrier systems *in vivo*.

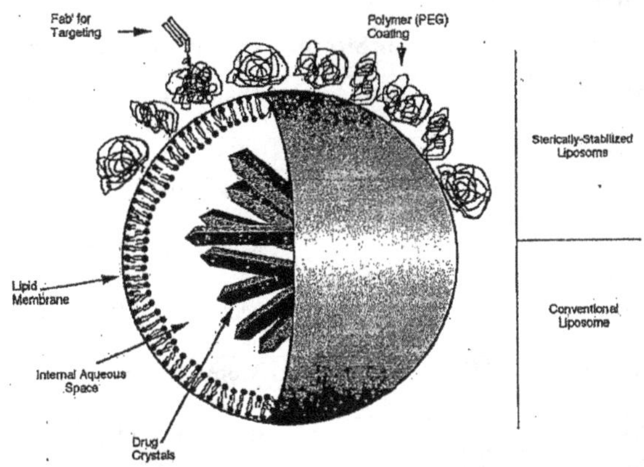

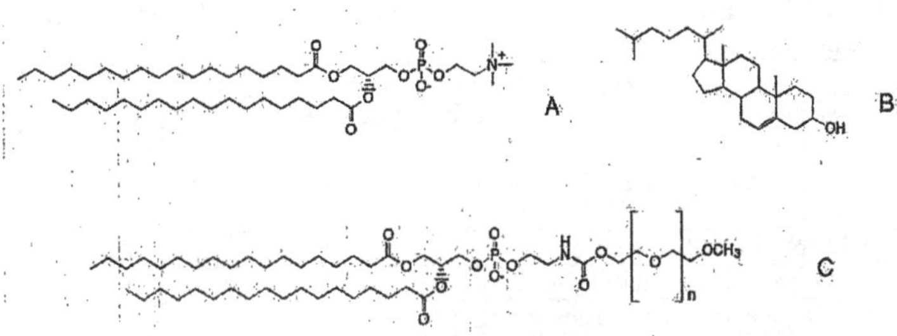

Figure: 2.8. Diagram of a drug-loaded liposome both with (SSL) and without (CL) a PEG coating. (A) or an equivalent, HSPC, is the primary phospholipid component, whereas Cholesterol (B) is the neutral lipid component. PEG-DSPE (C) is incorporated at concentrations of 4 to 6 mol% in SSL formulations.

Classification of Liposomes (Abdus Samad, Y et al., 2007)

Liposomes are classified on the basis of:

1. Structure.
2. Method of preparation.
3. Composition and application.
4. Conventional liposome.
5. Specialty liposome.

1. Classification Based on Structure

Table: 2.1.Vesicle Types with their Size and Number of Lipid Layers

Vesicle type	Abbreviation	Diameter size	No of Lipid bilayer
Unilamellar vesicle	UV	All size range	One
Small Unilamellar vesicle	SUV	20-100 nm	One
Medium Unilamellar vesicle	MUV	More than 100 nm	One
Large Lamellar vesicle	LUV	More than 100 nm	One
Giant Unilamellar vesicle	GUV	More than 1 micro meter	One
Oligolamellar vesicle	OLV	0.1-1 micro meter``	Aprrox. 5
Multilamellar vesicle	MLV	More than 1 micro meter	Multi compartmental structure

2. Based on Method of Preparation

Table: 2.2. Different Preparation Methods and the Vesicles Formed by these Methods

Preparation method	Vesicle type
Single or oligo lamellar vesicle made by reverse phase evaporation method	REV
Multi lamellar vesicle made by reverse phase evaporation method	MLV-REV
Stable pluri lamellar vesicle	SPLV
Frozen and thawed multi lamellar vesicle	FATMLV
Vesicle prepared by extrusion techniques	VET
Dehydration Rehydration method	DRV

3. Based on Composition and Application

Table: 2.3. Different Liposome with their Compositions

Type of Liposome	Abbreviation	Composition
Conventional liposome	CL	Neutral or negatively charge phospholipids and cholesterol
Fusogenic liposome	RSVE	Reconstituted sendai viriu envelops
pH sensitive liposomes	-	Phospholipids such as PER or DOPE with either CHEMS or OA
Cationic liposomes	-	Cationic lipid with DOPE
Long circulating liposomes	LCL	Neutral high temperature, cholesterol and 5- 10% PEG, DSP
Immuno liposomes	IL	CL or LCL with attached monoclonal antibody or recognition sequence

Based Upon Conventional Liposome

1- Stabilize natural lecithin (PC) mixtures
2- Synthetic identical, chain phospholipids
3- Glycolipids containing liposome

Based Upon Speciality Liposome

1- Bipolar fatty acid
2- Antibody directed liposome.
3- Methyl/ Methylene x- linked liposome.
4- Lipoprotein coated liposome.
5- Carbohydrate coated liposome.
6- Multiple encapsulated liposome.

Preparation of Liposomes

An important parameter to be considered when preparing the liposome is the rigidity of bi-layers. There are several groups of phospholipids that can be used for the liposome preparation which are as follows:

1. Phospholipids from natural source
2. Phospholipids modified from natural source
3. Semi synthetic phospholipids
4. Fully synthetic phospholipids and
5. Phospholipids with natural head groups

Dilauryl phosphotidyl choline (DLPC), Dimyristoyl phosphotidyl choline (DMPC), Dipalmitoyl phosphotidyl choline (DPPC), Distearoyl phosphotidyl choline (DSPC), Dioleolyl phosphotidyl choline (DOPC), Dilauryl phosphotidyl ethanolamine (DLPE), Dimyristoyl phosphotidyl ethanolamine (DMPE), Distearoyl phosphotidyl ethanolamine (DSPE), Dioleoyl phosphotidyl ethanolamine (DOPE), Dilauryl phosphotidyl glycerol (DLPG), Distearoyl phosphotidyl serine (DSPS) are the commonly used phospholipids for liposome preparation **(Table : 2.4).** Cholesterol can be added to the bilayer mixture for the following purposes:

1. Act as a fluidity buffer
2. Act as intercalator with phospholipids molecules

Alters the freedom of formation of carbon molecule in the acyl chain

3. Restrict the transformation of Trans to gauche conformation.

Table: 2.4. Phospholipids and Cholesterol which are Used for the Preparation of Liposome and their Transition Temperature (Tc) and Molecular Weights (Freise, J. et al., 1986)

Phospholipids	Abbreviation	Charge	Tc (°c)	Mol. Wt.
Brain Sphingomyellin	BSPM	0	32	814
Cholesterol	CH	0	--	387
Dimyristoyl phosphatidylcholine	DMPC	0	23	678
Dipalmitoyl phosphatidylcholine	DPPC	041		734
Distearoyl phosphatidylcholine	DSPC	0	58	790
Dioleyl phosphatidylcholine	DOPC	0	-22	786
Dilauryl phosphatidylglycerol	DLPG	-1	4	633
Dimyristoyl phosphatidylglycerol	DMPG	-1	23	689
Dipalmitoyl phosphatidylglycerol	DPPG	-1	41	745
Distearoyl phosphatidylglycerol	DSPG	-1	55	796
Phosphatidyl ethanolamine	PE	0	48	720
Dimyristoyl phosphatidyl ethanolamine	DMPE	0	--	636
Dipalmitoyl phosphatidyl ethanolamine	DPPE	0	60	692
Distearoyl phosphatidyl ethanolamine	DSPE	0	--	748
Dimyristoyl PA	DMPA	-2	51	618
Dipalmitoyl PA	DPPA	-2	67	649
Dioleoyl PA	DOPA	-2	--	701
Dipalmitoyl phosphatidyl serine	DPPS	--	48	758
Dicetyl phosphate	DCP	-1	--	547

Rajendran et al 1997 prepared liposome from egg lecithin by modified ether injection technique using stearylamine added dicetylphosphate as the charge inducing agent. The charged liposomes were larger in the size and showed better drug entrapment efficiency and were found more entrapped in the organs of the reticuloendothelial system than neutral liposome. It was also shown that cholesterol decreased the permeability coefficients of negative, neutral as well as positively charged membranes to Na+, K+, Cl- and glucose. Cholesterol also stabilized the membranes against temperature changes, leading to lower permeability at elevated temperatures. Cholesterol is essential for lowering membrane permeability, and imparting better stability. Cholesterol also modulates membrane- protein interactions. The polymorphic phase behavior of lipids is modulated by a variety of factors including hydration, temperature and divalent cations, degree of unsaturation of the acyl chains and the presence of other lipids such as sterols. *Lasic et al 1993* tried active trapping of amphipathic weak bases inside liposomes by using pH induced transmembrane potential establishment. Doxorubicin was used as a model drug. Triton X-100 has been observed to affect the physical properties of liposomes. Solubilizing effect of Triton X-100 on the membranes composed of different phospholipids and cholesterol has been evaluated. The measured changes indicated a drastic structure transformation into entities of fairly high dipolar moment leading to solubilization of phospholipids membranes. The three different strategies for the preparation of liposomes are as follows:

1. Mechanical methods
2. Methods based on replacement of organic solvent
3. Methods based on size transformation or fusion of prepared vesicle

1. Mechanical methods

A. Film Method

The original method of *Bangham et al 1965* is still the simplest procedure for the liposome formation but having some limitation because of its low encapsulation efficiency. In this technique liposome are prepared by hydrating the thin lipid film in an organic solvent and organic solvent is then removed by film deposition under vacuum. When all the solvent get removed, the solid lipid mixture is hydrated using aqueous buffer. The lipids spontaneously swell and hydrate to form liposome. This method yields a heterogeneous sized population of MLVs over 1 micro meter in diameter. *Nagarsenkar et al 1997* prepared lidocaine encapsulated liposome employing the conventional lipid film hydration technique. The prepared liposomal dispersions were investigated, the results showed that lidocaine incorporated into the liposomes got selectively partitioned and localized in the skin to a greater extent. A topical liposomal gel formulation containing 2% w/w lidocaine was prepared using cabopol-934 as the gelling agent. The liposome preparation of lidocaine gave a much longer duration of action compared to the conventional topical formulation. *Ridy et al 1997* prepared oxamniquine liposomes with different compositions and surface charge were prepared by the chloroform film method. The amount of oxamniquine entrapped was estimated. Negatively charged liposomes exhibited the highest percentage entrapment (23.09%). The maximum oxamniquine entrapment was achieved in liposomes prepared from phospholipid molar ratio (7:4:1). The chemoprophylactic effect of free and oxamiquine liposome formulations was estimated and showed that drug encapsulated in liposomes provided more efficient prophylaxis.

B. Ultrasonic Method

This method is used for the preparation of SUVs with diameter in the range of 15-25 μm. Ultrasonication of an aqueous dispersion of phospholipids is done by two types of sonicators i.e. either probe sonicators or bath sonicators. The probe sonicators are used for the small volume which requires high energy while the bath sonicators are employed for the large volume (Hwang, K.J. et al., 1987).

2. Methods Based on Replacement of Organic Solvents

In this method lipids are co-solvated in organic solution, which is then dispersed into aqueous phase containing material to be entrapped within the liposome. This method is of two types:

A. Reverse Phase Evaporation

The lipid mixture is added to a round bottom flask and the solvent is removed under reduced pressure by a rotary evaporator. The system is purged with nitrogen and lipids are re-dissolved in the organic phase which is the phase in which the reverse phase vesicle will form. Diethyl ether and isopropyl ether are the usual solvents of choice. After the lipids are redissolved the emulsion are obtained and than the solvent is removed from an emulsion by evaporation to a semisolid gel under reduced pressure. Non encapsulated material is then removed. The resulting liposomes are called reverse phase evaporation vesicles (REV). This method is used for the preparation of large uni-lamellar and oligo-lamellar vesicles formulation and it has the ability to encapsulate large macromolecules with high efficiency. *Pleumchitt et al. 2000* showed the physicochemical properties of phospatidylcholine cholesterol liposomes containing amphotericin B prepared by reverse phase evaporation method. The liposomes containing amphotericin B 2.0 mol % of total lipid demonstrated the highest percentage of drug entrapment. The highest drug entrapment efficiency (approx. 95%) with particle size range of 1307- 1451 nm was obtained with the formulation containing 1:1 molar ratio of phosphatidycholine to cholesterol.

B. Ether Vaporization Method

There are two method according to the solvent used:

1- Ethanol injection method.
2- Ether injection method.

In ethanol injection method, the lipid is injected rapidly through a fine needle into an excess of saline or other aqueous medium. In ether injection method the lipid is injected very slowly through a fine needle into an excess of saline or other aqueous medium.

3. Methods Based on Size Transformation or Fusion of Preformed Vesicle

A. Freeze Thaw Extrusion Method

The freeze thaw method is an extension of the classical DRV method. Liposomes formed by the film method are vortexed with the solute to be entrapped until the entire film is suspended and the resulted MLVs are frozen in luke warm water and than vortexed again. After two cycles of freeze thaw and vortexing the sample is extruded three times. This is followed by six freeze thaw cycle and addition eight extrusions. This process ruptures and defuses SUVs during which the solute equilibrates between inside and outside and liposome themselves fuse and increase in size to form large Unilamellar vesicle by extrusion technique (LUVET). For the encapsulation of protein this method is widely used. *Canto et al 1999* prepared liposomes of soya phosphatidylcholine, cholesterol and stearylamine (molar ratio 6/3/1) and 0.1 % ∝ tocopherol by the extrusion of multi-lamellar vesicles through 0.2 μm polycarbonate membrane. They analyzed free piroxicam at 4 mg/kg, piroxicam encapsulated in liposomes and added to 1.5% hydroxyethylcellulose (HEC) gel at 1.6 mg/kg, and piroxicam encapsulated in liposomes and added to HEC gel at 4 mg/kg. The inhibition of inflammation obtained was 21.1%, 32.8% and 47.4% respectively. These results showed that the encapsulation of piroxicam produced an increase of topical anti-inflammatory effect.

B. The Dehydration- Rehydration Method

In this method the empty buffer containing SUVs and rehydrating it with the aqueous fluid containing the material to be entrapped after which they are dried. This leads to a dispersion of solid lipids in finely subdivided form. Freeze drying is often the method of choice. The vesicles are than rehydrated. Liposomes obtained by this method are usually oligo lamellar vesicle. *Bhalerao et al 2003* prepared liposome by the conventional thin film hydration technique. The result showed that the formation of bi-layered liposomes in the particle size range of 0.2-0.8276 μm occurred with a maximum entrapment efficiency of 42.6%. The liposomes stored at 4-5oC showed maximum stability as compared to those stored at any other temperature.

Sizing of Liposomes

Size characteristic of liposome have a major effect on their fate i.e. for which application they can be used for. The therapeutic applications of liposome are dependent on physical integrity and stability of lipid bilayer structure. Therefore liposome production procedure must be predictable and reproducible with particle size distribution within a certain size range. Lipid based formulation can be devised as site specific drug delivery vesicles that are:

1. Relatively cleared by kupffer cells of liver and the macrophages
2. Evade detection of active substance by the reticuloendothelial system (RES) and efficiency deliver liposome incorporated material to target tissue, organ or tumor. Sizing of liposome are usually performed by sequential extrusion at relatively low pressure through polycarbonate membrane (PCM). The membrane extrusion technique can be used to process LUVs as well as MLVs to form LUVETs. The membrane (PCM) is of pore size 0.27 micrometer. The other procedure of sizing of the liposomes are gel chromatography , mainly used to size liposome but more typically used to remove encapsulated components by separation. Sonication is the third method of sizing of liposomes, but this method is related with following disadvantages:

- Exclusion of oxygen is difficult which result in per oxidation reaction
- Titanium probes shed metal particle resulting in contamination
- They can generate aerosols, which exclude them with from use with certain agents

These above problems are mainly related with the probe sonication but these problems can be removed by using the bath sonication.

Characterization of Liposomes

After preparation and before use in immunoassay the liposome must be characterized. Evaluation could be classified into three broad categories which are physical, chemical and biological methods. The physical methods include various parameters, which are size, shape, surface features, lamellarity phase behaviors and drug release profile.

Ma et al 1993 evaluated structural integrity of liposomal phospholipids membrane by a new technique of gamma-ray perturb angular correlation (PAC) spectroscopy. In this ^{111}In-label diethyene triamine penta acetic acid (DTPA) derivative dipalmitoyl phosphatidyl ethanolamine (DPPE) lipid were incorporated in the SUVs. This helped in the continuous non- invasive monitoring of the microenvironment of the lipid bilayer.

Kolchens et al 1993 used quasi elastic light scattering (QELS) or photon correlate spectroscopic (PCS) technique for determining distribution of vesicles prepared by freeze-thaw extrusion method. The influence of filter pore size, extrusion press and lipid concentration on the size and size distribution extruded vesicles was studied. Chemical characterization includes those studies which established the purity and potency of various liposomal constituents. Biological characterization is helpful in establishing the safety and suitability of formulation for the *in vivo* use for therapeutic application. The characteristics of the carrier through appropriate choice of membrane components, size and charge determines the final behavior of liposomes both *in vitro* and *in vivo* as well.

Jousma et al 1987 characterized the vesicles obtained by repetitive extrusion through polycarbonate membranes using freeze fracture electron microscopy, small angle X-ray scattering (SAXS), and encapsulated volume using 6-carboxy flurescein (6-CF) and ^{31}p-NMR as aqueous markers.

Characterization of Liposomes with their Quality Control Assays (Jones, G. R. et al 1989)

A. Biological characterization

• Characterization parameters	-Instrument for analysis
• Sterility	-Aerobic/anaerobic culture
• Pyrogenicity	-Rabbit fever response
• Animal toxicity	-Monitoring survival rats

B. Chemical characterization

• Characterization parameter	-Instrument for analysis
• Phospholipids concentration	-HPLC/Barrlet assay
• Cholesterol concentration	-HPLC / cholesterol oxide assay
• Drug concentration	-Assay method
• Phospholipids per oxidation	-UV observance
• Phospholipids hydrolysis	-HPLC/ TLC
• Cholesterol auto-oxidation	-HPLC/ TLC
• Anti-oxidant degradation	-HPLC/TLC
• PH	-PH meter
• Osmolarity	-Osmometer

C. Physical Characterization

• Characterization parameter	-Instrument for analysis
• Vesicle shape, and surface morphology	-TEM and SEM
• Vesicle size and size distribution	-Dynamic light scattering, TEM
• Surface charge	- Free flow electrophoresis
• Electrical surface potential and surface-pH sensitive probe	-Zeta potential measurement and pH

• Lamellarity	-P^{31}NMR
• Phase behavior	-DSC, freeze fracture electron Microscopy
• Percent capture	-Mini column centrifugation, gel Exclusion
• Drug release	-Diffuse cell/ dialysis

Stabilization of Liposome

The stability of liposome should meet the same standard as conventional pharmaceutical formulation. The stability of any pharmaceutical product is the capabilities of the delivery system in the prescribed formulation to remain within defined or pre established limits for predetermined period of time. Chemical stability involves prevention of both the hydrolysis of ester bonds in the phospholipids bilayer and the oxidation of unsaturated sites in the lipid chain. Chemical instability leads to physical instability or leakage of encapsulated drug from the bilayer and fusion and finally aggregation of vesicles. *Chen et al 1987* introduced the pro-liposome concept of liposome preparation to avoid physicochemical instability encountered in liposome suspension such as aggregation, fusion, hydrolysis, and/or oxidation. Approaches that can be taken to increase liposomal stability involve efficient formulation and lyophillization. Formulation involves the selection of the appropriate lipid composition, concentration of bilayer, aqueous phase ingredients such as buffers, antioxidant, metal chelators and cryoprotectants. Charge inducing lipid such as phosphotidyl glycerol can be incorporated into liposome bilayer to decrease fusion while cholesterol and sphingomyellin can be included in the formulation to decrease permeability and leakage of encapsulated drugs. Buffers at neutral pH can decrease hydrolysis; addition of antioxidant such as sodium ascorbate can decrease oxidation. Oxygen potential is kept to minimum during processing by nitrogen purging solution. In general successful formulation of stable liposomal drug product requires the following precautions:

1. Processing with fresh, purified lipids and solvents.
2. Avoidance of high temperature and excessive shear forces
3. Maintenance of low oxygen potential (Nitrogen purging)
4. Use of antioxidant or metal chelators
5. Formulating at neutral pH.
6. Use of lyoprotectant when freeze drying

2.2.7. Super critical fluid technology

Conventional preparation of liposomes unfortunately involves evaporation of organic solvent, preparation of vesicles by sonication, and dialysis to provide Unilamellar vesicles. Use of SCF CO_2 to provide a "clean" and effective alternative to traditional methods of drug processing, related to micronization, encapsulation, and impregnation of molecules of interest to pharmaceutical industry; formation of micronsized particles with SCF CO2 by rapid expansion of supercritical solutions (RESS) or phase separation by gas saturated solutions (PGSS), gas antisolvent (GAS) techniques by solubilizing the drug in an organic solvent and introducing SCF to solubilize the solvent and allow the drug to precipitate and also incorporating drugs into controlled matrices; based on these techniques, nanoparticles of cyclosporine A in phospholipid and ibuprofen nanoparticles in aqueous solution were made. In the gas antisolvent (GAS) technique, in which the gas is used as an antisolvent to reduce the solvating power of the organic solvent, the ability of the SCFs to dissolve and expand the organic solvents for precipitation of solids from organic solution is exploited (Udaya Sankar Kadimi et al., 2007). Conventional drug particle precipitation uses organic solvents as an antisolvent for precipitation or as emulsifiers for emulsion process. Traces of residual organic solvents, such as methylene chloride, that may still be in the drug particles have motivated researchers to find alternative methods for particle formation. Organic solvent use should be limited for pharmaceutical manufacturing operations, based on United States Pharmacopeia (USP) standards. An alternative to reduce this problem is to use supercritical carbon dioxide (CO_2) as an antisolvent to precipitate drug particles from solution since CO_2 is nonflammable, non-toxic, inexpensive, renewable, and environmentally benign (McHugh, M.A. et al., 1994).

Toxic, flammable, volatile, combustible, and expensive organic solvents are used in considerable amounts in many industrial processes. As a possible alternative to reduce health, environmental, and safety risks, supercritical or near critical fluids, especially carbon dioxide are considered. A substance is in its supercritical state at conditions above the critical temperature and pressure. The substance is then neither a gas nor a liquid but possesses properties of both. The density is liquid like, the viscosity is gaseous, and the diffusion coefficient lies between that of gas and liquid. In the supercritical state a change in the density of the fluid can be easily obtained by manipulation of pressure and/or temperature (Lene Frederiksen et al., 1997).

In order to successfully design a CO_2 antisolvent process, it is important to understand the effects of the operating parameters on particle characteristics. However, very few authors have explained experimental particle size and morphology results in light of current hydrodynamic, kinetic and thermodynamic theories (Bristow, S. et al., 2001). Furthermore, the development of unique methodologies for optimizing these parameters to control particle size is essential. Thus far very few authors have been able to analyze particle nucleation and growth inside the precipitation vessel due to the extremely short time scale of drug precipitation. Online monitoring techniques to understand the fundamental mechanisms of dense gas precipitation are limited by the high-pressure environment (Thiering, R. et al., 2001). The progression of the precipitation process is therefore hard to record and the effects of start-up and shut down of the process cannot be determined. This dissertation attempts to address these issues by demonstrating a technique for monitoring and determining the thermodynamic, fluid dynamic, and crystallization mechanisms that are important for designing and optimizing different CO_2 antisolvent processes for the formulation of small crystalline drug products. Furthermore, other applications for the use of CO_2 antisolvent process in improving drug crystallinity and drug encapsulation are presented.

Benefits of carbon dioxide as an antisolvent

Researchers have developed particle formation methods that utilize the unique properties of supercritical fluids. A fluid is said to be supercritical when the pressure and temperature are higher than its critical pressure (PC) and critical temperature (TC). Some of the most common inorganic used for supercritical technology are listed in **Table: 2.5.**

Table: 2.5. Critical parameters for some common inorganics used for supercritical technology

Gas	TC (K)	PC (kPa)	Tb (K at 100 kPa)
Helium	3.31	110	3.2
Nitrogen	126	3400	77.4
Carbon Dioxide	304	7380	(gas-solid)
Water	647	22100	373

Out of all the available supercritical fluids, carbon dioxide is the best processing medium in the pharmaceutical industries because it is non-toxic, affordable, has a relatively mild critical temperature (304 K) and low critical pressure (7.38 MPa) and a very high volatility. A representative phase diagram of the CO2 system is shown in a representative phase diagram of the CO_2 system is shown in **Figure: 2.9.**

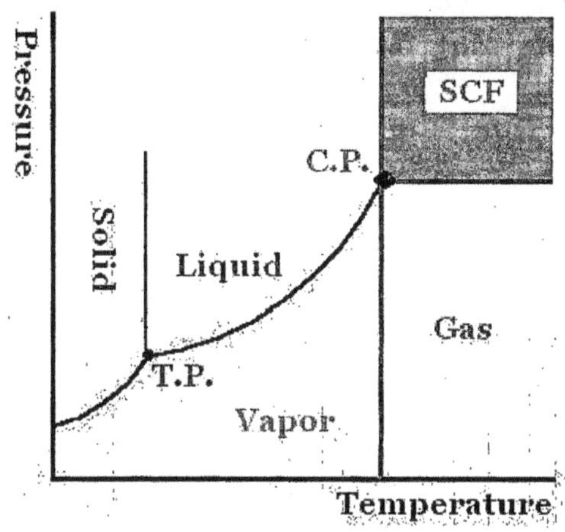

Figure: 2.9. Phase diagram of CO_2 system

A supercritical fluid (SCF) is characterized by physical and thermal properties that are between those of the pure liquid and gas. The fluid density is a strong function of the temperature and pressure. The diffusivity of SF is much higher than for a liquid and SCF readily penetrates porous and fibrous solids. Consequently, SCF can offer good catalytic activity.

Properties of Supercritical Fluids

There are drastic changes in some important properties of a pure liquid as its temperature and pressure is increased approaching the thermodynamic critical point. For example, under thermodynamic-equilibrium conditions, the visual distinction between liquid and gas phases, as well as the difference between the liquid and gas densities, disappear at and above the critical point. Similar drastic changes exist in properties of a liquid mixture as it approaches the thermodynamic critical loci of the mixture. Other properties of a liquid fuel that change widely near the critical region are thermal conductivity, surface tension, constant-pressure heat capacity and viscosity. In comparing a liquid sample with a supercritical fluid (SCF) sample of the same fuel both possessing the same density, thermal conductivity and diffusivity of a SF are higher than the liquid, its viscosity is much lower, while its surface tension and heat of vaporization have completely disappeared. These drastic changes make a supercritical fuel appreciably preferred over that of a liquid fuel with the same density. Further, it is expected that the combustion phenomena resulting from that of a supercritical fuel will be quite different from that of a liquid fuel. Applications of SCF include recovery of organics from oil shale, separations of biological fluids, bioseparation, petroleum recovery, crude de-asphalting and dewaxing, coal processing (reactive extraction and liquefaction), selective extraction of fragrances, oils and impurities from agricultural and food products, pollution control, combustion and many other applications

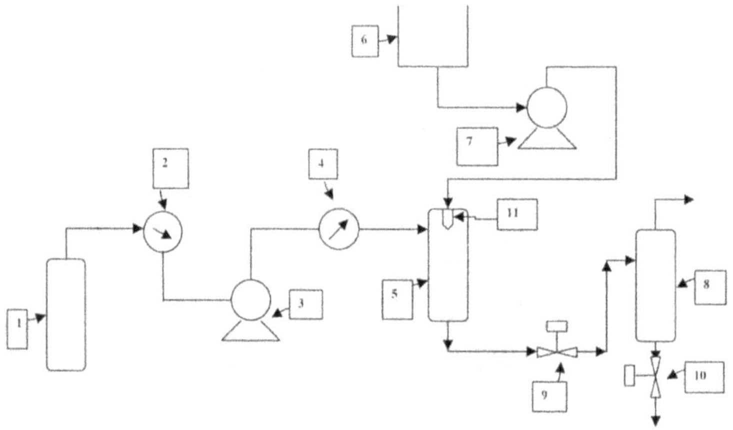

Figure: 2.10. Schematic diagram of Supercritical fluid particle former.

In addition to these advantages, supercritical CO_2 possesses fluid properties intermediate between liquid and gas. Around the critical point, properties such as density, viscosity, solvency, diffusivity can all be manipulated by changing either pressure or temperature (McHugh, M.A. et al., 1994). Supercritical CO_2 has both a gas-like viscosity and a liquid-like density. The low viscosity compared to other liquids such as water allows CO_2 to have a faster transport rate for particulate formation processes. The diffusion coefficient for CO_2 into solvent is very large compared to conventional liquid antisolvents. This results in rapid mixing to initiate nucleation inside the solvent droplets. A typical nucleation rate of a solute in a CO_2 antisolvent process is on the order of 10-5 to 10-4 s. Furthermore, for the application of particle design, supercritical fluids are desirable since they have controllable solvating power. By adjusting the pressure and temperature, CO_2 can extract the organic solvent and dry the particles in a continuous and single step process. Since supercritical CO_2 create non-oxidizing and non-degrading environments for sensitive compounds, the drying process causes less damage to drug particles compared to conventional solvent evaporation process.

Table: 2.6. Critical conditions of commonly used supercritical solvents (D. R. Lide, 1994)

Fluid	Tc (oC)	Pc (bar)
Ethylene	9.3	50.4
Carbon dioxide	31.1	73.8
Nitrous oxide	31.3	73.8
Ethane	32.3	48.8
Chlorodifluoromethane	96.0	51.9
Propylene	91.8	46.2
Propane	96.7	42.5
Ethanol	240.8	61.4
Water	374.1	217.7

Carbon dioxide antisolvent particle formation methods

There are many different processes that use CO_2 either as a solvent or an antisolvent for particle formation applications. This section will review these processes and the applications with which they are normally associated.

1. **Rapid expansion of supercritical solutions (RESS)**

The process of rapid expansion of supercritical solutions (RESS) produces particles by spraying a supercritical solution with the dissolved solute through a nozzle into atmospheric conditions to rapidly expand the supercritical fluid, resulting in a highly supersaturated solution and rapid precipitation. The resulting high-pressure drop creates very high jet velocity to atomize the droplets. A diagram of the process is seen in **Figure: 2.11.**

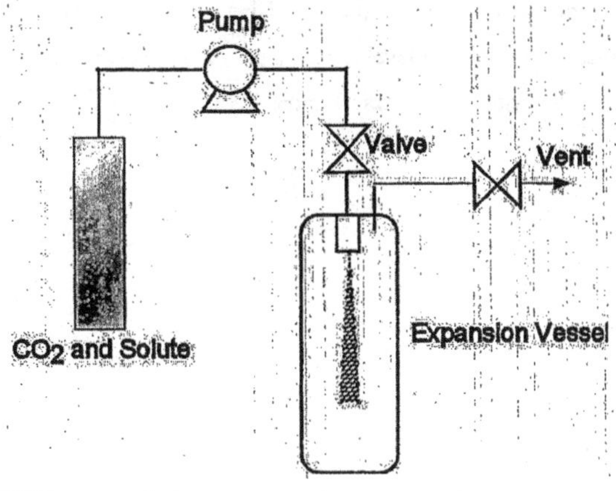

Figure: 2.11. RESS system design

There are many applications using this type of process for coatings (Chernyak, Y. et al., 2001), microparticles processing of polymers and drugs, and encapsulation of the drug with a polymer. The benefit of RESS is that it is fairly simple and requires only the use of one capillary nozzle for the expansion process. The major limitations of its use for pharmaceutical application are that the solute has to be able to dissolve in the supercritical fluid at appreciable amounts in order to be viable for manufacturing (Debenedetti, P.G. et al., 1993). A realistic assumption for the production rate of drugs would be around 90.7-1814 kg per annum, which equates to about 10-230 g/h. Typical solubility of a crystalline drug such as acetaminophen is only soluble up to 0.005486 kg/m3 in high pressure CO_2 with a density of 854.07 kg/m3, which will make the RESS process highly unprofitable. Since most small molecules, proteins, and biodegradable polymers are not very soluble in supercritical CO_2 (York, P. et al., 2004), there would be a need to use harmful organic co-solvents in order to enhance the solubility of the target drug. Furthermore, there has not been much success with the encapsulation of drugs in a polymer matrix with RESS due to the difficulty in dissolving two components in supercritical CO_2 and controlling the different time scales needed for sequential precipitation of the drug and polymer.

2. Particles from gas saturated solutions (PGSS)

The particles from gas saturated solutions or PGSS process involves injecting supercritical CO_2 into either a melted or liquid-suspended substance first, which leads to a gas saturated suspension. The suspension is then expanded through a nozzle to produce fine particles similar to spray drying. PGSS can formulate drugs that normally do not dissolve in CO_2, which expands the number of compounds that can be treated by this technique. This process however is more promising for making particles from materials that normally absorb CO_2 at high levels such as polymers (Reverchon, E. et al., 2001). A diagram of the PGSS system is shown in **Figure: 2.12.**

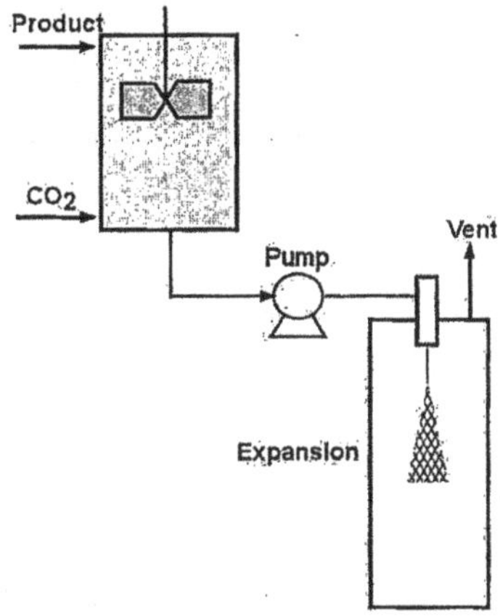

Figure: 2.12.PGSS system design

Sievers R E et al 1999 patented a similar process for preparation of protein particles that allows the proteins to dissolve in water without the use of organic solvents.

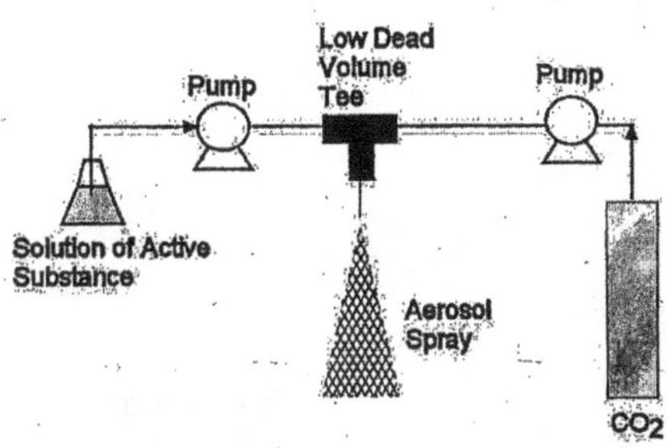

Figure: 2.13. *Sievers et al 1999* design for the production of proteins with PGSS without use of organic solvents

The CO_2 at high pressure is mixed with water at a low volume tee, which forms an emulsion before expanding to atmospheric pressure and high temperature to form drug particles. A problem with this design is that water under contact with CO_2 will form carbonic acid from CO_2 and lower the pH to as low as 3 (Holmes, J.D. et al., 1999) which may potentially denature proteins and other sensitive pharmaceutical compounds. Another problem is that this process prevents encapsulation of the drug since most biodegradable polymers are not water-soluble (McHugh, M.A. et al., 1994).

3. Gas antisolvent (GAS)

The gas antisolvent (GAS) process uses a dense gas such as CO_2 as an antisolvent to precipitate out the drug from a batch solution. In order for the process to work, CO_2 needs to be appreciably miscible with the solvent and the drug needs to be insoluble with CO_2 at the operating pressure and temperature range. The precipitator is initially filled with a solution at a certain drug concentration and temperature. The rapid injection of compressed CO_2 into the vessel mixes with the solution and causes a volumetric expansion of the system reducing the bulk density of the solution, which in turn lowers the solvating power of the solvent. Due to the rapid mass transfer of compressed CO_2 into the solvent, the mixing of the two fluids is very fast and results in smaller and more uniform particles as compared to conventional processes such as "salting out" that uses either electrolytes or non-electrolytes. Furthermore, the GAS process has also been shown to retain the biomolecular activity of proteins such as lysozyme, meaning that the process is suitable for sensitive biomolecules (Winters, M.A. et al., 1999). A diagram of the GAS process is shown in **Figure: 2.14.**

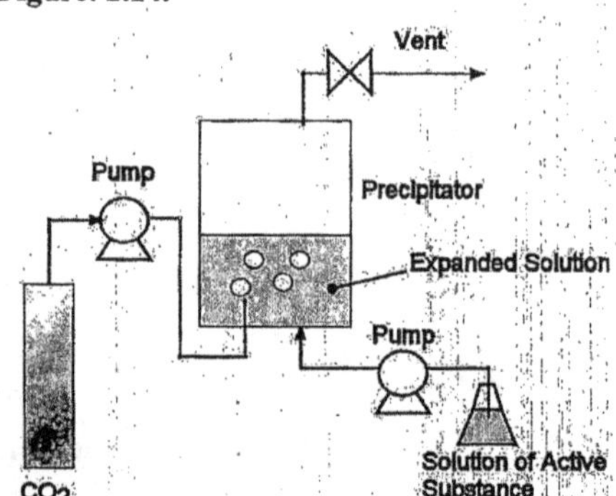

Figure: 2.14. GAS system design

GAS is more versatile than RESS since the process does not rely on the solubility of the compound in compressed CO_2. Particle formulations of a variety of drug and polymer compounds that are normally not significantly soluble in pure CO_2 have been demonstrated with the GAS process (Warwick, B. et al., 2000). Several works have also demonstrated GAS fractionation for different compounds ranging from small molecule drugs to macromolecules (Muhrer, G. et al., 2003). Very few authors have attempted to use GAS for encapsulation of drug in a biodegradable polymer because of the difficulty in controlling the time scales of precipitation of the drug and the polymer. GAS encapsulation has been done by either preparing the polymer separately from the drug precipitation or by using a semi-continuous GAS process, where the solution carrying the drug and polymers are sprayed into a CO_2-filled tank (Elvassore, N. et al., 2001). Since there is a lot of solvent inside the vessel, a major disadvantage of GAS is the long drying time to reduce organic solvents from the particles to satisfactory levels. The residual solvent in some instances may not be fully removed especially in the case for polymer and protein products (Muhrer, G. et al., 2003). A solution to the drying step has been proposed in which the system was injected with carbon dioxide in the two-phase region where there is liquid and vapor antisolvent present inside the vessel. Another problem to consider with GAS is the long loading and unloading time between each experiment.

4. Supercritical antisolvent process (SAS)

Supercritical antisolvent process (SAS) is a semi-continuous process in which the solution with the product is sprayed through a specially designed nozzle into condensed gas in a pressurized vessel (Bleich, J. et al., 1993). The nozzle in SAS disperses the solution into the condensed gas phase inside the vessel to enhance mixing and mass transfer. SAS is also referred to as aerosol solvent extraction system (ASES) or precipitation with compressed antisolvent (PCA). A diagram of the SAS process is shown in **Figure 2.15.**

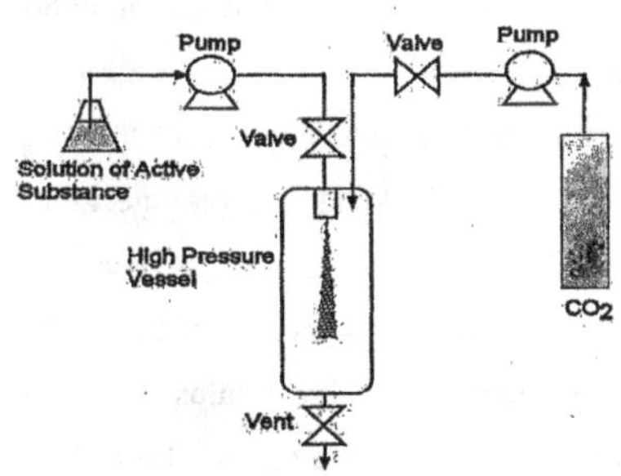

Figure 2.15. SAS system design

Similar to the GAS process, the CO_2 needs to be miscible with the solvent in order to precipitate the drug. Controlling how the solution disperses into compressed CO_2 to initiate precipitation is important in controlling the particle size and morphology. Some authors have designed either different nozzle configurations or added ultrasound vibration at the nozzle tip to enhance the mixing and diffusion of CO_2 into the solution to initiate precipitation (Chattopadhyay, P. et al., 2001). The CO_2 and solution can also mix inside a low volume area before being sprayed inside the vessel. The ease in changing the system configuration to tune the product characteristics is what makes SAS very attractive. Thus far in the literature, SAS seems to offer the best particle formation method due to its capability to produce smaller and more uniform particles compared to the GAS process as a result of the enhanced mixing between the antisolvent and drug solution (Fusaro, F. et al., 2005). The semi-continuous nature of the process allows for generation of large amounts of drug products without the need to stop the system, which makes SAS an attractive manufacturing process compared to GAS. Furthermore, the solvent inside the vessel is constantly extracted and removed from the system during the experiment to give SAS an added advantage to the more time consuming drying associated with the GAS process. The presence of less solvent inside the vessel during the SAS experiments compared to GAS generally results in less agglomeration of the particles. Both GAS and SAS are milder processes for preventing drug degradation and loss of activity for biomolecules as compared to conventional organic solvent "salting out" methods (Winters, M.A. et al., 1996). SAS has been used in processing different materials such as pigment powders [61], semiconductor precursors (Reverchon, E. et al., 1998) and inorganic crystals (Yeo, S.D. et al., 2000). Single component particle design for many pharmaceutical compounds have been widely studied with varying results with respect to morphology and particle size (Reverchon, E. et al., 2000). The particular focus for single component precipitation is in controlling polymer morphology and shape with SAS process for use in controlled release applications (Reverchon, E. et al., 1999). Due to the ease of separating the time scale of precipitation for the drug and the polymer by either changing the nozzle design or by adding multiple injection nozzles, many authors have shown that the drugs can be encapsulated in a single process at appreciable amounts.

5. Solution enhanced dispersion by supercritical fluids (SEDS)

Solution enhanced dispersion by supercritical fluids (SEDS) was developed by Hanna and York (Hanna, M. et al., 1994) to improve on the idea of SAS by changing the design of the nozzle to enhance mixing of the solution and to control microparticle formation. The system borrows from the benefits of SAS in that the drug of interest does not need to be dissolved in CO_2 and toxic solvents can be reduced or eliminated in a single continuous process. The uniqueness of SEDS rests in the design of the nozzle, which uses the idea of coaxial tube geometry to simultaneously deliver the solution and the antisolvent. A diagram of this configuration taken from experiments conducted in this dissertation is depicted in **Figure: 2.16.**

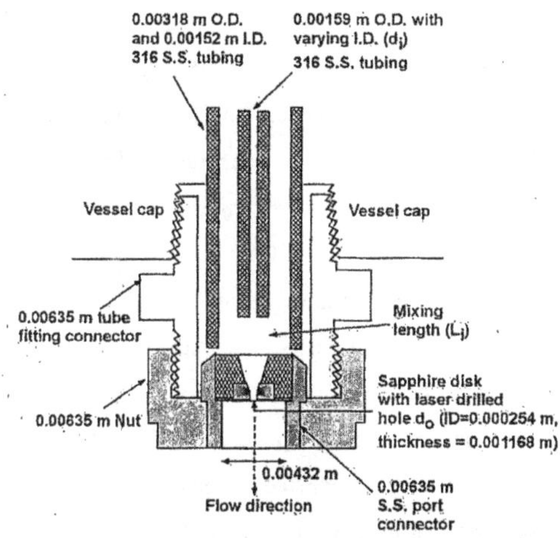

Figure: 2.16. SEDS coaxial tubing design used for the present study

Prior to spraying the particles into the pressurized precipitation vessel through a nozzle constriction, the solvent carrying the product mixes rapidly with the supercritical fluid in a small volume area called the mixing length (Li). The mixing length is believed to enhance mixing and initiate nucleation before the particles are sprayed into the collection vessel (Hanna, M. et al., 1994). Furthermore, Hanna and York explained that the design would allow for better control of parameters such as temperature, pressure, and flow rate at the point of nucleation inside the mixing length. Similar to other antisolvent processes, SEDS is a mild precipitation process for sensitive pharmaceutical compounds, such as proteins, that causes minimal loss of activity (Moshashaee, S., M. et al., 2000). The flexibility of SEDS lies in the fact that the coaxial tubing can be arranged in different configurations to allow for more flexibility in controlling encapsulation of biomolecules (Ghaderi, R. P. et al., 2000). SEDS has been shown to be able to control particle size of many drugs and polymers by adjusting the temperature, pressure, flow rate, and concentration (Ghaderi, R. P. et al., 2000).

Applications of Supercritical fluid technology for Particle Engineering

SCFs can be applied to a variety of other applications where nano- and micro dimensions of the drug material in excipients are important for drug release. These include the following.

Production of nanoparticles using supercritical fluid technology

Conventional methods such as solvent extraction-evaporation, solvent diffusion and organic phase separation methods require the use of organic solvents which are hazardous to the environment as well as to physiological systems. Therefore, the supercritical fluid technology has been investigated as an alternative to prepare biodegradable micro- and nanoparticles because supercritical fluids are environmentally safe. A supercritical fluid can be generally defined as a solvent at a temperature above its critical temperature, at which the fluid remains a single phase regardless of pressure. Supercritical CO_2 (SC CO2) is the most widely used supercritical fluid because of its mild critical conditions (Tc = 31.1 °C, Pc = 73.8 bars), non-toxicity, non-flammability, and low price. The most common processing techniques involving supercritical fluids are supercritical anti-solvent (SAS) and rapid expansion of critical solution (RESS). The process of SAS employs a liquid solvent, eg methanol, which is completely miscible with the supercritical fluid (SC CO_2), to dissolve the solute to be micronized; at the process conditions, because the solute is insoluble in the supercritical fluid, the extract of the liquid solvent by supercritical fluid leads to the instantaneous precipitation of the solute, resulting the formation of nanoparticles. *Thote and Gupta et al 2005* reported the use of a modified SAS method for formation of hydrophilic drug dexamethasone phosphate drug nanoparticles for microencapsulation purpose. RESS differs from the SAS process in that its solute is dissolved in a supercritical fluid (such as supercritical methanol) and then the solution is rapidly expanded through a small nozzle into a region lower pressure , Thus the solvent power of supercritical fluids dramatically decreases and the solute eventually precipitates. This technique is clean because the precipitate is basically solvent free. RESS and its modified process have been used for the product of polymeric nanoparticles. Supercritical fluid technology technique, although environmentally friendly and suitable for mass production, requires specially designed equipment and is more expensive (Mohanraj et al., 2006).

Polymer Foams

Since a fast removal of dissolved CO_2 can be achieved by rapid depressurization, this behavior can be used to create foams especially that of poly (lactide–co–glycolide) (PLGA) polymer, because CO_2 has a good solubility in this approved polymer. *Hile et al 2000* prepared PLGA foam capable of sustained release of basic fibroblast growth factor for tissue engineering applications. To prepare the foam, a water-in-oil microemulsion consisting of an aqueous protein phase (typical reverse micelle domain size of 5–10 nm) and an organic polymer solution was prepared. The microemulsion was filled in molds and then placed in a pressure vessel. Now, the pressure vessel was pressurized with supercritical CO_2, to extract the organic phase, causing the polymer to precipitate onto the protein droplets. Now the vessel is purged with more CO_2 to remove the solvent from the system. Finally, the vessel is depressurized in 10–12 sec causing rapid removal of the CO_2 that was dissolved in the polymer, making a porous foamy structure.

Liposomes

Liposomes, in which nanodomains of drug are stabilized using lipids, are useful drug carriers for both small and macromolecular drugs. Unfortunately, the conventional methods of making liposomes require large amounts of organic solvents and have difficulty with scale-up for hydrophilic drugs. Lipids actually have some solubility in supercritical CO_2, and this behavior has been used to form liposomes without using organic solvents. For example, *Fredereksen et al 1997* dissolved a phospholipid (1-palmitoyl-2-oleoylphosphatidylcholine) and cholesterol in supercritical CO2 using 7% ethanol cosolvent. The mixture is expanded into an aqueous state containing fluorescein isothiocyanate (FITC)–dextran at low pressure. Because of the sudden reduction in the solubility of the phospholipid and the cholesterol at the nozzle tip, liposome encapsulating FITC–dextran was formed. The process yielded 200-nm-size liposomes (termed as critical fluid liposomes) with 20% encapsulation efficiency. The main benefit of this process is the significantly reduced use of organic solvent. *Castor and Chu et al 1998* prepared liposomes containing hydrophobic drugs, such as paclitaxel, camptothecins, doxorubicin, vincristine, and cisplatin. These formulations including 150–250-nm paclitaxel liposomes are claimed to be more effective against tumors in animals compared to commercial formulations.

Inclusion Complexes

Inclusion compounds, such as inclusion of poorly water-soluble drugs in cyclodextrin, are useful in enhancing bioavailability. Basically, the lipophilic drug is included in the lipophilic interior of the cyclodextrin molecule. The exterior of the cyclodextrin molecule is hydrophilic, and hence the whole complex can be dissolved in water. Inclusion can be achieved when both the drug and the cyclodextrin molecules are in a dissolved state, i.e., have a higher molecular mobility as compared to the solid forms. In conventional technique, both are dissolved in an organic solvent and then the solvent is removed. Unfortunately, the concentration of the residual solvent is high in the final product (Lin, S.Y. et al., 1989). Supercritical CO_2 processes allow preparation of drug– cyclodextrin inclusion complexes without the use of organic solvents. This is because the interaction of supercritical CO_2 with solid cyclodextrin makes the cyclodextrin molecules more fluid. This interesting plasticizing effect of supercritical CO_2 has been well known for organic polymers, for which the glass transition or melting can be achieved at a lower temperature with SC CO_2. To make inclusion compounds, the physical solid mixture of the drug and cyclodextrin is exposed to supercritical CO_2, and then rapidly CO_2 is removed by depressurization.

Solid Dispersions

In many delivery applications, molecularly intimate mixtures (i.e., solid dispersion) of drug with excipients, such polymers are needed. An organic solvent, which can dissolve both, does bring the two in intimate contact while in solution. Unfortunately, when the solvent is removed by evaporation or by addition of a liquid antisolvent, the drug and the polymer phases precipitate out or separate. Hence, the dispersion of the two is poor in the solid state. Supercritical CO_2 antisolvent induces the precipitation about 100-fold faster than the liquid antisolvent, not allowing enough time for the drug and the polymer domains to separate out. Thus, supercritical CO_2 precipitation can provide a more dispersed solid mixture. Supercritical CO_2-based precipitation is superior to the liquid-based precipitation or the milling process. For example, a solid dispersion of carbamazepine in polyethyleneglycol (PEG)-4000, produced by CO_2method, increased the rate and the extent of dissolution of carbamazepine (Moneghini, M. et al., 2001). In this method, a solution of carbamazepine and PEG4000 in acetone was loaded in a pressure vessel, in which supercritical CO_2 was added from the bottom to obtain solvent-free particles.

Safety and Health Issues

When dealing with supercritical carbon dioxide, there are two safety and health issues that are to be kept in mind when designing and operating the extractor: (i) the high pressure involved requires that personnel is protected from the plant by proper isolating walls and (ii) if carbon dioxide is released in the closed atmosphere it can lead to asphyxiation, as it can replace the oxygen in the surroundings.

2.2.8. Polymer conjugates

Polymer conjugates, especially those prepared using N- (2-hydroxypropyl) methacrylate (HPMA) have been extensively studied for intracellular and cytoplasmic drug delivery. HPMA conjugated to oligonucleotides *via* lysosomally degradable spacers were shown to enter the cytoplasm and nucleus of the cells (Jensen, K.D. et al., 2003). The polymer conjugates offer the flexibility of attaching specific targeting molecules that enable their accumulation in specific intracellular compartments. For example, efficient cytoplasmic and nuclear accumulation of the HPMA conjugates can be obtained by attaching either a NLS (Nuclear localization sequences) or a TAT peptide to the conjugate (Jensen, K.D. et al., 2003).

Polymeric conjugates for angiogenesis targeting

Polymeric conjugates have been used for targeted delivery of drugs to tumor sites because the attachment of drugs to water soluble polymer increases their solubility, reduces the side effect, and overcomes multi-drug resistance; the large size of conjugates increases blood half life and significantly alters the drug properties and pharmacokinetics; the conjugates can be tailor-made (i.e., side-chain content, molecular weight, charge etc.) for specific targeting and delivery needs; they can be designed to passively (EPR) or actively target tumor sites; and site specific drug release can be achieved by designing biodegradable spacers that can be enzymatically cleaved or that are pH sensitive. The advantages have led to the development of a wide range of polymer-anti-cancer drug conjugates, some of which are currently in clinical trials.

Use of macromolecular carriers such as water-soluble polymer-drug conjugates has been recognized as a promising way to increase the therapeutic efficacy of low molecular weight drugs. The main concept is based on improving pharmacokinetic properties of low molecular weight drugs and targeting the diseased site. Conjugates of cytostatic drugs with polymeric carriers are being widely tested as potent new systems for cancer treatment. Although the idea of highly sophisticated polymeric systems is quite old, only few of them have reached the preclinical and clinical testing.

One of the most promising systems is based on water soluble N-(2-hydroxypropyl) methacrylamide (HPMA). HPMA homopolymer was originally developed by Kopecek and a colleague as plasma expander (Ruth Duncan et al., 2003) HPMA copolymers has been employed to modify the in vivo biodistribution of chemotherapeutics agents and enzymes. The advantage of HPMA copolymer over other water soluble polymers is that they can be tailor-made with simple chemical modification to regulate drug and targeting moiety content for biorecognization, internalization, or subcellular trafficking depending on specific therapeutics needs. The over all molecular weight of HPMA copolymers is determined by the polymerization conditions, particularly the concentration of initiator and chain transfer agents. Various side chain moieties (isotope cheater, targeting moieties and drug) may be directly linked to the polymer chain via a biodegradable or non-biodegradable spacer.

Advantage of HPMA copolymer:

Covalent binding of anticancer drugs to HPMA copolymers can:

- Simultaneously improve the solubility of the drugs.
- Prolong their blood circulation time.
- Increase accumulation in solid tumors as a result of enhanced permeability and a retention (EPR) effect.
- Overcome Glycoprotein-associated multidrug resistance and to have greater efficacy than the free drug.

In addition to the well-established targeting strategies, a rather new approach is to use receptor-binding epitopes as the biorecognition sites in HPMA copolymer conjugates that mediate specific interactions of the conjugates with receptor bearing cells. The design of macromolecular therapeutics must be based on a sound biological rationale. The HPMA copolymer-drug conjugate should be biorecognizable at two levels: at the plasma membrane to increase the recognition and internalization by a subset of target cells and intracellularly by lysosomal enzymes to release the drug from the carrier. The latter is a prerequisite for transport of the drug into the cytoplasm and nucleus resulting in biological activity.

The synthesis and characterization of N-(2- hydroxypropyl) methacrylamide (HPMA) copolymers for drug delivery are well established (Luet, Z.R. al., 2002). HPMA copolymers are biocompatible, nonimmunogenic and nontoxic water–soluble copolymers (Kpcecheke, J. et al., 2000). They can be used as a means to (1) restrict delivery of radionuclides and drugs to the vascular space; (2) carry multiple aVh3 selective ligands (RGD4C) to target tumor associated capillary beds; and (3) allow bioactive agents to kill the new vessels.

Mechanism of action of drug conjugates

Polymeric based delivery systems have been used as carriers for passive and active targeting of drugs in the treatment of various diseases and as novel imagine agents. Without a specific targeting ligand moderate-size (> 30 kD) polymer can passively (*via* EPR) accumulate in tumor tissues. The EPR effect has been used to deliver macromolecular bioactive agents to solid tumors including anti-angiogenic drugs.

There are number of important differences between small molecular weight drugs and polymeric conjugates of these small molecules. The advantages of polymer-based delivery system stem decreased extravasation in normal tissues because of the large molecular weight of the conjugates. Low extravasation of polymer conjugates in normal tissues generally results in reduced systemic toxicity. In this regard, predominant liver and kidney uptake of small RGD peptides has been identified as a significant disadvantage of targeting tumor angiogenesis with small peptides.

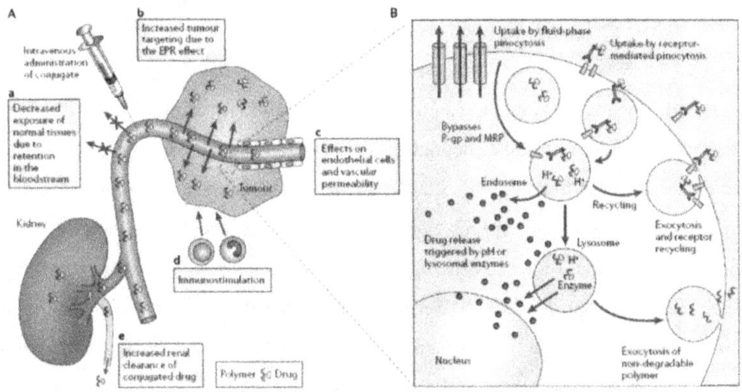

Figure: 2.17. **Current understanding of the mechanism of action of polymer–drug conjugates.**

[A] Hydrophilic polymer– drug conjugates administered intravenously can be designed to remain in the circulation — their clearance rate depends on conjugate molecular weight, which governs the rate of renal elimination.

(a) Drug that is covalently bound by a linker that is stable in the circulation is largely prevented from accessing normal tissues (including sites of potential toxicity), and biodistribution is initially limited to the blood pool.

(b) The blood concentration of drug conjugate drives tumor targeting due to the increased permeability of angiogenic tumor vasculature (compared with normal vessels), providing the opportunity for passive targeting due to the enhanced permeability and retention effect (EPR effect).

(c) Through the incorporation of cell-specific recognition ligands it is possible to bring about the added benefit of receptor-mediated targeting of tumor cells.

(d) It has also been suggested that circulating low levels of conjugate (slow drug release) might additionally lead to immuno stimulation.

(e) If the polymer–drug linker is stable in the circulation, for example, *N*-(2-hydroxypropyl) methacrylamide (HPMA) copolymer–Gly-Phe-Leu-Gly–doxorubicin, the relatively high level of renal elimination (whole body $t_{1/2}$ clearance >50% in 24 h) compared with free drug ($t_{1/2}$ clearance ~50% in 4 days) can increase the elimination rate. [B] On arrival in the tumor interstitium, polymer-conjugated drug is internalized by tumor cells through either fluid-phase pinocytosis (in solution), receptor-mediated pinocytosis following non-specific membrane binding (due to hydrophobic or charge interactions) or ligand–receptor docking. Depending on the linkers used, the drug will usually be released intracellularly on exposure to lysosomal enzymes (for example, Gly-Phe-Leu-Gly and polyglutamic acid (PGA) are cleaved by cathepsin B) or lower pH (for example, a hydrazone linker degrades in endosomes and lysosomes (pH 6.5–<4.0). The active or passive transport of drugs such as doxorubicin and paciltaxel out of these vesicular compartments ensures exposure to their pharmacological targets. Intracellular delivery can bypass mechanisms of resistance associated with membrane efflux pumps such as p-glycoprotein. If >10-fold, EPR-mediated targeting will also enable the circumvention of other mechanisms of drug resistance. Non-biodegradable polymeric platforms must eventually be eliminated from the cell by exocytosis. Rapid exocytic elimination of the conjugated drug before release would be detrimental and prevent access to the therapeutic target. In general, polymeric carriers do not access the cytosol Multidrug Resistance Protein (MRP).

Most of the anticancer-drug conjugates that have been tested clinically have used HPMA copolymers as the carrier **(Table: 2.7).**

Table: 2.7. Polymer–drug conjugates and polymeric micelles in clinical trials as anticancer agents

Compound	Name	Company	Linker	Status of development	References
HPMA copolymer–doxorubicin	PK1; FCE28068	CRC/Pharmacia	Amide	Phase II	Huang, P. S. et al. Vasey, P. et al.
HPMA copolymer–doxorubicingalactosamine	PK2; FCE28069	CRC/Pharmacia	Amide	Phase I/II	Seymour, L. W. et al. Duncan, R. et al.
HPMA copolymer–paclitaxel	PNU166945	Pharmacia	Ester	Phase I	Meerum Terwogt, J. M. et al.
HPMA copolymer–camptothecin	MAG-CPT, PNU166148	Pharmacia	Ester	Phase I	Schoemaker, N. E. et al.
HPMA copolymer–platinate	AP5280	Access	Malonate	Phase I	Gianasi, E. et al.

Peptide-targeted delivery has a basis in nature as many peptides are used as attachment ligands by bacteria and viruses. The use of peptides as ligands for receptor targeting has been investigated by several groups (Shadidi et al., 2003). Peptide ligands have a number of advantages. These include their lower antigenic potential, making them less likely to cause an immune reaction. They are also easier to synthesize and characterize. Their smaller size means multiple peptides could be attached to a single nanoparticles conferring multivalent attachment. The most widely investigated receptor family for targeting with peptide ligands is the integrin family. These receptors are expressed on the neo-vasculature of various tumors and are involved in adhesion and cell signaling (Vander et al., 1994). Their peptide ligands are defined as arginine-glycine-aspartic acid (RGD) peptides, and comprise a range of linear and cyclic peptides containing the RGD motif (Arap et al., 1998). *Arap et al 1998* found that mice treated with RGD-targeted doxorubicin had greater survival than mice treated with doxorubicin alone in a murine tumour model. Many other targets are being investigated with peptide ligands targeting the tumor vasculature, cancer cell surface and surface immunoglobulins (Shadidi et al., 2003).

A major objective in the design of functionalized polymer surfaces for tissue engineering applications has been the covalent attachment of peptides that regulate cell adhesion: specifically those that promote integrin-mediated cell attachment (Shakesheff, K.M. et al., 1998 and Rezania, A. et al., 1999). Since the vast majority of mammalian cells are anchorage-dependent, they must attach and spread on a substrate to proliferate and function normally (Madri, J.A. et al., 1988 and Baldwin, S.P. et al., 1998). By controlling the surface properties of the substrate, cell attachment and growth *in vitro* can be altered (Kim, B.S. et al., 1999). A great deal of work has focused on RGD containing peptides to regulate cell adhesion (Shakesheff, K.M. et al., 1998, Besselink, G.A.J, et al., 1998 and Chinn, J.A. et al., 1998). Peptides containing the RGD (R=arginine, G=glycine, D=aspartic acid) sequence are considered important small cell-adhesive ligands (Shakesheff, K.M. et al., 1998, Besselink, G.A.J, et al., 1998). This cell-binding sequence is present in adhesive proteins like fibrinogen, vitronectin, collagens, and fibronectin (Ruoslahti, E. et al., 1987). Membrane proteins of blood platelets, endothelial cells, and several other cell types can bind RGD-containing peptides whether the peptide is in solution or immobilized onto a solid surface (Hynes, R.O. et al., 1992 and Plow, E.F et al., 1986).

RGD-based therapeutics that function either as agonists to promote the interaction of cells and tissues with artificial matrices, or as antagonists to control the nature of cell-cell and cell-ECM interactions (Craig, W. S. et al., 1995). At this state of the art many different RGD peptides have been developed. Linear and cyclic RGD peptides, and chemically designed peptidomimeticsare currently being tested by researchers.

RGD peptide classification

Integrin superfamily

Integrins are a family of cell-adhesion receptors which interact with the extracellular matrix (ECM) and the cytosolic components. Integrins transfer signals bidirectionaly via so-called inside out and outside-in signaling. They are heterodimeric glycoproteins, consisting of an α and a β subunit. The schematic signaling pathway is activated by binding a ligand, clustering of integrins and cytoskeletal and lysosomal activation, shown in **Figure: 2.18** (Duong, L. T. et al., 2000). This RGD-binding site is involved in cell morphology, differentiation, proliferation and gene expression. Integrin signaling pathways are although responsible for the survival of the cell, and apoptosis seems to be linked to a disturbance of integrin function. The proteins that interact most with RGD-dependent integrins are fibronectin, vitronectin, bone sialoprotein, osteopontin, thrombospondin, fibrinogen, laminin, collagen, nectipepsin and other unknown molecules (Robey, P. G. et al., 1996 and Blancher, C. et al., 1996). A very interesting fact is the use of the RGD sequence by pathogenic microbes. Bacteria, viruses and yeasts use the RGD sequence to get into the host cell (Virji M. et al., 1996 and Goldman M. J. et al., 1995). *Humphries et al 1995* explored the RGD competitive sequence QAGDV and LDV in integrin binding. The integrin subunits have been identified on different type of cells. The integrins reported most commonly in the literature are $\alpha_V\beta_1$, $\alpha_2\beta_1$, $\alpha_1\beta_1$, and $\alpha_V\beta_3$, as shown in **Table: 2.8.**

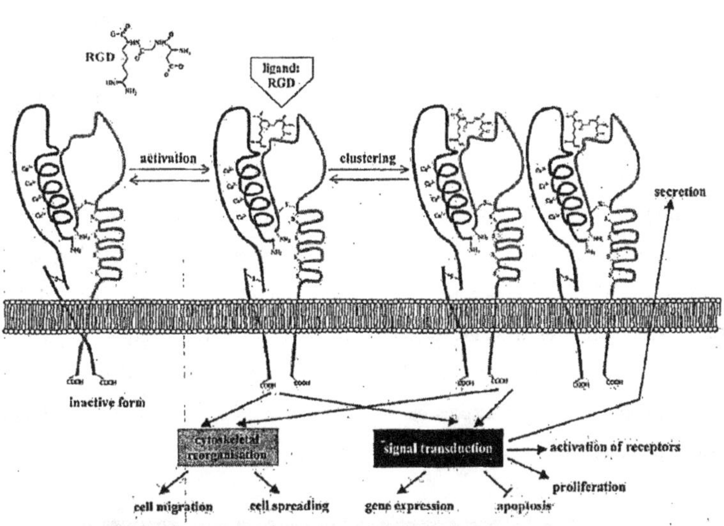

Figure: 2.18. Scheme of binding the RGD peptide to an integrin. Influence of RGD-peptide binding and possible ways into the cell.

Table: 2.8. Integrins and ligands.

Subunits		RGD dependence	Ligands	Cell type
β_1	α_1	+	LM, Col IV+I	LC; SM, ML, OB
	α_2	–(+)	LM, Col, FN	EC, LC, MC, NP, TC, OC, OB
	α_3	+/–	FN, LM, Col I,epiligrin	EC, LC, MC, ML, OB
	α_4	–	FN, V-CAM	LC, MC, OB
	α_5	+	FN, L1	EC, LC, MC, TC, OB
	α_6	–/+	LM	EC, LC, MC, TC
	α_7		LM	TB, MU, ME
	α_8		FN, VN, TN	
	α_9		TN	EP
	α_V	+	VN, FN, FG, L1, Col, LM, OP	ME, CA, ML, FB, OC, SM
β_2	α_L	–	ICAM-1, ICAM-2	LC, MC, NP
	α_M	+?	C3 bi, factorX, FG, ICAM-1 β-glucan, leishmania gp63	MC, NP
	α_X	?	FG, C3bi, β-glukan	MC, NP
β_3	α_{IIb}	+	FG, Fx, VN, FN, vWF, TS, fibrin, L1	MK, TC
	α_V	+	VN, FG, FN, vWF, TS, OP, BSP, PB, Col, L1, TN	EC, LC, MC, NP, TC, SM, OC, FB, OB
β_4	α_6	+/–	LM(?)	EP.
β_5	α_V	+	VN, vWF, FN, BSP, OP	OC, OB, SM
β_6	α_V	+	FN, VN	EC
$\beta_7(=\beta_p)$	α_4		FN, V-CAM, Md-CAM	
	α_5	–	Peyers patch, addressin, FN, VCAM-1	FB, LC
	α_{IEL}			
β_N	α_V		FN, Col	
β_8	α_V	+	VN, FN	

Ligands: BSP, bone sialoprotein; C3 bi, inactive type of C3b component of complement; factor X, coagulation factor X; FG, fibrinogen; FN, fibronectin; Fx, fragment x of FG; Col, Collagen; L1,: 6th Ig-similar domain of cell adhesion molecule L1; LM, laminin; OP, osteopontin; PB, penton base of adenovirus; TN, tenascin; TS, thrombospondin; VN, vitronectin; vWF, von Willebrand factor. Cell types: CA, carcinoma; EC, endothelial cells; EP, epithelial cells; FB, fibroblasts; LC, lymphocytes; MC, macrophages; ME, melanoma; MK, megacaryocytes; ML, melanocytes; MU, muscle cells; NP, neutrophil cells; OC, osteoclasts; SM, smooth muscle tissue; TB, cytotrophoblasts; TC, thrombocytes (Schaffner, P. et al., 2003).

Integrin-binding peptide sequence and classification

According to the above classification, integrins are selective toward their substratum ligands. The specificity is a central issue in the use of cell adhesion peptides and surface engineering. Whether peptide sequences that promote cell adhesion will in the future exhibit specificity for a single cell type remains unclear. Integrins showed different binding activity for RGD peptides. If one specific cell to the RGD sequence which is specific for the integrins it expresses. This opens a possibility to control binding of cells to RGD peptides and mediate specific cell attachment to surfaces.

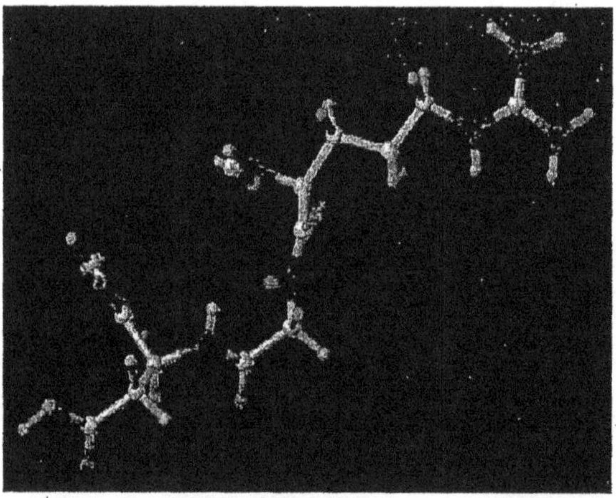

Figure 2.19. Molecular model of the RGD sequence conformation of the cyclic RGD peptide c(RGDfK) (Schaffner, P. et al., 2003).

The affinity of RGD peptides for their ligands may be affected by steric conformation of the peptide. Several peptides that contain RGD serve as ligands for integrins. It has been suggested that substrata composed of RGD not only promote cell attachment but may also enhance other fundamental cell functions (e.g. proliferation). The amino acid sequences flanking RGD also may affect the selectivity and affinity of peptides toward integrins. For initial cell adhesion, *Rezania et al 1999* proposed the collagen receptor $\alpha_2\beta_1$ for osteoblastlike cells. For spreading, cytoskeletal organization, focal contact formation and possibly migration they proposed $\alpha_V\beta_3$ (vitronectin receptor). An additional interesting point is the influence of RGD-mediated cell-matrix interactions in bone cell mechano transduction suggested by *Salter et al 1997.* Chemists synthesize RGD peptide amphiphiles to influence the specific binding of RGD peptides. Synthetic dialkyl lipid tails have been linked to the amino-terminus, carboxyl-terminus and both termini of the cell recognition sequence RGD to produce amino-coupled, carboxyl-coupled and looped RGD peptide amphiphiles. It has been established that amphiphiles are the most effective in influencing human melanoma cell response when the RGD sequence is made accessible through formation of a flexible loop conformation. According to these authors, future studies with new versions of RGD peptide amphiphiles that contain longer RGD sequences, both linear and cyclic, have the potential to further clarify the role of sequence accessibility and conformation in promoting specific cell responses. *Nicolaou et al 1998* describe a group of nonpeptide mimetics based on the structure of the RGD peptides. They tested binding selectivity and ability to inhibit cell adhesion among different integrins ($\alpha_V\beta_3$, $\alpha_V\beta_5$, $\alpha_{II}\beta_3$). The tested library showed excellent results for five nonpeptide mimetics generated.

Linear RGD peptides

The binding of RGD peptides to different integrins showed a different binding pattern which is influenced by chemical alteration of the side flanking amino acids. Examples of linear peptides and their origin are shown in **Table: 2.9.** Early studies with RGD peptides demonstrated the influence of stereochemistry and conformation on binding specificity in cell adhesion. In linear peptides, the fourth amino acid alters the binding specificity. *Hern et al 1998* showed in their in vitro re-endothelialization studies with YRGDS and GRGDS that the distance of the presented RGD sequence from a surface promotes specific cell adhesion. Cyclization of a peptide showed an increase in activity and a change in integrin specificity. The specificity changed from fibronectin to vitronectin. In linear peptides, the nature of residues flanking the RGD sequence could influence receptor affinity, receptor selectivity and other biological properties. Tetrapeptides RGDS, RGDV, RGDT were synthesized using an improved liquid-phase procedure. It was found that RGDV exhibits remarkable cell-attachment activity when tested on L-929 fibroblasts. The valine residue contributes to RGDX conformation to fit to the structure of receptor on the cell surface. A review by *Healy et al 1999* on biomimetic engineering of materials addressing the RGD peptide problem concludes with the following words: 'It is unlikely that materials modified only with the ubiquitous linear RGD signal will lead to controlled responses of a specific cell type in complex environments (e.g. *in vivo*)'. This limitation is one of the reasons for developing cyclic RGD peptides.

Table: 2.9. Linear peptides (Schaffner, P. et al., 2003).

Linear peptides	Integrins/proteins	
GRGDSY	$\alpha_v\beta_3/\alpha_v\beta_3$	VN
GRGDVY		
GRGESY = negative control		
RGDC	vasoactive peptide	
BRB10	$\alpha_v\beta_3/\alpha_v\beta_5$	BSP
BRB9		
BA3 = EPRGDNYRG		
EPRGDNYR	$\alpha_v\beta_3/\alpha_v\beta_5$	BSP
EPRGENYR = negative control		
RGDS	$\alpha_v\beta_3/\alpha_v\beta_5$	VN, FG
RGDV		
Ac-RGDV-NH_2		
Ac-RGDS-NH_2		
GRGESP = negative control		
GRGES = negative control		
GRGDdSP = negative control		
Ac-(CIT)GDS-NH_2 = negative control		
GdRGDSP	$\alpha_v\beta_3/\alpha_v\beta_5$	VN, FG
GRGDTP		
GRGDSP		
GRGDS		
GRADSP = negative control		
VTYAVTGRGDSPASSKP	$\alpha_v\beta_3/\alpha_v\beta_5$	FN,
TNIMEILRGDFSSANNR		FG,
TSSTSYNRGDSTFESKS		FG
ECKPQVTRGDVFTMPED		VN
VVTGSPERGDQSSWKSV		vWF
TVDTYDGRGDSVVYGLR		OP
G(Pen)GHRGDLRCA	$\alpha_{IIb}\beta_3$	
Pen substitutes		
R(Pmc) GHRGDLRCA		
Substitutes at position 3, −1, −2,		
combination of positions 1 and 3,		
= 48 different peptides! −		
$(GRGDSP)_4K$ = repeated linear P	$\alpha_v\beta_3$	FN

Cyclic RGD peptides

In cyclic peptides the RGD peptide sequence is flanked by other amino acids to build a ring system. These systems offer the possibility to present the RGD sequence in a specific conformation. Cyclic peptides are much more potent and more specific than their linear counterparts, and their advantage is their resistance against proteolysis. Table 3 shows different cyclic peptides and their origin. Cyclic RGD peptides have been developed for various purposes: fibrinogen receptor antagonists, selective $\alpha_V\beta_3$ integrin antagonists for treatments of human tumor metastasis and tumor-induced angiogenesis, phagocytosis of cells undergoing apoptosis, bone remodeling and osteoporosis, diabetic retinopathy and acute renal failure. Stereochemistry influence in c(RGDFV) of used D-amino acids was shown by *Müller et al 1992*. Each backbone amide bond of (RGDfV) was successively *N*-methylated to result in a series of five monomethylated cyclic pentapeptides. The authors propose five classes of cyclic peptides and their representative RGD arrangements with different integrin binding specificities. The influence of this *N*-methylation scan on biological activity revealed that (RGDf-N(Me)V) is one of the most active and selective $\alpha_V\beta_3$ integrin antagonists known (Dechantsreiter, M. A. et al., 1998).

Stereoisomerism has a great influence on biological activity of c(RGDfV). Studies on retro-inverso peptides showed that the backbone conformation, the side-chain topology of the peptides and the amide bond direction lead to drastically different inhibitory activities to the a_Vb_3 receptor (Dechantsreiter, M. A. et al., 1998). A structure of the peptide loops alters activity on receptor binding to fibrinogen. Loops were stabilized by building blocks with kanthene, phenoxazine and phenothiazine derivatives. The possibility of disulfide bonds at cysteine residues in the structure of cyclic RGD peptides alters the binding activity of the peptides (Assa-Munt, N. et al., 2001). *Bogdanowich-Knipp et al 1999* compared the solution stability of a linear and a cyclic RGD peptide as a function of pH and buffer concentration (Bogdanowich-Knipp, S. J et al., 1999). It appeared that the cyclic peptide is 30-fold more stable than the linear peptide at pH 7. The degradation mechanisms of both peptides primarily involved the aspartic acid residue. This degradation leads to the loss of biological activity (Geiger, T. et al., 1987 and Manning M. C. et al., 1989). It has been clearly demonstrated that the increase in stability of the cyclic peptide compared with the linear one is due to decreased structural flexibility imposed by the ring (Bogdanowich-Knipp, S. J et al., 1999). Cyclic RGD peptides react like native cell adhesion molecules, such as fibronectin, in binding specifically to an integrin (Gurrath, M. et al., 1992). This suggests that cyclic RGD peptides may function as more efficient mediators of osteoprogenitor-cell adhesion than linear peptides. Studies of cyclic RGD peptides immobilized on surfaces showed that such conformationally restrained peptides were more potent in promoting cell adhesion than their linear counterparts (Ivanov, B. et al., 1995 and Xiao, Y. et al., 1996).

Table: 2.10. Cyclic peptide (Schaffner, P. et al., 2003).

Cyclic peptides	Integrins /proteins	
(Pmc)GHRGDLRCR Ac-CIPRGD(Y-OMe)RCNH$_2$ Ac-CNPRGD(Y-OMe)RCNH$_2$	$\alpha_{IIb}\beta_3$	TC
Ac-G(dR)GDSPASSK-GGG(dR)LLLLLL(dR)NH$_2$= Peptide 2000 (Telios)[a]	$\alpha_V\beta_3$	FN
CBA4=DPA-EPRGDNYRCYS-NH$_2$	$\alpha_V\beta_3/\alpha_V\beta_5$	BSP
BSA-CM-A-DPA-EPRGDNYRCysNH$_2$=BSA-CNB DPA-EPRGDNYRCysNH$_2$=CNB Ac-DPA-EPRGDNYRCysNH$_2$=Ac-CNB EPRGDNYRCysNH$_2$=C-BC3 dYRGDNYRCysNH$_2$=C-CB1	$\alpha_V\beta_3/\alpha_V\beta_5$	BSP
G4120=cycRGD[b]	$\alpha_V\beta_3/\alpha_V\beta_5$	VN
CycGPenGRGDSPCA=peptide 2000 (Telios)[a]	$\alpha_V\beta_1$ $\alpha_V\beta_3/\alpha_V\beta_5$	LM VN
Ac-CGGNGEPRGDTRAY-NH$_2$	$\alpha_V\beta_3/\alpha_V\beta_5$	BSP
Ac-C(NMe)-RGD-PenNH$_2$=SK&F 106760[c] Ac-C(NMe)-RGN-PenNH$_2$=negative control	$\alpha_V\beta_3/\alpha_V\beta_5$	VN
XantheneRGDF XantheneARGDFP XantheneIARGDFPD XantheneRIARGDFPDD XantheneARIARGDFPDDR	flavoridin	
C(GRGDSPA) C(GRGD) C(RGDS) C(GRGDSP) C(GRGDS) C(RGDSP) C(RGDSPA)	$\alpha_V\beta_3$	FN
EMD 121974=c(RGDfK)[d]	$\alpha_V\beta_3/\alpha_V\beta_5$	VN
cRGDVGS-BTD-SGVA	$\alpha_V\beta_3/\alpha_V\beta_5$	VN
cRGDRGD	$\alpha_V\beta_3/\alpha_V\beta_5$	VN
cPRGD-Mamb[e]	$\alpha_V\beta_3/\alpha_V\beta_5$	VN
c(-N(Me)R-GDfV) c(R-Sar-DfV) c(RG-N(Me)D-fV) c(RGD-N(Me)f-V) c(RGDf-N(Me)V-)=EMD 121974[d]	$\alpha_V\beta_3/\alpha_V\beta_5$	VN
c(RGDFV) c(RADFV)	$\alpha_V\beta_3/\alpha_V\beta_5$	VN

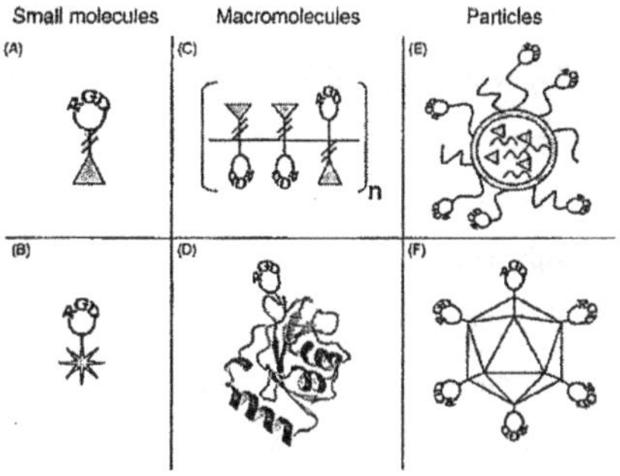

Figure: 2.20. Schematic representation of RGD-mediated drug delivery and imaging constructs. (Panels A and B) Small molecule conjugates. Organic drug molecules (A) have been conjugated to cyclic RGD-ligands via various linkers. As most drugs are inactive when coupled to the RGD-ligand, a biodegradable linkage is required between drug and RGD-peptide. In contrast, imaging agents (B) need stable linkages. (Panels C and D) Macromolecules. Synthetic and natural polymers (C) can be modified with multiple copies of both drug (affording a high drug/carrier ratio) and RGD(affording multivalent binding and internalization). Therapeutic proteins (D) have been equipped with RGD-motifs by recombinant means. (Panels E and F) Particulate systems. Synthetic particulate systems (E) like liposomes, Nanoparticles or non-viral gene vectors have been equipped with RGD mostly via extended PEG tethers, to prevent unwanted interactions with non-target cells. Adenoviral vectors (F) have been modified with RGD motifs to enhance infectivity. Viral carriers have been used to deliver genes and siRNA, or as oncolytic replicating systems. (Temming, K. et al, 2005).

Requirements of RGD-peptide as an $\alpha_V\beta_3$ -ligand

The RGD sequence is currently the basic module for a variety of RGD-containing peptides which display preferential binding to either $\alpha_V\beta_3$ integrin and related α_V-integrins, or to other types of integrins. For example, $\alpha_{IIb}\beta_3$ integrin is an integrin that has been investigated intensely in relation to platelet aggregation (Andronati et al., 2004). Since the RGD-sequence is conserved in all natural and new developed ligands, the relative affinity and specificity of the peptides and proteins are determined by other amino acid residues flanking the RGD-motif, especially at the two positions following the aspartic acid (Pierschbacher et al., 1987). Besides direct interactions between these residues and the integrin, flanking groups influence the folding of the peptide and thereby the conformational features of the RGD-motif. Cyclization is commonly employed to improve the binding properties of RGD-peptides. Since cyclization confers rigidity to structure, it greatly improves the selectivity of the promiscuous RGD-sequence for a specific integrin subtype. Indeed, all selective RGD-peptide ligands are cyclic, having at least one or more ring structures, as will be discussed. Furthermore, linear RGD-peptides proved highly susceptible to chemical degradation, which is due to the reaction of the aspartic acid residue (D) with the peptide backbone (Bogdanowich-Knipp et al., 1999). Since the rigidity conferred by cyclization prevents this, cyclic peptides are more stable. Lastly, non-natural peptide modifications such as the introduction of d-amino acids as well as replacement with peptidomimetic structures have yielded RGD-peptide ligands with increased specificity and nanomolar or higher affinity (Goodman et al., 2002). The elucidation of the crystal structure of $\alpha_V\beta_3$ integrin and subsequent docking studies on this template have aided in the design of novel RGD-ligands (Marinelli et al., 2003). One of the best studied RGD-peptide ligands for $\alpha_V\beta_3$ integrin is c(RGDf-N(Me)-V), which is also known as EMD121974 or Cilengitide (**Figure: 2.21 , structure 1).** This RGDpeptide affinity in the subnanomolar range in competing with biotinylated vitronectin or fibrinogen for binding to immobilized integrins. Furthermore, Cilengitide displays a 1000-fold preference for $\alpha_V\beta_3$ integrin over $\alpha_{IIb}\beta_3$ integrin (Dechantsreiter et al., 1999). These features were attributed to the constrained ring structure and the introduced d-amino acid residue that force the RGD-sequence into the proper conformation for binding to $\alpha_V\beta_3$ integrin. Cilengitide has reached phase II clinical trials for the treatment of malignancies including melanoma, glioblastoma and prostate cancer.

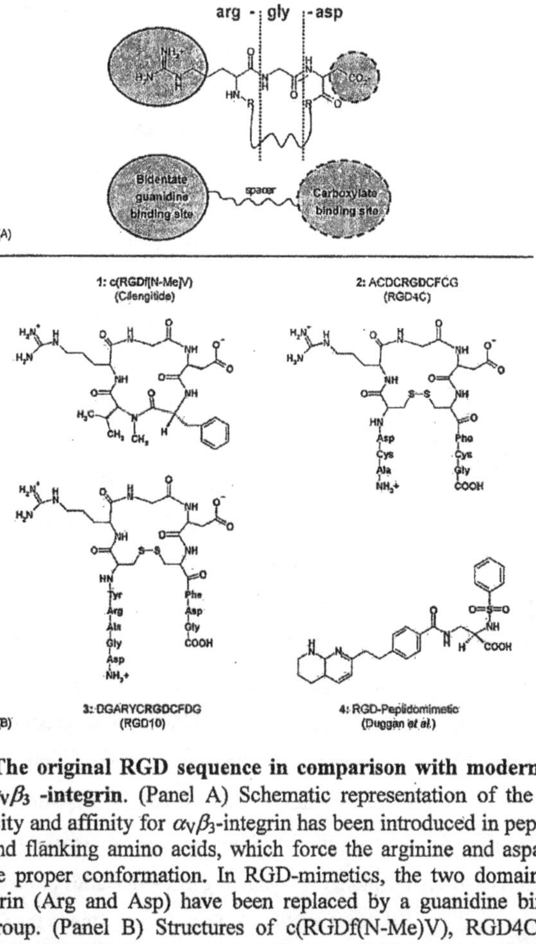

Figure:2.21. The original RGD sequence in comparison with modern high affinity ligands for $\alpha_V\beta_3$ -integrin. (Panel A) Schematic representation of the RGD binding motif. Specificity and affinity for $\alpha_V\beta_3$-integrin has been introduced in peptide ligands by ring closure and flanking amino acids, which force the arginine and aspartic acid side-chains into the proper conformation. In RGD-mimetics, the two domains that interact with the integrin (Arg and Asp) have been replaced by a guanidine binding site and carboxylate group. (Panel B) Structures of c(RGDf(N-Me)V), RGD4C, RGD10 and RGD-mimetic described by Duggan et al., which are all high affinity ligands for $\alpha_V\beta_3$ – integrin (Temming, K. et al, 2005).

Among the derivatives of this series, c(RGDfK) is one often used for the delivery of therapeutics, because the lysine residue (K) makes it an ideal building block for further chemical conjugation reactions. Several drug targeting and imaging constructs, bearing either one or more c(RGDfK) ligands, will be highlighted in the following sections of this review. Another RGD-ligand with high binding affinity and specificity for $\alpha_V\beta_3$ has been developed using phage display. Selection of RGD-peptide ligands from a cyclic peptide library afforded a structure that contained two disulfide bonds (ACDCRGDCFCG) **(Figure: 2.21, structure 2).** This so-called RGD4C peptide was at least 20-fold more potent than similar peptides with a single disulfide bond and 200-fold more potent than commonly used linear peptides (Koivunen et al., 1995). The RGD4C peptide has been exploited as targeting ligand for the delivery of cytostatic drugs; moreover it is especially suitable for incorporation into proteins and viruses by recombinant means. A disadvantage of RGD4C is that the peptide can fold into different cyclic structures. Apart from the preferred bicyclic structure, additional monocyclic and bicyclic structures can form, which demonstrated 10-fold less binding affinity (Assa-Munt et al., 2001). If one compares c(RGDfK) and RGD4C, c(RGDfK) is preferred for a chemical conjugation approach, due to its higher stability and relative ease of coupling. As mentioned, RGD4C is the best choice to equip a protein with a targeting moiety by recombinant means. RGD peptides with d-amino acids or other chemical modifications cannot be incorporated by this recombinant strategy.

Recently, a novel RGD-peptide with high affinity for $\alpha_V\beta_3$ was discovered by phage display technology (Holig et al., 2004). This peptide, RGD10 **(Figure: 2.21, structure 3)**, has only one disulfide bond, but the amino acids flanking the CRGDC core have similar physicochemical properties as the ones in RGD4C. RGD10 and RGD4C displayed similar binding properties. Several RGD peptidomimetics have been reported with further improved binding to α_V-integrins (Goodman et al., 2002). Most of these compounds contain a guanidine mimetic to replace arginine, while the aspartic acid of the RGD motif has been substituted by a carboxylic acid. These two essential groups have been linked together by various tethers and constraints, yielding compounds with low nanomolar or even picomolar affinities for $\alpha_V\beta_3$ integrin **(Figure: 2.21, structure 4).** Only few RGD-peptidomimetics have been exploited for targeting of therapeutics or diagnostics (Hood et al., 2002; Liu et al., 2003; Winter et al., 2003). This is partly due to the fact that they lack groups suitable for the coupling of drug or drug carriers. Likely, peptidomimetics will be applied more often as a targeting moiety, since their excellent binding properties as well as their stability can be regarded ideal for drug delivery. The affinity as well as the pharmacokinetic properties of RGD-ligands can be improved by coupling them to a carrier system. The multivalent RGD-protein conjugates synthesized by *Kok et al 2002* showed subnanomolar affinity for $\alpha_V\beta_3$ expressing human umbilical cord endothelial cells (HUVEC), which is a 250-fold increase versus the single RGD-peptide. Furthermore, multivalency not only greatly improves affinity but also facilitates internalization (Boturyn et al., 2004; Schraa et al., 2002a). Carrier systems like liposomes, nanoparticles, proteins and other polymers bearing multiple RGD-peptides are therefore more likely to be internalized via receptor-mediated endocytosis than single peptide constructs. Several other common advantages are attributable to RGD-equipped macromolecular carriers even though they represent a diverse group.

1. More drug molecules can be delivered per internalizing receptor/targeted molecule.
2. Higher affinity and internalization are facilitated by multivalent RGD-ligands, as mentioned above.
3. Renal filtration is inhibited since the higher molecular size of the carrier prevents glomerular filtration. This may lead to prolonged blood circulation times and longer presentation of the ligand to target receptors within the tissue (Schraa et al., 2002b).
4. Shielding of drugs from receptors or enzymes in the blood circulation renders targeting more predictable.
5. The high molecular weight of most carriers leads to passive retention in a tumor, via the so-called enhanced permeability and retention (EPR) phenomenon. For example, RGD4C equipped polymers accumulated in a s.c. prostate carcinoma in the course of 3 days, while radioactivity in other organs decreased (Mitra et al., 2005). This resulted in a 50:1 tumor:blood ratio at day 3. The control polymer without RGD-targeting motif accumulated in the tumor to a lesser extent, demonstrating the contribution of RGD-mediated targeting to the EPR effect. The need for appropriate control to prove the actual role of RGD/integrin recognition has to be mentioned. The substitution of only one amino acid had been demonstrated to abolish interaction with the integrin (Pierschbacher et al., 1987). Most researchers apply RAD or RGE peptides for this purpose. A control construct prepared with such peptides would bear identical structural changes as compared to the RGD modified construct. Comparison in effectiveness of both constructs demonstrates the role of the RGD mediated targeting.

2.3. Breast Cancer

Cancer is a general term that refers to cells that grow and multiply out of control and possibly spread to other parts of the body. There are many different types of breast cancer. Each may have different characteristics, and each one may require a different treatment. Cancer can cause harm in different ways. Cancer cells take nutrition and space away from normal cells. A lump of cancer cells, called a tumor, can invade or destroy normal tissue. Cancer cells can also spread to other parts of the body. This is called metastasis. Breast cancer is a common cancer among women in the United States and second only to skin cancer, affecting about 178,480 women in the United States in 2007. Most breast cancer begins in the milk ducts. These ducts connect the milk-producing glands (called lobules) to the nipple. Some breast cancer begins in the lobules themselves, and the rest begins in other tissues. The diagram shows where these body parts are within the breast.

2.3.1. Introduction of breast cancer

Breast cancers are potentially life-threatening malignancies that develop in one or both breasts. The structure of the female breast is important in understanding this cancer:

- The interior of the female breast consists mostly of fatty and fibrous connective tissues.
- It is divided into about 20 sections called lobes.
- Each lobe is further subdivided into a collection of lobules, structures that contain small milk-producing glands.
- These glands secrete milk into a complex system of tiny ducts. The ducts carry the milk through the breast and converge in a collecting chamber located just below the nipple.
- Breast cancer is either noninvasive (referred to as *in situ*, confined to the site of origin) or invasive (spreading).

Noninvasive breast cancers include

- Ductal carcinoma in situ (also called intraductal carcinoma or DCIS). DCIS consist of cancer cells in the lining of the duct. DCIS is a non-invasive, early cancer, but if left untreated, it may sometimes progress to an invasive, infiltrating ductal breast cancer. DCIS is the most common type of noninvasive breast cancer.
- Lobular carcinoma in situ, or LCIS. Although it is technically not a cancer, lobular carcinoma in situ is a marker for an increased risk of invasive cancer the same or both breasts.

A diagnosis of these early cancers (DCIS and LCIS) is made when there is no evidence of invasion.

Invasive Breast Cancer

Invasive cancer occurs when cancer cells spread beyond the basement membrane, which covers the underlying connective tissue in the breast. This tissue is rich in blood vessels and lymphatic channels that are capable of carrying cancer cells beyond the breast. Invasive breast cancers include the following:

- Invasive (also called infiltrating) ductal carcinoma. This is invasive breast cancer that penetrates the wall of a milk-passage duct. It comprises between 70 - 80% of all breast cancer cases.
- Invasive (also called infiltrating) lobular carcinoma. This invasive cancer has spread through the wall of a milk-producing lobule. It accounts for 10 - 15% of all breast cancers. It may sometimes appear in both breasts, sometimes in several separate locations.

How is the breast designed?

The breasts sit on the chest muscles that cover the ribs. Each breast is made of 15 to 20 lobes. Lobes contain many smaller lobules. Lobules contain groups of tiny glands that can produce milk. Milk flows from the lobules through thin tubes called ducts to the nipple. The nipple is in the center of a dark area of skin called the areola. Fat fills the spaces between the lobules and ducts.

The breasts also contain lymph vessels. These vessels lead to small, round organs called lymph nodes. Groups of lymph nodes are near the breast in the axilla (underarm), above the collarbone, in the chest behind the breastbone, and in many other parts of the body. The lymph nodes trap bacteria, cancer cells, or other harmful substances.

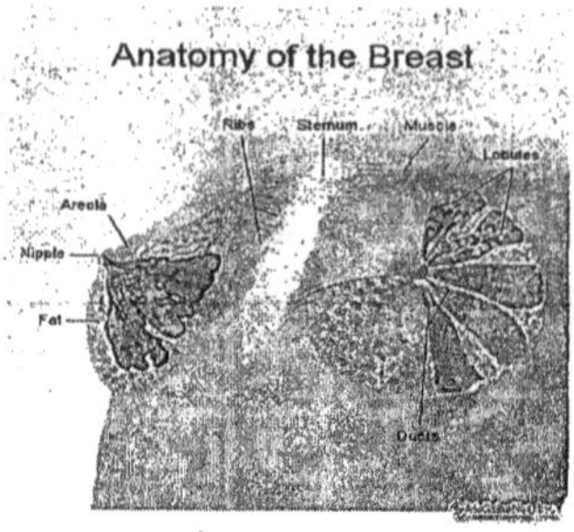

Figure: 2.22. Anatomy of the breast cancer

2.3.2. Risk Factors

About 12% of women develop breast cancer in their lifetime. Each year in the United States, about 180,000 women are diagnosed with invasive breast cancer and about 68,000 women are diagnosed with pre-invasive breast cancer. (Although breast cancer in men is rare, about 2,000 American men are diagnosed each year with invasive breast cancer. About 40,000 American women die from breast cancer each year. Breast cancer death rates have declined significantly since the 1990s, especially for women younger than age 50. The earlier breast cancer is diagnosed, the earlier the opportunity for treatment. In the United States, there are currently more than 2.5 million breast cancer survivors.

Risk factors for breast cancer include:

Age

Most cases of breast cancer occur in women older than age 60. According to the American Cancer Society, about 1 in 8 cases of invasive breast cancer are found in women younger than age 45, while 2 in 3 cases of invasive breast cancer occur in women age 55 and older.

Race and Ethnicity

Breast cancer is slightly more common among white woman than African-American, Asian, Latina, or Native American women. However, African-American women tend to have more aggressive types of breast cancer tumors and are more likely to die from breast cancer than women of other races. It is unclear whether this is mainly due to biologic or socioeconomic reasons. Social and economic factors make it less likely that African-American women will be screened, so they are more likely to be diagnosed at a later stage. They are also less likely to have access to effective treatments. Breast cancer is also more prevalent among Jewish women of Eastern European (Ashkenazi) descent (see Genetic Factors).

Family and Personal History

Women who have a family history of breast cancer are at increased risk for developing breast cancer themselves. Having a first-degree relative (mother, sister, or daughter) who has been diagnosed with breast cancer doubles the risk for developing breast cancer. Women who have had ovarian cancer are at increased risk for developing breast cancer. And, a personal history of breast cancer increases the risk of developing a new cancer in the same or other breast.

Genetic Factors

About 5 - 10% of breast cancer cases are due to inherited genetic mutations.

BRCA Genes. Inherited mutations in genes known as BRCA1 or BRCA2 are responsible for most cases of hereditary breast cancers, ovarian cancers, or both in families with a history of these cancers. BRCA gene mutations are present in only about 0.5% of the overall population. However, certain ethnic groups -- such as Jewish women of Eastern European (Ashkenazi) descent -- have a higher prevalence (2.5%) of BRCA gene mutations. BRCA gene mutations are also seen in some African-American and Hispanic women.

Screening Guidelines for BRCA Genes. The U.S. Preventive Services Task Force (USPSTF) recommends that women at high risk should be tested for BRCA genes, but does not recommend routine genetic counselling or testing in low-risk women (no family history of BRCA 1 or 2 genetic mutations). Risk assessment is based on a woman's family history of breast and ovarian cancer (on both the maternal and paternal sides). The relevance of the inherited BRCA1 or BRCA2 mutations to survival is controversial. Some studies have suggested that these mutations are linked to less lethal breast cancer. Others suggest that they do not change prognosis or may worsen it. Women with these genetic mutations do have a greater risk for a new cancer to develop. Patients with BRCA1 mutations tend to develop tumors that are hormone receptor negative, which can behave more aggressively.

Other Genetic Mutations. Other genes associated with increased hereditary breast cancer risk include p53, CHEK2, ATM, and PTEN.

Exposure to Estrogen

Because growth of breast tissue is highly sensitive to estrogens, the more estrogen a woman is exposed to over her lifetime, the higher her risk for breast cancer.

Duration of Estrogen Exposure. Early age at menarche (first menstrual period) or later age at menopause may slightly increase a woman's risk for breast cancer.

Pregnancy. Women who have never had children or who had their first child after age 30 may have a slightly increased breast cancer risk. Having children at an early age, and having multiple pregnancies, reduces breast cancer risk. Evidence does not show an association between abortion and increased breast cancer risk. Studies have been mixed on whether breast-feeding decreases breast cancer risk. Breast-feeding reduces a woman's total number of menstrual cycles and thereby estrogen exposure, which may account for its possible protective effects. Some studies suggest that the longer a woman breast-feeds, the lower her risk.

Oral Contraception. Although studies have been conflicting about whether estrogen in oral contraception increases the chances for breast cancer, the most recent research indicates that current or former oral contraceptive use does not significantly increase breast cancer risk. Women who have used oral contraceptives may have slightly more risk for breast cancer than women who have never used them, but this risk declines once a woman stops using birth control pills.

Hormone Replacement Therapy. Many studies have reported a higher risk for breast cancer in postmenopausal women who take combination hormone replacement therapy (HRT), which contains both estrogen and progestin. A combination of estrogen and testosterone also increases breast cancer risk. Several studies of women who had a hysterectomy indicate that estrogen alone does not increase overall breast cancer risk when the drug is used for 7 years or less. However, women who take estrogen for 10 - 15 years or more do have an increased risk, especially women who are already at higher risk for breast cancer. In addition, HRT increases breast cancer density, making mammograms more difficult to read. This can cause cancer to be diagnosed at a later stage. Women who take estrogen HRT should be aware that they need frequent mammogram screenings. The North American Menopause Society recommends that women who are at risk for breast cancer should avoid hormone therapy and try other options to manage menopausal symptoms such as hot flashes. Most doctors recommend that women use HRT only for short-term relief of menopausal symptoms.

Infertility and Infertility Treatments. Despite some concerns that infertility treatments using the drug clomiphene may increase the risk for breast cancer, most studies do not show an association. Some studies indicate that ovulation induction with clomiphene may actually decrease breast cancer risk. (Clomphine is related to tamoxifen, a drug that is used for breast cancer prevention in high-risk women.)

2.3.3. Breast Abnormalities

Abnormalities or Breast Conditions Suggesting a higher Risk. Certain factors and breast conditions may increase the risk for breast cancer:

- Dense breast tissue is associated with a higher risk for breast cancer. Studies suggest that women with highly dense tissue have 2 - 6 times the risk of women with the least dense tissue. Genetic factors play a large role in breast density. Hormone replacement therapy also increases breast density. In addition, dense breasts make mammograms more difficult to read, which increases the likelihood of missing early signs of cancer.
- Benign proliferative breast disease, or unusual cell growth known as atypical hyperplasia, is a significant risk factor for breast cancer.

Some common benign breast abnormalities that pose few or no risks include the following:

- Cysts. These mostly occur in women in their middle-to-late reproductive years and can be eliminated simply by aspirating fluid from them.

Physical activity contributes to health by reducing the heart rate, decreasing the risk for cardiovascular disease, and reducing the amount of bone loss that is associated with age and osteoporosis. Physical activity also helps the body use calories more efficiently, thereby helping in weight loss and maintenance. It can increase basal metabolic rate, reduces appetite, and helps in the reduction of body fat.

Dietary Factors

Despite much research on the association between diet and breast cancer, there is still little consensus. The best advice is to eat a well-balanced diet and avoid focusing on one "cancer-fighting" food. The American Cancer Societies dietary guidelines for cancer prevention recommend that people:

- Choose foods and amounts that promote a healthy weight.
- Eat 5 or more servings of fruits and vegetables each day.
- Choose whole grains instead of refined grain products.
- Limit consumption of processed and red meat.
- Women should limit alcohol consumption to 1 drink per day (women at high risk for breast cancer should consider not drinking alcohol at all).

For breast cancer survivors, the American Cancer Society recommends diets that include lots of fruits and vegetables, low amounts of saturated fat (from meat and high-fat dairy products), moderation in soy foods, and moderate or no alcohol consumption. Here are results from recent studies evaluating diet and breast cancer, for preventing both the development of cancer and its recurrence:

Fats. Research is still mixed on the role that fats, and which specific types of fats, play in breast cancer risk and prevention. Several studies have indicated that red meat, which is high in saturated fat, may increase breast cancer risk when eaten in large quantities on a daily basis. (Red meat is also high in iron, which in itself may increase breast cancer risk.) According to results from the Women's Health Initiative study of dietary fat and breast cancer, there is no definite evidence that a low-fat diet will help prevent breast cancer. However, the study suggested that women who normally eat a very high-fat diet may benefit by reducing their fat intake. In the study, the low-fat diet reduced blood estrogen levels by 15%. The low-fat diet also appeared to reduce the risk for developing progesterone receptor-negative tumors.

Fruits and Vegetables. Fruits and vegetables are important sources of antioxidants, which may help protect against the tissue damage linked to increased cancer risk. Antioxidants include vitamin C, vitamin E, and carotenoids such as beta-carotene and lycopene. Richly colored fruits and vegetables -- not supplements -- are the best sources for these nutrients. These fiber-rich foods are an essential part of a healthy diet. However, it is not clear whether fruits and vegetables can specifically prevent breast cancer development or recurrence.

Calcium and Vitamin D. Eating lots of foods rich in calcium and vitamin D (such as yogurt and milk) may modestly reduce the risk of breast cancer for premenopausal women. Low-fat or non-fat dairy products are a healthier choice than high-fat ones.

Soy. Soy is an excellent low-fat protein alternative to meat. Soy contains phytoestrogens, which are estrogen-like plant chemicals. In particular, soy contains a type of phytoestrogen called isoflavones. Because many soy foods (such as tofu) are eaten in Asian countries where women tend to have a lower incidence of breast cancer, research has focused on whether soy may have a protective effect. To date, the evidence does not indicate that soy foods or supplements can reduce breast cancer risk. In addition, some studies suggest that high intakes of soy may actually increase the risk of estrogen-responsive cancers such as breast cancer. Some animal studies have suggested that the isoflavone compound genistein may reduce the protective properties of tamoxifen, a drug used to prevent breast cancer in high-risk women. The American Cancer Society recommends that women with breast cancer eat only moderate amounts of soy foods and avoid taking dietary supplements that contain high amounts of isoflavones.

Specific Preventive Measures for High-Risk Women

Lifestyle Factors. Premenopausal women at higher risk, usually because of family history, should take as many preventive measures as possible, starting at an early age. The following lifestyle choices may be beneficial:

- Exercising and eating healthily is the first essential rule.
- High-risk premenopausal women may choose alternatives to oral contraceptives and, if feasible, consider having children early in their life.
- High-risk postmenopausal women may want to forego hormone replacement therapy.
- Any woman at high risk for breast cancer should consider avoiding alcohol or drink it very sparingly.

Tamoxifen and Raloxifene. Drugs known as selective estrogen-receptor modulators (SERMs) act like estrogen in some tissues but behave like estrogen blockers (anti-estrogens) in others. Two SERMs -- tamoxifen (Nolvadex) and raloxifene (Evista) -- are approved for breast cancer prevention for high-risk women. Tamoxifen and raloxifene are not recommended as prevention for women at low risk for breast cancer or its recurrence. Women at high risk for breast cancer should discuss with their doctors the risks and benefits of SERMs. Tamoxifen (Nolvadex) is the most studied of these drugs. It is currently used to treat breast cancer and was the first drug approved for prevention. Evidence strongly suggests that it halves the risk for estrogen receptor-positive cancers in high-risk women, including those with BRCA2 mutations (although possibly not BRCA1). It also helps prevent recurrence in women who have been treated for breast cancers. However, it has no protective effects against estrogen receptor-negative (hormone-insensitive) cancers. Tamoxifen can increase the risk for uterine (endometrial) cancers. It can also increase the risk for blood clots, strokes, and endometriosis. Less serious side effects include hot flashes and vaginal discharge. Raloxifene (Evista) was approved in 2007 for prevention of breast cancer in postmenopausal women with osteoporosis and postmenopausal women at high risk for invasive breast cancer. Raloxifene was previously approved for prevention and treatment of osteoporosis in postmenopausal women. Studies indicate that it works as well as tamoxifen in reducing the risk of invasive breast cancer. One of raloxifenes main benefits is that it has a lower risk than tamoxifen of causing uterine cancer and blood clots. However, women with a history of blood clots in the legs, lungs, or eyes should not take raloxifene. Although studies indicate raloxifene does not increase the risk of stroke, it can increase the risk of dying from a stroke. Women with a history of or current risk factors for stroke or heart disease should discuss with their doctors whether raloxifene is an appropriate choice. Less serious side effects of raloxifene include hot flashes, leg cramps, swelling of the legs and feet, flu-like symptoms, joint pain, and sweating. Raloxifene can cause birth defects and is approved only for postmenopausal women. It should not be taken with the cholesterol-lowering drug cholestyramine (Questran) or with estrogens.

Investigational Drugs for Breast Cancer Prevention .Aromatase inhibitors such as anastrazole (Armidex), letrozole (Femara), and exemestane (Aromasin) are effective treatments for postmenopausal women with hormone-receptor positive breast cancer. Like tamoxifen, these drugs are also being investigated for protection in high-risk women. However, aromatase inhibitors may decrease bone mineral density and cognitive function, and increase the risk for falls.

2.3.4. Symptoms

Breast cancers in their early stages are usually painless. Often the first symptom is the discovery of a hard lump. Fifty percent of such masses are found in the upper outer quarter of the breast. The lump may make the affected breast appear elevated or asymmetric. The nipple may be retracted or scaly. Sometimes the skin of the breast is dimpled like the skin of an orange. In some cases there is a bloody or clear discharge from the nipple. Many cancers, however, produce no symptoms and cannot be felt on examination. They can be detected only with a mammogram.

Monthly breast self-exams should always include: visual inspection (with and without a mirror) to note any changes in contour or texture, and manual inspection in standing and reclining positions to note any unusual lumps or thicknesses.

2.3.5. Diagnosis

Breast Examination by a Health Professional. Women ages 20 - 49 should have a physical examination by a health professional every 1 - 2 years. Those over age 50 should be examined annually.

Self-Examinations. Women have been encouraged to perform self-examination each month, but some studies have reported no difference in mortality rates between women who do self-examination and those who do not. This does not mean women should stop attempting self-examinations, but they should not replace the annual examination done by a health professional.

Monthly Self-Examination

1. Pick a time of the month that is easy to remember and perform self-examination at that time each month: The breast has normal patterns of thickness and lumpiness that change within a monthly period, and a consistently scheduled examination will help differentiate between what is normal from abnormal. Many doctors recommend breast awareness rather than formal monthly self-examinations.

2. Stand in front of a mirror: Breasts should be basically the same size (one may be slightly larger than the other). Check for changes or redness in the nipple area. Look for changes in the appearance of the skin. With hands on the hips, push the pelvis forward and pull the shoulders back and observe the breasts for irregularities. Repeat the observation with hands behind the head. Move each arm and shoulder forward.

3. Lie down on the back with a rolled towel under one shoulder: Apply lotion or bath oil over the breast area. The finger action should be as follows: Using the 2nd, 3rd, and 4th finger pads (not tips) held together, make dime-sized circles. Press lightly first to feel the breast area, and then press harder using a circular motion.

Using this motion, start from the collarbone and move downward to underneath the breast. Shift the fingers slightly over, slightly overlapping the previously checked region, and work upward back to the collarbone. Repeat this up-and-down examination until the entire breast area has been examined. Be sure to cover the entire area from the collarbone to the bottom of the breast area and from the middle of the chest to the armpits. Move the towel under the other shoulder and repeat the procedure.

Examine the nipple area, by gently lifting and squeezing it and checking for discharge.

4. Repeat step 3 in an upright position: (The shower is the best place for this, using plenty of soap.)

Note: A lump can be any size or shape and can move around or remain fixed. Of special concern are specific or unusual lumps that appear to be different from the normal varying thicknesses in the breast. Monthly breast self-exams should always include: visual inspection (with and without a mirror) to note any changes in contour or texture, and manual inspection in standing and reclining positions to note any unusual lumps or thicknesses.

Mammograms

Current Recommendations for Screening. Mammograms are very effective low-radiation screening methods for breast cancer. At this time, the U.S. Preventive Services Task Force recommends screening mammograms, with or without breast examination, every 1 - 2 years for all women over age 40. Guidelines from the American College of Physicians (ACP), however, debate whether women with a low risk for breast cancer should begin mammogram screening at age 40. The 2007 guidelines, instead, recommend that women in their 40s ask their doctor when they should begin having the test. In contrast, the American Cancer Society and the U.S. National Cancer Institute continue to endorse annual screening for women age 40 and older. Supporters of the ACP guidelines believe that their recommendations reflect some of the risks involved in screening younger women. These risks include radiation exposure and unnecessary biopsies. Mammographies in younger women produce a relatively high rate of false-positive results (when the test falsely indicates breast cancer). Scientists are working on new technologies to improve mammography's accuracy, but more work is needed. Opponents of the ACP guidelines argue that mammograms help catch tumors while they are in their earliest and most treatable stages, and that the most deadly types of breast cancer tend to occur in women in their 40s. After age 50, all guidelines recommend annual screenings. As a woman ages, her risk for developing breast cancer increases. (Women over age 65 account for most new cases of breast cancer.) Women with risk factors for breast cancer, including a close family member with the disease, should consider having annual mammograms starting 10 years earlier than the age at which the relative was diagnosed.

Other Imaging Techniques

Magnetic Resonance Imaging and Ultrasound. Magnetic resonance imaging (MRI) and ultrasound techniques can detect very small tumors (less than half an inch). However, they are expensive and time-consuming procedures, and ultrasound may yield more false-positive results. Nevertheless, some doctors believe they are important in identifying small tumors missed on mammography in women who are receiving lumpectomy or breast-conserving surgeries. Such findings allow surgeons to remove the optimal amount of abnormal tissue. Ultrasound may be particularly helpful for women with dense breast tissue who show signs of breast cancer. In 2007, the American Cancer Society recommended that high-risk women have an MRI of their breast with their annual mammogram, including those who have:

- A BRCA1 or BRCA2 mutation
- A first-degree relative (parent, sibling, child) with a BRCA1 or BRCA2 mutation, even if they have yet to be tested themselves
- A lifetime risk of breast cancer that has been scored at 20 - 25% or greater based on various risk assessment tools that evaluate family history and other factors
- Had radiation to the chest between ages 10 - 30
- Li-Fraumeni syndrome, Cowden syndrome, or Bannayan-Riley-Ruvalcaba syndrome, or may have one of these genetic syndromes based on a history in a first-degree relative

For women who have had cancer diagnosed in one breast, MRIs can also be very helpful for detecting hidden tumors in the other breast. An important study reported that MRI scans of women who were diagnosed with cancer in one breast detected over 90% of cancers in the other breast that had been previously missed by mammography or clinical breast exam. Currently, few women who are diagnosed with cancer in one breast are offered an MRI of the other breast. Some doctors advocate MRIs for all women newly diagnosed with breast cancer; others oppose this view. MRI scans may be most useful for younger women with breast cancer who have dense breast tissue that may obscure tumors from mammography readings. MRIs are less likely to be helpful for older women with early tumors in one breast and clear mammography readings in the other.

It is very important that women have MRIs at qualified centres that perform many of these procedures each year. MRI is a complicated procedure and requires special equipment and experienced radiologists. MRI facilities should also be able to offer biopsies when suspicious findings are detected.

Scintimammography. In scintimammography, a radioactive chemical is injected into the circulatory system, which is then selectively taken up by the tumor and revealed on mammograms. This method is used for women who have had abnormal mammograms or for women who have dense breast tissue. It is not used for regular screening or as an alternative to mammography.

Biopsy

A definitive diagnosis of breast cancer can be made only by a biopsy (a microscopic examination of a tissue sample of the suspicious area).

- When a lump can be felt and is suspicious for cancer on mammography, an excisional biopsy may be recommended. This biopsy is a surgical procedure for removing the suspicious tissue and typically requires general anesthetic.

A core biopsy involves a small incision and the insertion of a spring-loaded hollow needle that removes several samples. The patient only requires local anesthetic.

- A wire localization biopsy may be performed if mammography detects abnormalities but there is no lump. With this procedure, using mammography as a guide, the doctor inserts a small wire hook through a hollow needle and into the suspicious tissue. The needle is withdrawn, and the hook is used by the surgeon to locate and remove the lesion. The patient may receive local or general anesthetic.
- A vacuum-assisted device may be used for some biopsies. This uses a single probe through which a vacuum is used to draw out tissue. It allows several samples to be taken without having to remove and re-insert the probe.

Final analysis of the breast tissue may take several days.

Lymphadenectomy

If breast cancer has been determined, the next diagnostic step is to find out how far it has spread. To do this, the doctor performs a procedure called an *axillary lymphadenectomy*, which partially or completely removes the lymph nodes in the armpit beside the affected breast (called *axillary* lymph nodes). It may require a hospital stay of 1 - 2 days. Once the lymph nodes are removed, they are analyzed to determine whether subsequent treatment needs to be more or less aggressive:

- If no cancer is found in the lymph nodes, the condition is referred to as *node negative* breast cancer. The chances are good that the cancer has not spread and is still local.
- If cancer cells are present in the lymph nodes, the cancer is called *node positive.* Their presence increases the possibility that the cancer has spread microscopically to other areas of the body. In such cases, however, it is still not known if the cancer has metastasized beyond the lymph nodes or, if so, to what extent. The doctor may perform further tests to see if the cancer has spread to the bone (bone scan), lungs (x-ray or CT scan) or brain (MRI or CT scan).

Side effects of the procedure may include increased risk for infection and pain, swelling in the arm from fluid build-up, and impaired sensation and restricted movement in the affected arm.

Sentinel Node Biopsy

Sentinel node biopsy is a less invasive alternative to axillary lymph node dissection. This procedure can help determine if cancer has spread beyond the nodes. If the doctor finds no evidence of cancer, the patient may not need to have a complete axillary lymphadenectomy.

Sentinel node biopsy involves:

- The procedure uses an injection of a tiny amount of a tracer, either a radioactively-labeled substance (radioisotope) or a blue dye, into the tumor site.
- The tracer or dye then flows through the lymphatic system into the sentinel node. This is the first lymph node to which any cancer would spread.
- The sentinel lymph node and possibly one or two others are then removed.
- If they do not show any signs of cancer, it is highly likely that the remaining lymph nodes will be cancer free, making further surgery unnecessary.

Patients who have a sentinel node biopsy tend to have better arm function and a shorter hospital stay than those who have an axillary node biopsy. The American Society of Clinical Oncology's guidelines recommend sentinel node biopsy instead of axillary lymph node dissection for women with early stage breast cancer who do not have nodes that can be felt during a physical exam. It is still not known if the sentinel node biopsy has any survival advantages compared to standard lymph node removal procedures.

2.3.6. Prognosis

Breast cancer is the second most lethal cancer in women. (Lung cancer is the leading cancer killer in women.) The good news is that early detection and new treatments have improved survival rates. The 5-year survival rate for women diagnosed with cancer is 80%. About 88% of women diagnosed with breast cancer will survive at least 10 years. Unfortunately, women in lower social and economic groups still have significantly lower survival rates than women in higher groups.

Several factors are used to determine the risk for recurrence and the likelihood of successful treatment. They include:

- Location of the tumor and how far it has spread
- Whether the tumor is hormone receptor-positive or -negative
- Tumor markers
- Gene expression
- Tumor size and shape
- Rate of cell division

The good news is that women are living longer with breast cancer. Due to better treatment options, breast cancer mortality rates declined by about 25% since 1990. However, survivors must live with the uncertainties of possible recurrent cancer and some risk for complications from the treatment itself. Recurrences of cancer usually develop within 5 years of treatment. About 25% of recurrences and half of new cancers in the opposite breast occur after 5 years.

Location of the Tumor

The location of the tumor is a major factor in outlook:

- If the cancer is ductal carcinoma in situ (DCIS) or has not spread to the lymph nodes (node negative), the 5-year survival rates with treatment are up to 98%.

- If the cancer has spread to the lymph nodes or beyond the primary site (node positive), the 5-year survival rate is about 84%.
- If the cancer has spread (metastasized) to other sites (most often the lung, liver, and bone), the average 5-year survival rate is 27%. New drug therapies, particularly aromatase inhibitors, have helped prolong survival for women with metastatic cancer.

The location of the tumor within the breast is an important predictor. Tumors that develop toward the outside of the breast tend to be less serious than those that occur more toward the middle of the breast.

Hormone Receptor-Positive or -Negative

Breast cancer cells may contain receptors, or binding sites, for the hormones estrogen and progesterone. Cells containing these binding sites are known as hormone receptor-positive cells. If cells lack these connectors, they are called hormone receptor-negative cells. About 75% of breast cancers are estrogen receptor-positive (ER-positive, or ER+). About 65% of ER-positive breast cancers are also progesterone receptor-positive (PR-positive, or PR+). Cells that have receptors for one of these hormones, or both of them, are considered hormone receptor-positive. Hormone receptor-positive cancer is also called "hormone sensitive" because it responds to hormone therapy such as tamoxifen or aromatase inhibitors. Hormone receptor-negative tumors are referred to as "hormone insensitive" or "hormone resistant." Women have a better prognosis if their tumors are hormone receptor-positive because these cells grow more slowly than receptor-negative cells. In addition, women with hormone receptor-positive cancer have more treatment options. (Hormone receptor-negative tumors can be treated only with chemotherapy.) Recent declines in breast cancer mortality rates have been most significant among women with estrogen receptor-positive tumors, due in part to the widespread use of post-surgical hormone drug therapy.

Tumor Markers

Tumor markers are proteins found in blood or urine when cancer is present. Although they are not used to diagnose cancer, the presence of certain markers can help predict how aggressive a patient's cancer may be and how well the cancer may respond to certain types of drugs.

Tumor markers relevant for breast cancer prognosis include:

HER2. The American Cancer Society recommends that all women newly diagnosed with breast cancer get a biopsy test for a growth-promoting protein called HER2/neu. HER2-positive cancer usually occurs in younger women and is more quickly-growing and aggressive than other types of breast cancer. The HER2 marker is present in about 20% of cases of invasive breast cancer. Two types of tests are used to detect HER2:

- Immunohistochemistry (IHC)
- Fluorescence in-situ hybridization (FISH)

Some doctors think that FISH is a more accurate test than IHC. According to 2006 HER2 testing guidelines from the American Society of Clinical Oncology and the College of American Pathologists, either test may be used as long as it is performed by an accredited laboratory. Tests that are not clearly positive or negative should be repeated. Treatment with trastuzumab (Herceptin) or lapatinib (Tykerb) may help women who test positive for HER2. In 2008, the FDA approved a new genetic test (Spot-Light) that can help determine which patients with HER2-positive breast cancer may be good candidates for trastuzumab treatment.

Other Markers. Other markers that may be evaluated include CA 15-3, CA 27.29, CEA, ER, PgR, uPA, and PAI-1.

Gene Expression Profiling

Gene expression profiling tests (Oncotype DX, MammaPrint) examine a set of genes in tumor tissue to determine the likelihood of breast cancer recurrence. These tests are also used to help determine whether adjuvant (following surgery) drug treatments should be given. The American Society of Clinical Oncology and the National Comprehensive Cancer Network now recommend that gene expression profiling tests be administered to newly diagnosed patients with node-negative, estrogen-receptor-positive breast cancer. Based on the results, a doctor can decide whether a patient who has had surgery may benefit from chemotherapy.

Other Factors for Predicting Outlook

Tumor Size and Shape. Large tumors pose a higher risk than small tumors. Undifferentiated tumors, which have indistinct margins, are more dangerous than those with well-defined margins.

Rate of Cell Division. The more rapidly a tumor grows, the more dangerous it is. Several tests measure aspects of cancer cell division and may eventually prove to predict the disease. For example, the mitotic index (MI) is a measurement of the rate at which cells divide. The higher the MI, the more aggressive the cancer. Other tests measure cells at a certain phase of their division.

Effect of Emotions and Psychological Support

Recent evidence has not supported early reports of survival benefits for women with metastatic breast cancer who engage in support groups. However, some studies have suggested that psychotherapy, group support, or both may relieve pain and reduce stress, particularly in women who are suffering emotionally. Stress has been ruled out as a risk factor either for breast cancer itself or for its recurrence.

Treatment

The three major treatments of breast cancer are surgery, radiation, and drug therapy. No one treatment fits every patient, and combination therapy is usually required. The choice is determined by many factors, including the age of the patient, menopausal status, the kind of cancer (ductal verses lobular), its stage, and whether or not the tumor contains hormone-receptors.

Breast cancer treatments are defined as local or systemic:

- *Local Treatment.* Surgery and radiation are considered local therapies because they directly treat the tumor, breast, lymph nodes, or other specific regions. Surgery is usually the standard initial treatment.
- *Systemic Treatment.* Drug treatment is called systemic therapy, because it affects the whole body. Drugs may include either chemotherapy or hormone therapy. Drug therapy may be used as primary therapy for patients for whom surgery or

radiation therapy is not appropriate, neoadjuvant therapy (before surgery or radiation) to shrink tumors to a size that can be treated with local therapy, or as adjuvant therapy (following surgery or radiation) to reduce the risk of cancer recurrence. For metastatic cancer, drugs are used not to cure but to improve quality of life and prolong survival.

Any or all of these therapies may be used separately or, most often, in different combinations. For example, radiation alone or with chemotherapy or hormone therapy may be beneficial before surgery, if the tumor is large or not easily removed at prevention. Surgery followed by radiation and hormone therapy is usually recommended for women with early-stage, hormone-sensitive cancer. There are numerous clinical trials investigating new treatments and treatment combinations. Patients, especially those with advanced stages of cancer, may wish to consider enrolling in a clinical trial.

2.3.7. Cancer Stage and Treatment Options

Treatment strategies depend in part on the stage of the cancer.

Stage 0 (Carcinoma in Situ): Stage 0 breast cancer is considered non-invasive (in situ"), meaning that the cancer is still confined within breast ducts or lobules and has not yet spread to surrounding tissues. Stage 0 cancer is classified as either:

- Ductal carcinoma in situ (DCIS). These are cancer cells in the lining of a duct that have not invaded the surrounding breast tissue.
- Lobular carcinoma in situ (LCIS). These are cancer cells in the lobules of the breast. LCIS rarely develops into invasive breast cancer, but having it in one breast increases the risk of developing cancer in the other breast.

Treatment options for DCIS include:

- Breast-conserving surgery and radiation therapy (followed by hormone therapy for women with hormone-sensitive cancer). Many doctors recommend this approach.
- Total mastectomy (followed by hormone therapy for women with hormone-sensitive cancer)
- Breast-conserving surgery without radiation therapy

Treatment options for LCIS include:

- Regular exams and mammograms to monitor any potential changes (observation treatment)
- Hormone therapy to prevent development of breast cancer (for women with hormone-sensitive cancer)
- Mastectomy of both breasts was previously used as treatment, but is now rarely recommended

Stage I and II (Early-Stage Invasive): In stage I cancer, cancer cells have not spread beyond the breast and the tumor is no more than 2 cm (about 3/4 of an inch) across.

Stage II cancer is classified as either stage IIA or stage IIb.

In stage IIA cancer the tumor is either:

- No more than 2 centimeters and has spread to the underarm lymph nodes (axillary lymph nodes)
- Between 2 - 5 centimeters and has not spread to the underarm lymph nodes

In stage IIB cancer the tumor is either:

- Larger than 2 centimeters and less than 5 centimeters and has spread to 1 - 3 axillary lymph nodes
- Larger than 5 centimeters but has now spread to lymph nodes

Treatment options for stage I and stage II breast cancer may include:

- Breast-conserving surgery (such as lumpectomy) followed by radiation therapy
- Modified radical mastectomy with or without breast reconstruction
- Post-surgical therapy (adjuvant therapy), including radiation of lymph nodes, chemotherapy, or hormone therapy
- Trastuzumab (Herceptin) given along with or following adjuvant chemotherapy for women with HER2-positive cancer

Stage III (Locally advanced): Stage III breast cancer is classified into several sub-categories: Stage IIIA, stage IIIB, and stage IIIC (operable or inoperable).

In stage IIIA breast cancer, the tumor is either:

- Not more than 5 centimeters and has spread to 4 - 9 axillary lymph nodes
- Larger than 5 centimeters and has spread to 1 - 9 axillary nodes or to internal mammary nodes.

Treatment options for stage IIIA breast cancer are the same as those for stages I and II.

In stage IIIB breast cancer, the tumor has spread to either:

- Tissues near the breast (including the skin or chest wall)
- Lymph nodes within the breast or under the arm

Stage IIIB treatment options may include:

- Chemotherapy, and possibly hormone therapy (sometimes in combination with chemotherapy)
- Chemotherapy followed by surgery (breast-conserving surgery or total mastectomy) with lymph node dissection followed by radiation therapy and possibly more chemotherapy or hormone therapy
- Clinical trials

Stage IIIC breast cancer is classified as either operable or inoperable.

In operable stage IIIC, the cancer may be found in:

- 10 or more of the underarm lymph nodes
- Lymph nodes beneath the collarbone and near the neck on the same side of the body as the affected breast
- Lymph nodes within the breast as well as underarm lymph nodes

Treatment options for operable stage III breast cancer are the same as those for stage I and II breast cancers.

In inoperable stage III breast cancer, the cancer has spread to lymph nodes above the collarbone and near the neck on the same side of the body as the affected breast. Treatment options are the same as those for stage IIIB.

Stage IV (Advanced Cancer): In stage IV, the cancer has spread (metastasized) from the breast to other parts of the body. In about 75% of cases, the cancer has spread to the bone. The cancer at this stage is considered to be chronic and incurable, and the usefulness of treatments is limited. The goals of treatment for stage IV cancer are to stabilize the disease and slow its progression, as well as to reduce pain and discomfort.

Treatment options for stage IV cancer include:

- Surgery or radiation for any localized tumors in the breast.
- Chemotherapy, hormone therapy, or both. Targeted therapy with trastuzumab (Herceptin) or lapatinib (Tykerb) should be considered for women with HER2-positive cancer.
- Cancer that has spread to the brain may require radiation and high-dose steroids.
- Cancer that has spread to the bone may be helped by radiation or bisphosphonate drugs. Such treatments can relieve pain and help prevent bone fractures.
- Clinical trials of new drugs or drug combinations, or experimental treatments such as high-dose chemotherapy with stem cell transplant.

Post-Treatment Care

The American Society of Clinical Oncology (ASCO) recommends follow-up care for patients who have been treated for breast cancer:

- Visit your doctor every 3 - 6 months for the first 3 years after your first cancer treatment, every 6 - 12 months during the fourth and fifth year, and once a year thereafter.
- Have a mammogram 1 year after the mammogram that diagnosed your cancer (but no earlier than 6 months after radiation therapy), and every 6 - 12 months thereafter.
- Perform a breast self-exam every month (however, this is no substitute for a mammogram).
- See your gynecologist regularly (women taking tamoxifen should be sure to report any vaginal bleeding).
- A year after diagnosis, you can either continue to see your oncologist or transfer your care to your primary care physician.

- If you are on hormone therapy, discuss with your oncologist how often to schedule follow-up visits for re-evaluation of your treatment.

ASCO does not recommend the use of laboratory blood tests (complete blood counts, carcinoembryonic antigen) or imaging tests (bone scans, chest x-rays, liver ultrasound, FDG-PET scan, CT scan) for routine breast cancer follow-up.

Genetic counselling may be helpful if you have:

- Ashkenazi Jewish heritage
- Personal or family history of ovarian cancer
- Personal or family history of cancer in both breasts
- Any first-degree female relative (mother, sister, daughter) diagnosed with breast cancer before age 50
- Two or more first-degree or second-degree (grandparent, aunt, uncle) diagnosed with breast cancer
- History of breast cancer in a male relative

Pregnancy after Breast Cancer Treatment. There are no definite recommendations on how long a woman should wait to become pregnant after breast cancer treatment. Because of the connection between estrogen levels and breast cancer cell growth, some doctors recommend delaying pregnancy until 2 years after treatment in order to reduce the risk of cancer recurrence and improve odds for survival. However, other studies indicate that conceiving 6 months after treatment does not negatively affect survival. Discuss with your doctor your risk for recurrence, and when it may be safe to attempt pregnancy.

Recurrent Breast Cancer

Recurrent breast cancer is considered to be an advanced cancer. In such cases, the disease has come back in spite of the initial treatment. Most recurrences appear within the first 2 - 3 years after treatment, but breast cancer can recur many years later. Treatment options are based on the stage at which the cancer reappears, whether or not the tumor is hormone responsive, and the age of the patient. Between 10 - 20% of recurring cancers are local. Most recurrent cancers are metastatic. All patients with recurring cancer are candidates for clinical trials.

Because most breast cancer recurrences are discovered by patients in between doctor visits, it is important to notify your doctor if you experience any of the following symptoms. These symptoms may be signs of breast cancer recurrence:

- New lumps in the breast
- Bone pain
- Chest pain
- Abdominal pain
- Shortness of breath or difficulty breathing
- Persistent headaches or coughing
- Rash on breast
- Nipple discharge

Surgery

Surgery forms a part of nearly every patient's treatment for breast cancer. The initial surgical intervention is often a lumpectomy, the removal of the tumor itself. In the past, mastectomy (the removal of the breast) was the standard treatment for nearly all breast cancers. Now, many patients with early-stage cancers can choose breast-conserving treatment, or lumpectomy followed by radiation, with or without chemotherapy.

For invasive breast cancer, studies indicate that lumpectomy or partial mastectomy combined with radiation therapy works as well as a modified radical mastectomy.

Breast-Conserving Procedures

Breast-conserving procedures are now appropriate and as successful as mastectomy in most women with early stage breast cancer. All women should discuss these options fully with their doctor. Recurrence rates with conservative surgery are highest in women under age 45. Some women choose mastectomy over breast-conserving treatment even if the latter is appropriate because it gives them a greater sense of security and allows them to avoid radiation therapy.

Lumpectomy. Lumpectomy is the removal of the tumor, often along with lymph nodes in the armpit. It serves as an opportunity for biopsy, a diagnostic tool, and a primary treatment for small local breast tumors. If invasive cancer is found, the doctor will decide to proceed with breast radiation therapy, to remove additional tissue (should the margins of the specimen show signs of cancer), or to perform a mastectomy. Lumpectomy followed by radiation therapy is appropriate and as effective as mastectomy for most women with Stage I or II breast cancers.

Breast-Conserving Surgery (Quadrantectomy). Breast-conserving surgery (sometimes referred to as quadrantectomy) removes the cancer and a large area of breast tissue, occasionally including some of the lining over the chest muscles. It is less invasive than a full mastectomy, but the cosmetic results are less satisfactory than with a lumpectomy. Studies have found that breast-conserving surgeries plus postoperative radiotherapy offer the same survival rates as radical mastectomy in women with early breast cancer.

Mastectomy

Surgery to remove the breast (mastectomy) is important for women with operable breast cancer who are not candidates for breast conserving surgeries. There are different variations on the procedure:

- A total mastectomy involves removal of the whole breast and sometimes lymph nodes under the armpit.
- A radical mastectomy removes the breast, chest muscles, all of the lymph nodes under the arm, and some additional fat and skin. (A modified radical mastectomy removes the entire breast and armpit lymph nodes, with the underlying chest wall muscle.) For most patients, there are no survival advantages from radical mastectomy compared to less invasive mastectomies.

Complications and Side Effects of Surgery. Short-term pain and tenderness occur in the area of the procedure, and pain relievers may be necessary.

The most frequent complication of extensive lymph node removal is lymphedema, or swelling, of the arm. The likelihood of edema can be lessened by removing only some of the lymph nodes instead of all of them.

Infrequent complications include poor wound healing, bleeding, or a reaction to the anesthesia.

After mastectomy and lymph node removal, women may experience numbness, tingling, and difficulty in extending the arm fully. These effects can last for months or years afterward.

Breast Reconstruction

After a mastectomy, some women choose a breast prosthesis or opt for breast reconstruction, which can be performed during the mastectomy itself, if desired. Several studies have indicated that women who take advantage of cosmetic surgery after breast cancer have a better sense of well-being and a higher quality of life than women who do not choose reconstructive surgery. The breast is reshaped using a saline implant or, for a more cosmetic result, a muscle flap is taken from elsewhere in the body. Muscle flap procedures are more complicated, however, and blood transfusions may be required. (It should be noted that implants, including silicone implants, do not appear to put a woman at risk for breast cancer recurrence.) If the nipple is removed, it is rebuilt from other body tissues and color is applied using tattoo techniques. It is nearly impossible to rebuild a breast that is identical to its partner, and additional operations may be necessary to achieve a desirable effect.

Radiation

Radiation therapy uses high-energy x-rays to kill cancer cells or to shrink the size of a tumor in the breast or surrounding tissue. It is used for several weeks following lumpectomy or partial mastectomy, and sometimes after full mastectomy. Radiation therapy can help reduce the chance of breast cancer recurrence in the breast and chest wall. Radiation is also important in advanced stages of cancer for relief of symptoms and to slow progression. Research shows that radiation therapy is helpful for women of all ages, including those over age 65.

Administration of Radiation Therapy

Radiation is generally administered in the following ways:

External Beam Radiation. This type of radiation is administered 4 - 6 weeks after surgery and delivered externally by an x-ray machine that targets radiation to the whole breast. It may be delivered to the chest wall in high-risk patients (large tumors, close surgical margins, or lymph node involvement). The treatment is generally given daily (except for weekends) for about 6 weeks. Some hospitals offer a shortened course of 3 weeks of radiation for patients with early-stage breast cancer.

Brachytherapy. Less commonly, radiation is delivered in implants (called brachytherapy). Implants are most often used as a radiation boost after whole breast radiation.

Side Effects of Radiation Therapy

Side effects of radiation include:

- Fatigue is very common and increases with subsequent treatments, but most women are able to continue with normal activities. Exercise may be helpful.
- Nausea and lack of appetite may develop and worsen as treatment progresses.
- Skin changes and burns can occur on the breast skin. Using a cream that contains a corticosteroid, such as mometasone furoate (MMF), may be helpful. After repeated sessions, the skin may become moist and "weepy." Exposing the treated skin to air as much as possible helps healing. Washing the affected skin with soap and water is not harmful.
- Uncommonly, the breast may change color, size, or become permanently firm.
- Rarely, the nearest arm may swell and develop impaired mobility or even paralysis.

Long-Term Complications

Future complications include:

- Radiation to the left breast may increase the long-term risk for developing heart disease and heart attacks.
- There is a very small risk (less than 1%) of lung irritation and scarring.
- Some studies have reported a higher risk for future cancer in the opposite breast in younger women who have been given radiation to the chest wall.
- Radiation therapy can increase the risk of developing other cancers, such as soft tissue malignancies known as sarcomas.

Current advanced imaging techniques use precise radiation that reduces exposure. These newer techniques are likely to reduce the risks for heart disease and other serious complications.

Chemotherapy

Chemotherapy drugs are "cytotoxic" (cell-killing) drugs. They are given orally or by injection. They work systemically by killing cancer cells throughout the body. (Unfortunately, they also kill normal cells, which accounts for many of their side effects.) Chemotherapy is always used for advanced breast cancer, but may also be used to treat types of early-stage breast cancer. Newer biologic drugs target specific proteins involved in cancer. Because they do not work as systemically as chemotherapy or hormone therapy drugs, they tend to cause fewer widespread side effects, although they also carry risks of their own Chemotherapy needs to be tailored to the type of cancer involved. Women require different treatments depending on whether the tumor is node-negative or -positive, hormone receptor-positive or -negative, or HER2-positive or -negative. Different treatment approaches are also used for early-stage cancer and advanced cancer. In general, women with hormone receptor-negative cancers respond better to chemotherapy than women with hormone receptor-positive cancer. However, some women with hormone receptor-positive cancer do benefit from chemotherapy, as well as from hormone therapy. Adjuvant chemotherapy is administered following surgery and before radiation therapy. Delaying chemotherapy until more than 12 weeks after surgery may increase the risk for breast cancer recurrence and reduce the odds for survival.

Chemotherapy Drug Classes

Many different types of chemotherapy drugs are used to treat breast cancer. Common types of chemotherapy drug classes include:

- Anthracyclines include doxorubicin (Adriamycin) and epirubicin (Ellence). Anthracycline-based combination regimens are often used to treat early-stage breast cancer, as well as advanced cancer.
- Taxanes include paclitaxel (Taxol) and docetaxel (Taxotere). These drugs may be particularly helpful for node-positive breast cancer. A newer formulation of paclitaxel (Abraxane) is used as a secondary treatment for advanced breast cancer.

- Platinum-based drugs include oxaliplatin (Eloxatin) and carboplatin (Paraplatin). These drugs may be used in combination regiments for advanced cancer or for cancers associated with BRCA genes.

Chemotherapy Regimens for Early-Stage Breast Cancer

Some of the abbreviations used for chemotherapy drug combinations (regimens) refer to drug classes rather than drug names. For example, regimens that contain an anthracycline drug (such as doxorubicin) use the letter "A," and regimens that contain a taxane drug (such as docetaxel) use the letter "T." Cyclophosphamide (Cytoxan), fluorouracil (5-FU), and methotrexate (MTX) are standard cancer drugs used in many breast cancer chemotherapy regimens.

Chemotherapy regimens usually consist of 4 - 6 cycles of treatment given over 3 - 6 months. Common chemotherapy regimens for early-stage breast cancer include:

- AC (Doxorubicin and cyclophosphamide)
- AC followed by T (Doxorubicin and cylophosphamide followed by paclitaxel)
- CAF (Cyclophosphamide, doxorubicin, and 5-FU)
- CMF (Cyclophosphamide, methotrexate, and 5-FU)
- TAC (Docetaxel, doxorubicin, and cyclophosphamide)

Targeted Therapy for Early-Stage HER2-Positive Breast Cancer

Trastuzumab (Herceptin). Trastuzumab is a monoclonal antibody that targets the HER2 protein on cancer cells. HER2-positive cancers account for 15 - 25% of early-stage breast cancer and are associated with more aggressive disease. Younger women tend to be most affected. In 2006, the Food and Drug Administration approved trastuzumab for treatment of HER2-positive, early-stage breast cancer (cancer confined to the breasts or lymph nodes that has been surgically removed).

Trastuzumab is given along with other chemotherapy drugs following lumpectomy or mastectomy. Research indicates that trastuzumab can help prevent cancer recurrence and death among women with early-stage breast cancer, but it increases the risk of heart problems. Trastuzumab can cause heart failure. Women who have heart failure or weak heart muscle (cardiomyopathy) should not use this drug. Women who take trastuzumab need to have regular heart monitoring, especially if they have already have heart problems.

Chemotherapy for Advanced (Metastatic) Cancer

Patients who develop metastatic disease (cancer that spreads throughout the body) are generally not curable. New advances in drug therapies, however, can help shrink tumors, prolong survival, and improve quality of life. Chemotherapy regimens for advanced cancer may use a single drug or a combination of drugs. Many chemotherapy regimens used for early-stage breast cancer are also used for advanced breast cancer. Some specific combinations for advanced cancer include:

- Gemcitabine and paclitaxel. In 2004, the Food and Drug Administration approved the antimetabolite drug gemcitabine (Gemzar) for use in combination with paclitaxel (Taxol) as a first-line treatment option for women with metastatic breast cancer.
- Capecitabine (Xeloda) and docetaxel (Taxotere). Capecitabine is an oral drug that is chemically related to 5-FU. It is also being studied in combination with many other drugs. In 2007, the FDA approved a new type of drug, ixabepilone (Ixempra), for use in combination with capecitabine in patients with advanced breast cancer that have not responded to other types of chemotherapy.

Numerous chemotherapy drugs and drug combinations are being tested in clinical trials. Patients with advanced breast cancer may also receive other types of drug treatments. Bisphosphonate drugs, such as zoledronic acid (Zometa) and pamidronate (Aredia), are important supportive drugs for preventing fractures and reducing pain in people whose cancer has spread to the bones.

Targeted Therapy for Advanced HER2-Positive Breast Cancer

Three targeted therapy drugs are approved for the treatment of HER2-positive advanced breast cancer

- Trastuzumab (Herceptin) was approved in 1998 for treatment of metastatic breast cancer. It is used in adjuvant chemotherapy, along with drugs such as paclitaxel.

- Lapatinib (Tykerb) was approved in 2007 for patients who have not been helped by other cancer drugs, including an anthracycline, a taxane, or trastuzumab. Lapatinib is used in combination with capecitabine (Xeloda). Research suggests it may have fewer risks for heart problems than trastuzumab.
- Bevacizumab (Avastin) was approved in 2008 for treatment of patients who have not received chemotherapy for metastatic HER2-negative breast cancer. Studies indicate that bevacizumab does not help prolong overall survival, but may help slow tumor growth. Bevacizumab is used in combination with paclitaxel. Bevacizumab targets vascular endothelial growth factor (VEGF), a protein involved in tumor blood vessel formation (angiogenesis).

Investigational Drugs

Promising new treatments for breast cancer include:

- Zoledronic acid (Zometa) is an intravenous bisphosphonate drug that is used to help prevent or delay bone fractures in patients with breast cancer that has spread to the bones. Recent research suggests that the drug may also help reduce the risk for cancer recurrence in patients with early-stage breast cancer.

Side Effects of Chemotherapy

Side effects occur with all chemotherapeutic drugs. They are more severe with higher doses and increase over the course of treatment.

Common side effects include:

- Nausea and vomiting. Drugs such as ondansetron (Zofran) and aprepitant (Emend) can help relieve these side effects.
- Diarrhea
- Temporary hair loss
- Weight loss
- Fatigue
- Depression

Serious short- and long-term complications can also occur and may vary depending on the specific drugs used. They include the following:

- Anemia. Chemotherapy-induced anemia is usually treated with erythropoiesis-stimulating drugs, which include epoietin alfa (Epogen, Procrit) and darberpetin alfa (Aranesp). Erythropoiesis-stimulating drugs should not be used unless a patient's hemoglobin level drops to below 10 g/dL. These drugs may pose serious health risks when they are used to achieve a hemoglobin level of 12 g/dL or greater. Doctors need to follow strict dosing guidelines when administering these drugs. Patients should discuss the risks and benefits of erythropoiesis-stimulating drugs with their oncologists.
- Increased chance for infection from severe reduction in white blood cells (neutropenia). The addition of a drug called granulocyte colony-stimulating factor (filgrastim and lenograstim) is very helpful in reducing the risk for severe infection.
- Liver and kidney damage.
- Abnormal blood clotting (*thrombocytopenia*).
- Allergic reaction, particularly to platinum-based drugs.
- Menstrual abnormalities and infertility. Premature menopause occurs in about 30% of women, particularly in those over 40. A natural hormone medication called a gonadotropin-releasing hormone analogue, which puts women in a temporary pre-pubescent state during chemotherapy, may preserve fertility in some women. Women may also wish to consider embryo cryopreservation -- the harvesting of eggs, followed by in vitro fertilization and freezing of embryos for later use. The American Society of Clinical Oncology recommends that women being treated for cancer see a reproductive specialist to discuss all available fertility preservation options.
- Sexual dysfunction.
- Rarely, secondary cancers such as leukemia.
- A quarter to a third of women report problems in concentration, motor function, and memory, which can be long-term.
- Heart problems. Trastuzumab (Herceptin) may increase the risk for heart failure, particularly in women with pre-existing risk factors. Cumulative doses of

anthracyclines (doxorubicin, epirubicin) can also damage heart muscles over time and increase the risk for heart failure.

- Taxanes can cause a drop in white blood cells and possible problems in the heart and central nervous system. Allergic reactions can occur, more often in taxol than taxotere. Taking a steroid before taxane administration can help prevent such reactions. Taxane therapy may also cause severe joint and muscle pain in some patients, relievable with corticosteroids.

High-Dose Chemotherapy with Bone Marrow or Peripheral-Blood Stem Cell Transplantation

High-dose chemotherapy along with peripheral-blood stem cell rescue or bone marrow transplantation procedures have been used for cancer that has metastasized and, in some cases, for earlier stages of breast cancer in high-risk patients. The objective of this treatment is to be able to give patients very high toxic doses of cell-killing drugs.

Transplantation procedures are based on *stem cells*, which are produced in the bone marrow. Stem cells are the early forms for all blood cells in the body (including red, white, and immune cells). Cancer treatments can harm these growing cells as well as cancer cells.

Despite the initial enthusiasm over the use of transplantation therapy for treatment of high risk breast cancer, this approach is no longer generally recommended and is rarely used outside of a clinical trial setting.

Hormone Therapy

The goal of hormone therapy is to prevent estrogen from stimulating breast cancer cells. It is recommended for women whose breast cancers are hormone-receptor positive (either estrogen or progesterone), regardless of the size of the tumor and whether or not it has spread to the lymph nodes. Like chemotherapy, hormone therapy works systemically.

Hormone therapy works by blocking estrogen that causes cell proliferation. It is used only for patients with hormone receptor-positive tumors. Different types of hormone therapy work in different ways by:

- Blocking estrogen receptors in cancer cells (Tamoxifen)
- Suppressing estrogen production in the body (Aromatase inhibitors)
- Destroying ovaries, which produce estrogen (Ovarian ablation)

Tamoxifen was the first widely used hormonal therapy drug, but it has been replaced by aromatase inhibitors for some women. Aromatase inhibitors are used only to treat postmenopausal women. Tamoxifen is mainly used as adjuvant therapy for premenopausal women with hormone-sensitive breast cancer.

Tamoxifen and Selective Estrogen Receptor Modulators (SERMs)

Tamoxifen (Nolvadex) has been the standard hormonal drug used for breast cancer. It belongs to a class of compounds called selective estrogen receptor modulators (SERMs). SERMs chemically resemble estrogen and trick the breast cancer cells into accepting it in place of estrogen. Unlike estrogen, however, they do not stimulate breast cancer cell growth. Because SERMs block estrogens effects on cancer cells, they are sometimes referred to as "anti-estrogen" drugs.

Tamoxifen is used for all cancer stages in women of all ages with hormone receptor-positive cancers. In addition, it is used to prevent breast cancer in high-risk women. Another SERM drug, toremifene (Fareston), is an option for women with advanced cancer, but this drug is rarely used in the United States. A third drug, fulvestrant (Faslodex), works in a similar anti-estrogen way to tamoxifen but belongs to a different drug class. Fulvestrant is approved only for postmenopausal women with hormone-sensitive advanced breast cancer in which tamoxifen or aromatase inhibitors no longer work. To prevent cancer recurrence, women should take tamoxifen for 5 years following surgery and radiation. Tamoxifen is an effective cancer treatment, but it can cause unpleasant side effects and has small (less than 1%) but serious risks for blood clots and uterine (endometrial) cancer. Immediately report any signs of vaginal bleeding to the doctor, as this may be a symptom of uterine cancer. Less serious, but discomforting, side effects include hot flashes and mood swings. According to one study, nearly 25% of women stop taking tamoxifen within 1 year because of these symptoms. By 3.5 years, over 33% stop treatment. Taking tamoxifen for fewer than 5 years, however, increases the risk for cancer recurrence and death. Talk with your doctor about antidepressants or other therapies that may help you cope with tamoxifens side effects.

Many doctors now recommend that postmenopausal women switch to an aromatase inhibitor after 2 - 3 years of tamoxifen therapy. Several recent studies have indicated that switching from tamoxifen to an aromatase inhibitor significantly improves survival rates and reduces the risk of death from breast cancer as well as other causes. Endometrial cancer is a cancerous growth of the endometrium (lining of the uterus). It is the most common uterine cancer.

Aromatase Inhibitors

Aromatase inhibitors block aromatase, an enzyme that is a major source of estrogen in many major body tissues, including the breast, muscle, liver, and fat. Aromatase inhibitors work differently than tamoxifen. Tamoxifen interferes with tumors ability to use estrogen by blocking their estrogen receptors. Aromatase inhibitors reduce the overall amount of estrogen in the body. Because these drugs cannot stop the ovaries of premenopausal women from producing estrogen, they are recommended only for postmenopausal women. There are currently three aromatase inhibitors approved for treating early-stage, hormone receptor-positive breast cancer in postmenopausal women:

- Anastrazole (Armidex) for treatment after surgery
- Exemestane (Aromasin) for women who have taken tamoxifen for 2 - 3 years
- Letrozole (Femara) for treatment after surgery or for women who have completed 5 years of tamoxifen therapy

All of these drugs are also approved for women with advanced (metastatic) hormone-sensitive breast cancer. Studies indicate that the introduction of aromatase inhibitors has helped greatly in prolonging survival for women with advanced cancer. Compared to tamoxifen, aromatase inhibitors are less likely to cause blood clots and uterine cancer. However, these drugs are more likely to cause osteoporosis, which can lead to bone loss and fractures. In general, recent studies indicate that aromatase inhibitors are better than tamoxifen in improving survival and reducing the risk of cancer recurrence. Unfortunately, like tamoxifen, they can cause hot flashes, as well as joint pain.

Ovarian Ablation

Ovarian ablation literally shuts down estrogen production from the ovaries. Medications can accomplish ovarian ablation. Destroying the ovaries with surgery or radiation can also shut down estrogen production. (Osteoporosis is one serious side effect of this approach, but several therapies are available to help prevent bone loss.)

Chemical Ovarian Ablation. Drug treatment (non-chemotherapy drugs) to block ovarian production of estrogen is called chemical ovarian ablation. It is often reversible. The primary drugs used are luteinizing hormone-releasing hormone (LHRH) agonists, such as goserelin (Zoladex). (They are also sometimes called GnRH agonists). These drugs block the release of the reproductive hormones LH-RH, therefore stopping ovulation and estrogen production.

Bilateral Oophorectomy. Bilateral Oophorectomy, the surgical removal of both ovaries, may modestly improve breast cancer survival rates in some premenopausal women whose tumors are hormone receptor-positive. In these women, combining this procedure with tamoxifen may improve results beyond those of standard chemotherapies. Oophorectomy does not benefit women after menopause, and its advantages can be blunted in women who have received adjuvant chemotherapy. The procedure causes sterility and can have a major negative emotional impact on younger patients.

2.4. Drug Profile of Docetaxel

Docetaxel

Docetaxel is a clinically well established anti-neoplastic medication used mainly for the treatment of breast, ovarian and non-small cell lung cancer. Docetaxel has an approved claim for treatment of patients, who have locally advanced, or metastatic breast or non small-cell lung cancer that have undergone anthracycline-based chemotherapy and failed to stop cancer progression or relapsed. Administered as a one-hour infusion every three weeks generally over a ten cycle course, docetaxel is considered better than doxorubicin, paclitaxel and flurouracil as a cytotoxic antimicrotubule agent. Docetaxel is marketed under the name Taxotere® (docetaxel) Injection Concentrate by Sanofi-Aventis U.S. LLC.

Chemical formula: $C_{43}H_{53}NO_{14}$

Molecular weight: 807.879 g/mol

Chemical structure:

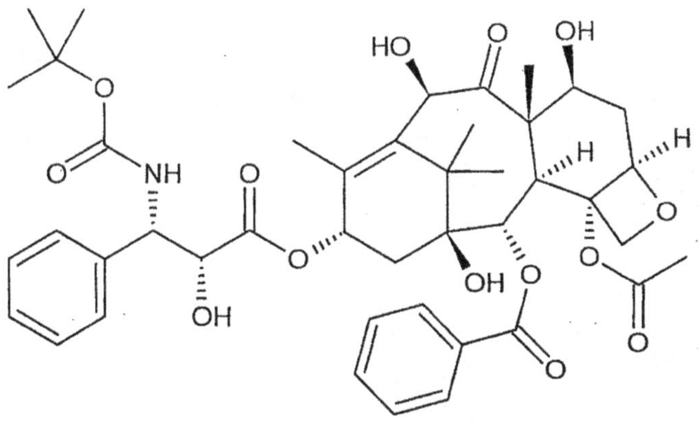

Systematic (IUPAC) name:

(2*R*,3*S*)-*N*-carboxy-3-phenylisoserine, *N*-tert-butyl ester, 13-ester with 5, 20-epoxy-1, 2, 4, 7, 10, 13-hexahydroxytax-11-en-9-one 4-acetate 2-benzoate, trihydrate

Chemical Structure, Nature and Composition Nature

Docetaxel is of the chemotherapy drug class; taxane, and is a semi-synthetic analogue of paclitaxel (Taxol), an extract from the rare Western yew tree Taxus brevifolia. Due to scarcity of paclitaxel, extensive research was carried out leading to the formulation of docetaxel - an esterified product of 10-deacetyl baccatin III, which is extracted from the renewable and readily available European yew tree.

Docetaxel differs from paclitaxel at two positions in its chemical structure. It has a hydroxyl functional group on carbon 10, whereas paclitaxel has an acetate ester and a tert-butyl substitution exists on the phenyl propionate side chain. The carbon 10 functional group change causes docetaxel to be more lipid soluble than paclitaxel.

Active regions

A model based on electron crystallographic density and nuclear magnetic resonance deconvolution has been proposed to explain the binding of docetaxel to β-tubulin. In this T-shaped/butterfly model, a deep hydrophobic cleft exists near the surface of the β-tubulin where three potential hydrogen bonds and multiple hydrophobic contacts bind to docetaxel. The hydrophobic pocket walls contain helices H1, H6, H7 and a loop between H6 and H7 that form hydrophobic interactions with the 3'-benzamido phenyl, 3'-phenyl, and the 2-benzoyl phenyl of docetaxel. 3'-phenyl also has contact with β-sheets B8 and B10. The C-8 methyl of docetaxel has van der Waals interactions with two residues, Thr-276 and Gln-281 near the C-terminal end of β-tubulin. Docetaxel's O-21 experiences electrostatic attraction to Thr-276 and the C-12 methyl has proximity with Leu-371 on the loop between B9 and B10.

Mechanism of action

Molecular target

Docetaxel binds to microtubules reversibly with high affinity and has a maximum stoichiometry of 1 mole docetaxel per mole tubulin in microtubules. This binding stabilises microtubules and prevents depolymerisation from calcium ions, decreased temperature and dilution, preferentially at the plus end of the microtubule. Docetaxel has been found to accumulate to higher concentration in ovarian adenocarcinoma cells than kidney carcinoma cells, which may contribute to the more effective treatment of ovarian cancer by docetaxel. It has also been found to phosphorylate oncoprotein bcl-2, which is apoptosis blocking in its oncoprotein form.

Modes of action

The cytotoxic activity of docetaxel is exerted by promoting and stabilising microtubule assembly, while preventing physiological microtubule depolymerisation/disassembly in the absence of GTP. This leads to a significant decrease in free tubulin, needed for microtubule formation and results in inhibition of mitotic cell division between metaphase and anaphase, preventing further cancer cell progeny.

Because microtubules do not disassemble in the presence of docetaxel, they accumulate inside the cell and cause initiation of apoptosis. Apoptosis is also encouraged by the blocking of apoptosis-blocking bcl-2 oncoprotein. Both in vitro and in vivo analysis show the anti-neoplastic activity of docetaxel to; be effective against a wide range of known cancer cells, cooperate with other anti-neoplastic agents activity, and have greater cytotoxicity than paclitaxel, possibly due to its more rapid intracellular uptake.

The main mode of therapeutic action of docetaxel is the suppression of microtubule dynamic assembly and disassembly, rather than microtubule bundling leading to apoptosis, or the blocking of bcl-2.

Cellular responses

Docetaxel exhibits cytotoxic activity on breast, colorectal, lung, ovarian, gastric, renal and prostate cancer cells. Docetaxel does not block disassembly of interphase microtubules and so does not prevent entry into the mitotic cycle, but does block mitosis by inhibiting mitotic spindle assembly. Resistance to paclitaxel or anthracycline doxorubicin does not necessarily indicate resistance to docetaxel. Microtubules formed in the presence of docetaxel are of a larger size than those formed in the presence of paclitaxel, which may result in improved cytotoxic efficacy. Abundant formation of microtubules and the prevention to replicate caused by the presence of docetaxel leads to apoptosis of tumor cells and is the basis of docetaxel use as a cancer treatment. It is unknown if pathophysiological interactions with docetaxel exist at this stage, however tumor type has been shown to have efficacy on cellular activity. Docetaxel activity is significantly greater in ovarian and breast tumors than for lung tumors.

Pharmacokinetics

Absorption and distribution

Intravenous administration of docetaxel results in 100% bioavailability and absorption is immediate. Oral bioavailability has been found to be 8% ± 6% on its own and when co-administered with cyclosporine, bioavailability increased to 90% ± 44%. In practice, docetaxel is administered intravenously only to increase dose precession. Evaluation of docetaxel pharmacokinetics in phase II and III clinical studies were with 100 mg/m2 dosages given over one-hour infusions every three weeks. The main plasma proteins docetaxel binds are lipoproteins, alpha1 acid glycoprotein and albumin. Alpha1 acid glycoprotein is the most variable of these proteins inter-individually, especially in cancer patients and so is the main determinant docetaxel plasma binding variability. Docetaxel interacted little with erythrocytes and was unaffected by the polysorbate 80 in its storage medium.

The concentration-time profile of docetaxel was consistent with a three compartment pharmacokinetic model. An initial, relatively rapid decline, with an α half-life of mean 4.5 minutes is representative of distribution to peripheral compartments from the systemic circulation. A β half-life of mean 38.3 minutes and a relatively slow γ half-life of mean 12.2 hours represent the slow efflux of docetaxel from the peripheral compartment.

Administration a 100 mg/m2 dose over a one hour infusion gave a mean total body clearance of 21 L/h/m2 and a mean steady state volume of distribution of 73.8 L/m2 or 123 L based on the mean BSA (body surface area) of 1.68 m2. Area under the plasma concentration-time curve had a mean value of 2.8 mg.h/L. The Cmax of docetaxel was found to be 4.15 ±1.35 mg/L. Increased dose resulted in a linear increase of the area under the concentration-time curve and so it is concluded that dose is directly proportional to plasma concentration.

Metabolism and excretion

Docetaxel is mainly metabolised in the liver by the cytochrome P450 CYP3A4 and CYP3A5 subfamilies of isoenzymes. Metabolism is principally oxidative and at the tert-butylpropionate side chain, resulting first in an alcohol docetaxel (M2), which is then cyclised to three further metabolites (M1, M3 and M4). M1 and M3 are two diasteromeric hydroxyoxazolidinones and M4 is an oxazolidinedione. Phase II trials of 577 patients showed docetaxel clearance to be related to body surface area and; hepatic enzyme and alpha1 acid glycoprotein, plasma levels. The following model is agreed to represent docetaxel clearance in humans:

$$\mathbf{CL = BSA\,(22.1 - 3.55AAG - 0.095AGE + 0.2245ALB)\,.\,(1 - 0.334HEP12)}$$

Where CL is total body clearance (L/h), AAG and ALB represent alpha1 acid glycoprotein and albumin plasma concentrations (g/L) respectively, BSA is total body surface area (m2) and AGE is the patients age (years). HEP12 represents a measure of hepatic dysfunction, affecting clearance of docetaxel. This final model accounted for a modest proportion of patients and identified most of the patients varying from the model (population median of CL = 35.6 L/h) as having hepatic dysfunction, indicating hepatic function as the most unpredictable factor with regards to clearance variability.

Patients with significant hepatic dysfunction had an approximately 30% decrease in clearance of docetaxel and were also at a higher risk of toxicity poisoning from docetaxel treatment. Clearance has been shown from population pharmacokinetic studies to decrease significantly with age, increased alpha1 acid glycoprotein and albumin concentrations and decreased body surface area.

Renal impairment is unlikely to affect metabolism or excretion of docetaxel as renal excretion contributes less than 5% of elimination. Limited data is available for docetaxel use in children with dosage between 55 and 75 mg/m2. Two pediatric studies have taken place that shows a mean clearance of 33 L/h/m2 and concentration-time profiles best fitted by a two-compartmental model of distribution and elimination. Mean distribution half-life was 0.09 hours and mean elimination half-life was 1.4 hours in pediatric studies.

Biodistribution of 14C-labelled docetaxel in three patients showed the bulk of the drug to be metabolized and excreted in bile to the faces. Of the radioactively labeled docetaxel administered, 80% was eliminated to the faces with 5% in the urine over seven days, an indication that urinary excretion of docetaxel is minimal. Saliva contributed minimal excretion and no excretion was detected through pulmonary means. The terminal half-life of docetaxel was determined as approximately 86 hours, through prolonged plasma sampling, contrary to the clinically stated terminal half-life of 10-18 hours.

Therapeutic Applications and Effects

Therapeutic applications

The main use of docetaxel is the treatment of a variety of cancers after the failure of anthracycline-based chemotherapy. Marketing of docetaxel as Taxotere® is mainly towards the treatment of breast, prostate and other non-small cell cancers. Clinical data has shown docetaxel to have cytotoxic activity against breast, colorectal, lung, ovarian, prostate, liver, renal and gastric cancer and melanoma cells. In the treatment of breast cancer, eight phase II studies were carried out in patients with either locally advanced or metastatic breast cancer. Taxotere® was administered over a one-hour infusion every three weeks for these trials. The 75 mg/m2 cohort showed an overall response rate of 47% and 9% complete responses. Duration of response and the time to progression (treatment failure) had median values of 34 weeks and 22 weeks, respectively. Patients with two or fewer organs involved had a response rate of 58.6%, whereas patients with three or more organs involved showed 29.4% response.

Previously untreated patients in the 100 mg/m2 cohort had an overall response rate of 56% and 9.4% complete responses. The previously treated population had an overall response of 48.6% and 3.6% complete responses. Median duration of response and time to progression was 30 weeks and 21 weeks for the previously untreated population and 28 weeks and 19 weeks for the previously treated patients. The 100 mg/m2 cohort showed higher toxicity. Previously untreated patients with three or more organs involved had a 54.3% response rate and previously treated patients had a 55.8% response rate.

Two randomized phase III studies of 326 alkylating agent failure and 392 anthracycline failure metastatic breast cancer patients have been carried out with 100 mg/m2 dosages administered over a one-hour infusion every three weeks for seven and ten cycles respectively. While no significant differences in median time to progression or survival were observed between docetaxel and doxorubicin in alkylating agent failure patients, anthracycline failure patients showed increased response rate to docetaxel. Median time to progression and median overall survival were also improved with docetaxel.

The following table is the results of a comparative, open-label, randomized phase III study of docetaxel and paclitaxel assigned randomly to 449 patients with advanced breast cancer. Docetaxel was administered as a one-hour infusion of 100 mg/m2 Taxotere® every three weeks and paclitaxel as a three-hour infusion of 175 mg/m2 paclitaxel every three weeks.

Clinical studies have taken place for the treatment of non-small cell lung cancer and prostate cancer. Patients treated for non-small cell lung cancer in phase II studies with 100 mg/m2 docetaxel showed an overall response rate of 26.9% for previously untreated patients (n=160) and 17% for previously treated patients (n=88). Median survival time for previously untreated patients was nine months and for previously treated patients, eight months.

The TAX 327 trial was a phase III study that showed significant survival benefit from docetaxel in androgen-independent metastatic prostate cancer. Compared with mitoxantrone treatment, docetaxel treated patients showed a 12% overall response rate and mitoxantrone showed a 7% overall response rate. Another large advantage of docetaxel was increased quality of life. Docetaxel showed a 22% response and mitoxantrone had a 13% response. Used in conjunction with prednisone for pain management, docetaxel had a 35% response and Mitoxantrone had a 22% response. This trial leads docetaxel to be a preferred method of treatment to Mitoxantrone where possible.

Specific outcomes and benefits of treatment

Treatment with docetaxel has the specific outcome of increasing survival time in patients with certain types of cancer. While some clinical trials show median survival times to be increased by approximately only three months, the range of survival time is large. Many patients survive beyond five years with treatment from docetaxel, however it is difficult to attribute these findings directly to treatment with docetaxel. Improved median survival time and response indicates that docetaxel slows metastatic cancer progression and can lead to disease-free survival. Conjunctive treatment of prednisone with docetaxel has been shown to lead to improved survival rate as well as improved quality of life and reduction of pain compared with treatments with mitoxantrone. Docetaxel has been shown to improve survival as an adjuvant therapy with doxorubicin and cyclophosphamide for the treatment of node-positive breast cancer and so docetaxel has the benefit of aiding other treatments.

Monitoring and combination of with other drugs

Docetaxel is administered via a one-hour infusion every three weeks over ten or more cycles. Treatment is given under supervision from an oncologist and takes place in a hospital, where vital signs are monitored during infusion. Strict monitoring of blood cell counts, liver function, serum electrolytes, serum creatinine, heart function and fluid retention is required to track the progression of tumor cells, response, adverse reactions and toxicity so that treatment can be modified or terminated if necessary.

Premedication with corticosteroids is recommended before each administration of docetaxel to reduce fluid retention and hypersensitive reactions. Oral dexamethasone is given before docetaxel treatment for prostate cancer. Docetaxel is typically used for the treatment of carcinoma on its own. Other medications will often be given to aid pain management and other symptoms. The treatment of breast cancer with doxorubicin and cyclophosphamide is enhanced by adjuvant treatment with docetaxel. Docetaxel is also used in combination with capecitabine, a DNA synthesis inhibitor.

Side-effects/contraindications/drug interactions

Positive side-effects

As well as inhibiting mitosis, docetaxel has been found to phosphorylate the oncoprotein bcl-2, which leads to apoptosis of cancer cells that had previously blocked the apoptotic inducing mechanism, leading to tumor regression. Enhanced effects of radiation therapy when combined with docetaxel have been observed in mice. Docetaxel has also been found to have greater cellular uptake and is retained longer intracellularly than paclitaxel allowing docetaxel treatment to be effective with a smaller dose, leading to fewer and less severe adverse effects.

Adverse effects

Docetaxel is a chemotherapeutic agent and is a cytotoxic compound and so is effectively a biologically damaging drug. As with all chemotherapy, adverse effects are common and many varying side-effects have been documented. Because docetaxel is a cell cycle specific agent, it is cytotoxic to all dividing cells in the body. This includes tumor cells as well as hair follicles, bone marrow and other germ cells. For this reason, common chemotherapy side effects such as alopecia occur. Incidence of commonly experienced non-haematological adverse effects reported for treatment with docetaxel. Data from 40 phase II and phase III studies (n=2045) with patients undergoing a one-hour infusion of 100 mg/m2 docetaxel once every three weeks.

Enlarge

Incidence of commonly experienced non-haematological adverse effects reported for treatment with docetaxel. Data from 40 phase II and phase III studies (n=2045) with patients undergoing a one-hour infusion of 100 mg/m2 docetaxel once every three weeks. Haematological adverse effects include Neutropaenia (95.5%), Anaemia (90.4%), Febrile neutropaenia (11.0%) and Thrombocytopaenia (8.0%). Deaths due to toxicity accounted for 1.7% of the 2045 patients and incidence was increased (9.8%) in patients with elevated baseline liver function tests (liver dysfunction). Observations of severe side effects in the above 40 phase II and phase III studies were also recorded. Incidence of severe adverse effects reported in patients treated with docetaxel. Data from 40 phase II and phase III studies with patients undergoing a one-hour infusion of 100 mg/m2 docetaxel once every three weeks.

Enlarge

Incidence of severe adverse effects reported in patients treated with docetaxel. Data from 40 phase II and phase III studies with patients undergoing a one-hour infusion of 100 mg/m2 docetaxel once every three weeks. Many more side effects have been reported for conjunctive and adjuvant treatment with docetaxel as well as rare post-marketing events.

Dosage

Adults: I.V. infusion: Refer to individual protocols:

Note: Premedicate with corticosteroids, beginning the day before docetaxel administration, (administer for 1-5 days) to reduce the severity of hypersensitivity reactions and pulmonary/peripheral edema.

Breast cancer: Locally-advanced or metastatic: 60-100 mg/m^2 every 3 weeks; patients initially started at 60 mg/m^2 who do not develop toxicity may tolerate higher doses. Operable, node-positive (adjuvant treatment): 75 mg/m^2 every 3 weeks for 6 courses (in combination with doxorubicin and cyclophosphamide)

Nonsmall cell lung cancer: 75 mg/m^2 every 3 weeks (as monotherapy or in combination with cisplatin).

Prostate cancer: 75 mg/m^2 every 3 weeks (in combination with prednisone)

Gastric adenocarcinoma: 75 mg/m^2 every 3 weeks (in combination with cisplatin and fluorouracil)

Head and neck cancer: 75 mg/m^2 every 3 weeks (in combination with cisplatin and fluorouracil) for 3 or 4 cycles, followed by radiation therapy

Dosing adjustment for toxicity:

Note: Toxicity includes febrile neutropenia, neutrophils? 500/mm^3 for >1 week, severe or cumulative cutaneous reactions; in nonsmall cell lung cancer, this may also include platelets <25,000/mm^3 and other grade 3/4 nonhematologic toxicities.

Breast cancer: Patients dosed initially at 100 mg/m^2; reduce dose to 75 mg/m^2; **Note:** If the patient continues to experience these adverse reactions, the dosage should be reduced to 55 mg/m^2 or therapy should be discontinued; discontinue for peripheral neuropathy ? Grade 3.

Breast cancer, adjuvant treatment: TAC regimen should be administered when neutrophils are? 1500 cells/mm^3. Patients experiencing febrile neutropenia should receive G-CSF in all subsequent cycles. Patients with persistent febrile neutropenia (while on G-CSF) or patients experiencing severe/cumulative cutaneous reactions or moderate neurosensory effects (signs/symptoms) should receive a reduced dose (60 mg/m^2) of docetaxel. Patients who experience grade 3 or 4 stomatitis should also receive a reduced dose (60 mg/m^2) of docetaxel. Discontinue therapy with persistent toxicities after dosage reduction.

Nonsmall cell lung cancer: Monotherapy: Patients dosed initially at 75 mg/m^2 should have dose held until toxicity is resolved, then resume at 55 mg/m^2; discontinue for peripheral neuropathy ? grade 3.

Combination therapy (with cisplatin): Patients dosed initially at 75 mg/m^2 should have the docetaxel dosage reduced to 65 mg/m^2 in subsequent cycles; if further adjustment is required, dosage may be reduced to 50 mg/m^2

Prostate cancer: Reduce dose to 60 mg/m^2; discontinue therapy if toxicities persist at lower dose.

Gastric cancer, head and neck cancer: **Note:** Cisplatin may require dose reductions/therapy delays for peripheral neuropathy, ototoxicity, and/or nephrotoxicity. Patients experiencing febrile neutropenia, documented infection with neutropenia or neutropenia >7 days should receive G-CSF in all subsequent cycles. For neutropenic complications despite G-CSF use, further reduce dose to 60 mg/m^2. Neutropenic complications in subsequent cycles should be further dose reduced to 45 mg/m^2. Patients who experience grade 4 thrombocytopenia should receive a dose reduction from 75 mg/m^2 to 60 mg/m^2. Discontinue therapy for persistent toxicities.

Gastrointestinal toxicity for docetaxel in combination with cisplatin and fluorouracil for treatment of gastric cancer or head and neck cancer:

Drug interaction

Drug interactions may be the result of altered pharmacokinetics or pharmacodynamics due to one of the drugs involved. Cisplatin, dexamethasone, doxorubicin, etoposide and vinblastine are all potentially co-administered with docetaxel and did not modify docetaxel plasma binding in phase II studies Cisplatin is known to have a complex interaction with some CYPs and has in some events been shown to reduce docetaxel clearance by up to 25%. Anticonvulsants induce some metabolic pathways relevant to docetaxel. CYP450 and CYP3A show increased expression in response to the use of anticonvulsants and the metabolism of docetaxel metabolite M4 is processed by these CYPs. A corresponding increase in clearance of M4 by 25% is observed in patients taking phenytoin and phenobarbital, common anticonvulsants.

Common and/or likely drug-drug combinations and known side effects from drug interactions	
Drug Interacting with Docetaxel	**Adverse Effects from Interaction**
Cisplatin	Increased risk of delayed neuropathy
Cyclosporine, Dalfopristin, Erythromycin, Itraconazole, Ketoconazole, Quinupristin, Terfenadine, Troleandomycin	Increased risk of docetaxel toxicity including some or all of; anaemia, leucopoenia, thrombocytopenia, fever, diarrhoea
Doxorubicin Hydrochloride	Cholestatic jaundice and pseudomembranous colitis
Doxorubicin Hydrochloride Liposome	Increased doxorubicin exposure

Vaccinations for; Bacillus of Calmette and Guerin, Measles, Mumps, Poliovirus, Rotavirus, Rubella, Smallpox, Typhoid, Varicella, Yellow Fever	Increased risk of infection by live vaccine
Thalidomide	Increased risk of venous thromboembolism

Erythromycin, ketoconazole and cyclosporine are CYP3A4 inhibitors and therefore inhibit the metabolic pathway of docetaxel. When used with anticonvulsants, which induce CYP3A4, an increased dose of docetaxel may be required. Pre-treatment with corticosteroids has been used to decrease hypersensitivity reactions and oedema in response to docetaxel and has shown no effect on the pharmacokinetics of docetaxel. The efficacy of docetaxel was improved by treatment with oral capecitabine and after more than 27 months follow-up, the survival benefit has been confirmed. Doxorubicin was combined with docetaxel in one study of 24 patients and resulted in an increased AUC of docetaxel by 50 to 70%, indicating doxorubicin may affect the disposition of docetaxel. Etoposide has also been shown to decrease docetaxel clearance; thought patient numbers for this observation have been low.

Prednisone given with docetaxel led to improved survival, quality of life and pain management in patients with hormone-refractory prostate cancer.

2.5. References

Abdus Samad, Y. et al, 2007, Liposomal Drug Delivery Systems: An Update Review, Current Drug Delivery, **297 (4)**, 297-305.

Alexis, F. et al, 2005, Factors affecting the degradation and drug-release mechanism of poly(lactide acid and poly(lactic acid-co-glycolic acid). Polymer, International, **54**, 36-46.

Amitava Mitraa et al, 2005, Targeting tumor angiogenic vasculature using polymer–RGD Conjugates, Journal of Controlled Release, **102**, 191–201 and microencapsulation for sustained release, Nanomedicine: Nanotech. Biology Medicine, **1**, 85-90.

Andronati, S.A. et al, Peptidomimetics–antagonists of the fibrinogen receptors: molecular design, structures, properties and therapeutic applications, Curr. Med. Chem., **11**, 1183–1211.

Arwyn, T. Jones et al, 23 -24 June 2001, Intracellular Drug Delivery. Workshop Report from the 28th International Symposium on Controlled Release of Bioactive Materials, San Diego, **2**, 917-920.

Assa-Munt, N. et al, 2001, Solution structures and integrin binding activities of an RGD peptide with two isomers, Biochemistry, **40**, 2373–2378.

Bae, Y. et al, 2005, Preparation and characterization of polymeric miceller drug carriers with intracellular pH-trigerred drug release property: tumor permeability, controlled subcellular distribution, and enhanced in-vivo antitumor efficacy, Bioconjug. Chem., **16,** 122-130.

Baldwin, S.P. et al, 1998, Materials for protein delivery in tissue engineering, Advanced Drug Delivery Reviews, **33**, 71-86.

Bangham, A.D. et al, 1965, J. Mol. Biol., **13**, 238.

Berg, W.A. et al, 2008, Combined screening with ultrasound and mammography vs mammography alone in women at elevated risk of breast cancer, JAMA, **14;299(18),** 2151-63.

Besselink, G.A.J. et al, Affinity-binding of cells to sephadex derivatized with peptides and proteins, in Frontiers in biomedical polymer applications, Technomic: Lancaster, 201-213.

Bhalerao, S.S. et al, 2003, Drug. Dev. Ind. Pharm., **29**, 451.

Bio-Alliance Pharma, 2006, Products & Technology - Drug Delivery Technologies - Transdrug®.
[cited 22th November 2007], http://www.bioalliancepharma.com/products_transdrug.asp.

Blancher C. et al, 1996, Nectinepsin: a new extracellular matrix protein of the pexin family. Characterization of a novel cDNA encoding a protein with an RGD cell binding motif, J. Biol. Chem., **271**, 26220–26226.

Bleich, J. et al, 1993, "Aerosol Solvent Extraction System-A New Microparticle Production Technique", International Journal of Pharmaceutics, **97(1-3),** 111-117.

Bogdanowich-Knipp et al, 1999, Solution stability of linear vs. cyclic RGD peptides, J. Pept. Res., **53**, 530–541.

Boturyn, D. et al, 2004, Template assembled cyclopeptides as multimeric system for integrin targeting and endocytosis, J. Am. Chem. Soc., **126**, 5730–5739.

Boyd, N.F. et al, 2007, Mammographic density and the risk and detection of breast cancer, N. Engl. J. Med. **18; 356(3),** 227-236.

Bristow, S.T. et al, 2001, Analysis of the Supersaturation and Precipitation Process with Supercritical CO2. Journal of Supercritical Fluids, **21**, 257-271.

Brittain, H.G. et al, 1991, Physical characterization of pharmaceutical solids, Pharm. Res. **8**, 963-973.

Canto, G.S. et al, 1999, Drug Dev. Ind. Pharm., **25(12)**, 1253.

Calvo, P. et al, 1997, Chitosan and chitosan/ethylene oxide-propylene oxide block copolymer nanoparticles as novel carriers for proteins and vaccines, Pharm. Res., **14(10)**, 1431-6.

Casey, P.M. et al, 2008, Oral contraceptive use and risk of breast cancer, Mayo Clin Proc., **83(1)**, 86-90.

Castor, T.P. et al, 1998, Methods and apparatus for making liposomes containing hydrophobic drugs. U.S. Patent 5,776,486.

Chattopadhyay, P. et al, 2001, "Production of Antiobiotic Nanoparticles Using Supercritical CO2 as Antisolvent with Enhanced Mass Transfer". Industrial and Engineering Chemistry Research, **40**, 3530-3539.

Chen, C.M. et al, 1987, J. Pharm. Sci., **76(5)**, 419.

Chernyak, Y. et al, 2001, "Formation of Perfluoropolyether Coatings by the Rapid Expansion of Supercritical Solutions (RESS) Process. Part 1: Experimental Results", Industrial & Engineering Chemistry Research, 40(26), 6118-6126.

Chia, S.K. et al, 2007, The impact of new chemotherapeutic and hormone agents on survival in a population-based cohort of women with metastatic breast cancer, Cancer, **23; 110(5)**, 973-979.

Chinn, J.A. et al, 1998, Blood and tissue compatibility of modified polyester: Thrombosis, inflammation, and healing, J. Biomed. Mater. Res., **39**, 130-140.

Cohen, H. et al, 2000, Sustained delivery and expression of DNA encapsulated in polymeric nanoparticles. Gene. Ther., **7**, 1896-1905.

Coombes, R.C. et al, 2007, Survival and safety of exemestane versus tamoxifen after 2-3 years' tamoxifen treatment (Intergroup Exemestane Study): a randomised controlled trial, Lancet, **17; 369** , 559-70.

Corveleyn S. et al, 1996, Maltodextrins as lyoprotectnats in the lyophilization of a model protein, LDH. Pharm. Res., **13**, 146-150.

Couvreur, P. et al, 1980, Tissue distribution of antitumor drugs associated with polyalkylcyanoacrylate nanoparticles, J. Pharm. Sci., **69**, 199-202.

Couvreur, P. et al, 2006, Nanotechnology: intelligent design to treat complex disease, Pharm. Res., **23**, 1417-1450.

Craig W. S. et al, 1995, Concept and progress in the development of RGD-containing peptide pharmaceuticals, Biopolymers, **37**, 157–175.

Daryl, C. et al, 1999, Optimizing Liposomes For Delivery of Chemotherapeutic Agents to Solid Tumors, Pharmacological Reviews, **51**(4), 691-732.

De Jaeghere, F. et al, 1999, In the Encyclopedia of control drug delivery. (E. Mathiowitz ed.) John Wiley & Sons, Inc. New York, **2**, 641- 664.

Debenedetti, P.G. et al, 1993, Rapid Expansion of Supercritical Solutions (RESS): Fundamentals and Applications". Fluid Phase Equilibria, **82**, 311-321.

Dechantsreiter, M. A. et al, 1999, N-Methylated cyclic RGD peptides as highly active and selective $\alpha_v\beta_3$ integrin antagonists, J. Med. Chem., **42**, 3033–3040.

Decher, G. et al, 1997, Fuzzy nanoassemblies: toward layered polymeric multicomposites, Science, **277**, 1232-1237.

Diminsky D et al, 1999, Physical, chemical and immunological stability of CHO-derived hepatitis B surface antigen (HBs Ag) particles, Vaccine,**18**, 3-17.

Dubernet, C. et al, 1995, Thermoanalysis of microspheres, Thermochim Acta, **248**, 259-269.

Duncan, R. et al, 1986, Fate of N-(2-hydroxypropyl) methacrylamide copolymers with pendant galactosamine residues after intravenous administration to rats, Biochim. Biophys. Acta, **880**, 62–71.

Dunne, M et al, 2000, Infulence of particle size and dissolution conditions on the degradation properties of PLGA particles, Biomaterials, **21**, 1659-1668.

Duong L. T. et al, 2000, Integrins and signaling in osteoclast function, Matrix Biol., **19**, 97–105.

Elvassore, N. A. et al, 2001, " Production of Insulin-Loaded Poly(ethylene glycol)/Poly(l-lactide) (PEG/PLA) Nanoparticles by Gas Antisolvent Techniques". Journal of Pharmaceutical Sciences, **90(10),** 1628-1636.

Ferguson, T. et al, 2007, Taxanes for adjuvant treatment of early breast cancer, Cochrane Database Syst Rev., **4,** CD004421.

Florence, A.T. et al, 1997, The oral absorption of micro- and nanoparticulates: neither exceptional nor unusual, Pharm. Res., **14,** 259-266.

Frederiksen, L. et al, 1997, Preparation of liposomes encapsulating water-soluble compounds using supercritical carbon dioxide, J. Pharm. Sci., **86(8)**,921–928.

Fukumori, Y. et al, 2006, Nanoparticles for cancer therapy and diagnosis, Adv. Powder. Technol., **17,** 1-28.

Fusaro, F. et al, 2005, "Dense Gas Antisolvent Precipitation: A Comparative Investigation of the GAS and PCA Techniques", Industrial & Engineering Chemistry Research, **44,** 1502-1509.

Galindo-Rodriguez, S.A. et al, 2005, Comparative scale-up of three methods for producing ibuprofen-loaded nanoparticles, Eur. J. Pharm. Sci., **25,** 357-367.

Garcia-Garcia, E. et al, 2005, Colloidal carriers and blood-brain barrier (BBB) translocation: a way to deliver drugs to the brain, Int. J. Pharm. **298,** 274-292.

Geiger, A.M. et al, 2007, Recurrences and second primary breast cancers in older women with initial early-stage disease, Cancer, **1; 109(5),** 966-974.

Geiger, T. et al, 1987, Deamidation, isomerization, and racemization at asparaginyl and aspartyl residues in peptides. Succinimide-linked reactions that contribute to protein degradation, J. Biol. Chem., **262,** 785–794.

Ghaderi, R.P. et al, 2000, "A New Method for PreparingBiodegradable Microparticles and Entrapment of Hydrocortisone in DL-PLG Microparticles Using Supercritical Fluids". European Journal of Pharmaceutical Sciences, **10,** 1-9.

Ghosh, S. et al, 2004, Recent research and development in synthetic polymer-based drug delivery systems. Journal of Chemical Reaserach, 241-246.

Gianasi, E. et al, 2002, HPMA copolymers platinates containing dicarboxylato ligands. Preparation, characterisation and in vitro and in vivo evaluation, J. Drug Targeting, **10,** 549–556.

Goldman M. J. et al, 1995, Expression of $\alpha_v\beta_5$ integrin is necessary for efficient adenovirus-mediated gene transfer in the human airway, J. Virol., **69,** 5951–5958.

Goodman, S.L. et al, 2002, Nanomolar small molecule inhibitors for $\alpha_v\beta_6$, $\alpha_v\beta_5$, and $\alpha_v\beta_3$ integrins, J. Med. Chem., **45,** 1045–1051.

Grislain, L. et al, 1983, Pharmacokinetics and distribution of a biodegradable drug-carrier, Int. J. Pharm., **15**, 335- 345.

Gurrath, M. et al, 1992, Conformation/activity studies of rationally designed potent anti-adhesive RGD peptides, Eur. J. Biochem., **210**, 911–921.

Hanna, M. et al, 1994, "Method and Apparatus for the Formation of Particles". World Intellectual Property Organization, Patent WO95/01121.

Hans, M L. et al, 2002, Biodegradable nanoparaticles for drug delivery and targeting. Curr. Opin. Solid State Mater. Sci., **6**, 319-327.

Healy, K. E. et al, 1999, Designing biomaterials to direct biological responses, Ann. N. Y. Acad. Sci., **87**, 24–35.

Hern, D. L. et al, 1998, Incorporation of adhesion peptides into nonadhesive hydrogels useful for tissue resurfacing, J. Biomed. Mater. Res., **39**, 266–276.

Hile, D.D. et al, 2000, Active growth factory delivery from poly(D,L-lactide-co-glycolide) foams prepared in supercritical CO2, J. Control. Rel. **66(2–3)**, 177–185.

Holig, P. et al, 2004, Novel RGD lipopeptides for the targeting of liposomes to integrin-expressing endothelial and melanoma cells, Protein Eng. Des. Sel., **17**, 433–441.

Holmes, J.D. et al, 1999, "Buffering the Aqueous Phase pH in Water-in-CO2 Microemulsions". Journal of Physical Chemistry B, **103**, 5703-5711.

Hong, L. et al, 2000, "Precipitation of Microparticulate Organic Pigment Powders by a Supercritical Antisolvent Process", Industrial & Engineering Chemistry Research, **39**, 4882-4887.

Hood, J.D. et al, 2002, Tumor regression by targeted gene delivery to the neovasculature. Science, **296**, 2404–2407.

Huang, P. S. et al, 2001, Drug-targeting strategies in cancer therapy, Curr. Opin. Genet. Dev., **11**, 104–110.

Humphries M. J. et al, 1995, The LDV peptide motif: its role in integrin- ligand binding, Top. Mol. Med., **1**, 27–35.

Hwang, K.J. et al, 1987, Biochim. Biophys. Acta, **88**, 901.

Hynes, R.O. et al, Integrins: Versatility, modulation, and signaling in cell adhesion, Cell, **69**, **53**, 11-25.

Illum, L. et al, 1982, Blood clearance and organ deposition of intravenously administered colloidal particles, The effects of particle size, nature and shape. Int. J. Pharm. **12**, 135-146.

Ivanov, B. et al, 1995, Synthesis and use of a new bromoacetyl-derivatized heterotrifunctional amino acid for conjugation of cyclic RGD-containing peptides derived from human bone sialoprotein, Bioconjug. Chem., **6**, 269–277.

Jain, R. K. et al, 1998, *Nat. Med.* **4**, 655–657.

Jayanth Panyama et al, 2003, Biodegradable Nan particles for drug and gene delivery to cells and tissue, Advanced Drug Delivery Reviews, 55,329–347.

Jensen, K.D. et al, 2003, J.Control. Release, **87**, 89-105.

Jeong, J.H. et al, 2003, Novel intracellular delivery system of antisense oligonucleotide by self assembled hybrid micelles composed of DNA/PEG conjugate and cationic fusogenic peptide, Bioconjug. Chem., **14**, 473-79.

Jones, G. R. et al, 1989, Liposome A Practical Approach, New R.R.C Ed, OIRLS press: Oxford.

Jousma, H. et al, 1987, Int. J. Pharm., **35**, 263.

Kadimi, U.S. et al, 2007, In vitro studies on liposomal amphotericin B obtained by supercritical carbon dioxide–mediated process, Nanomedicine: Nanotechnology, Biology, and Medicine, **3**, 273–280.

Kai Temming et al, 2005, RGD-based strategies for selective delivery of therapeutics and imaging agents to the tumour vasculature, Drug Resistance Updates, 381–402.

Kim, B.S. et al, 1999, Engineered smooth muscle tissues: Regulating cell phenotype with the scaffold. Experimental Cell Research, **251**, 318-328.

Koivunen, E. et al, 1995, Phage libraries displaying cyclic peptides with different ring sizes: ligand specificities of the RGD-directed integrins, Bio-Technology, **13**, 265–270.

Kok, R.J. et al, 2002, Preparation and functional evaluation of RGD-modified proteins as $\alpha_v\beta_3$ integrin directed therapeutics, Bioconjug. Chem., **13**, 128–135.

Kolchens, S. et al, 1993, Chem. Phys. Lipids, **1**, 65.

Kopecek, J. et al, 2000, HPMA copolymer–anticancer drug conjugates: design, activity and mechanism of action, Eur. J. Pharm. Biopharm., **50**, 61– 81.

Kreuter, J. et al, 1994, Nanoparticles, in Encyclopedia of Pharmaceutical Technology, J. Swarbrick and J.C. Boylan, editors. Marcel Dekker Inc.: New York, **10**, 165-190.

Kumaresh S. S. et al, 2001, Review Biodegradable polymeric nanoparticles as drug delivery devices, Journal of Controlled Release, **70**, 1–20.

Kunath, K. et al. 2003, Lowmolecular-weight polyethylenimine as a non-viral vector for DNA delivery: comparison of physicochemical properties, transfection efficiency and in vivo distribution with high-molecular-weight polyethylenimine. J. Control Release, **89**, 113–25.

Lasic, D.D. et al, 1993, Liposome Biophysics to Application, Elsevier: New York.

Lene Frederiksen, X. et al, 1997, Preparation of Liposomes Encapsulating Water-Soluble Compounds Using Supercritical Carbon Dioxide, Journal of Pharmaceutical Sciences, **86 (8)**, 921-928.

Li B et al. 2000, Lyophilization of cationic lipid-protamine-DNA(LPD) complexes, J. Pharm. Sci., **89**, 355-364.

Lide. R. et al, 1994, H. P. R. Frederikse (Eds.), CRC Handbook of Chemistry and Physics, 75 editon., D. CRC Press, Inc., Boca Raton, FL.

Lin, S.Y. et al, 1989, Solid particulates of drug-β-cyclodextrin inclusion complexes directly prepared by a spray-drying technique, Int. J. Pharm., **56**, 249–259.

Lu, Z.R et al, 2002, Design of novel bioconjugates for targeted drug delivery, J. Control. Release, **78**, 165–173.

Ma, W. et al, 1993, Pharm. Res., **10(2)**, 252.

Madri, J.A. et al, 1988, Endothelial cell-extracellular matrix interactions: Matrix as a modulator of cell function, in Endothelial cell biology in health and disease, Plenum Press: New York, 167-188.

Maeda, H. et al, 2000, Tumor vascular permeability and the EPR effect in macromolecular therapeutics. A review. J. Control Release, **65**, 271-84.

Manning, M. C. et al, 1989, Stability of protein pharmaceuticals, Pharm. Res., **6**, 903–918.

Marinelli, L. et al, 2003, Docking studies on $\alpha_v\beta_3$ integrin ligands: pharmacophore refinement and implications for drug design, J. Med. Chem., **46**, 4393–4404.

McHugh, M.A. et al, 1994, Supercritical Fluid Extraction, 2nd ed., Newton, MA: Butterworth-Heinemann.

Meerum Terwogt, J. M. et al, 2001, Phase I clinical and pharmacokinetic study of PNU166945, a novel water soluble polymer-conjugated prodrug of paclitaxel, Anticancer Drugs, **12**, 315–323.

Miller, N. et al, 1995, FASEB J. **9**, 190–199.

Mitra, A. et al, 2005, Targeting tumor angiogenic vasculature using polymer- RGD conjugates, J. Controlled Release, **102**, 191–201.

Moghimi, S.M. et al, 2001, Long-circulating and target-specific nanoparticles: Theory to practice. Pharmacological Reviews, **53**, 283-318.

Mohanraj, V.J. et al, 2006, Nanoparticles – A Review, Trop. J. Pharm. Res, **5 (1)**, 561-573.

Moneghini M. et al, 2001, Processing of carbamazepine-PEG 4000 solid dispersions with supercritical carbon dioxide: preparation, characterization, and in vitro dissolution, Int. J. Pharm., **222(1)**, 129–138.

Morishita, M. et al, 2006, Is the oral route possible for peptide and protein drug delivery? Drug. Discov. Today, **11**, 905-910.

Moshashaee, S.M. et al, 2000, "Supercritical Fluid Processing of Proteins I: Lysozyme Precipitation From Organic Solution", European Journal of Pharmaceutical Sciences, **11**, 239-245.

Mudit Tyagi et al, 2001, Marco, Internalization of HIV-1 Tat Requires Cell Surface Heparan Sulfate Proteoglycans, J. Biol. Chem., **276**, 3254-3261.

Mueller, G. et al, 1992, Dynamic forcing, a method for evaluating activity and selectivity profiles of RGD (Arg-Gly-Asp) peptides, Angew. Chem. Int. Ed. Engl., **31**, 326.

Muhrer, G. et al, 2003, "Precipitation of Lysozyme Nanoparticles from Dimethyl Sulfoxide Using Carbon Dioxide as Antisolvent". Biotechnology Progress, **19(2)**, 549-556.

Nagarsenker, M.S. et al, 1997, Drug. Dev. Ind. Pharm., **23(12)**, 1159.

Nakache, E. et al, 2000, In the Handbook of nanostructured materials and nanotechnology. (E: Nalwa, H.S. ed.) Academic Press, **5**, 577-635.

Nicolaou, K. C. et al, 1998, Design, synthesis and biological evaluation of nonpeptide integrin antagonists, Bioorg. Med. Chem., **6**, 1185–1208.

Oh, I. et al. 1999, Release of adriamycin from poly([gamma]-benzyl glutamate0/poly(ethylene oxide) nanoparticles. Int. J. Pharm., **181**, 107-115.

Page-Clisson, M.E. et al, 1998, Development of ciprofloxacin-loaded nanoparticles: physicochemical study of the drug carrier, J. Control. Release, **56**, 23-32.

Panagi, Z. et al, 2001, Effect of dose on the biodistribution and pharmacokinetics of PLGAand PLGA-mPEG nanoparticle, Int. J. Pharm., **221**, 143-152.

Panyam, J. et al, 2003, Biodegradable nanoparticles for drug and gene delivery to cells and tissue, Adv. Drug. Deliv. Rev., **55**, 329-347.

Pierschbacher, M.D. et al, 1987, Influence of stereochemistry of the sequence Arg-Gly-Asp-Xaa on binding specificity in cell adhesion, J. Biol. Chem., **262**, 17294–17298.

Pinto Reis, C. et al, 2006, Nanoencapsulation Methods for preparation of drug-loaded polymeric nanoparticles, Nanomedicine, **2**, 8-21.

Pleumchitt, R. et al, 2000, Drug Dev. Ind. Pharm., **29(1)**, 31.

Plow, E.F. et al, 1986, Biochemistry of platelets, Academic: Orlando, 225-226.

Rajendran, D. et al, 1997, Drug. Dev. Ind. Pharm., **23(11)**, 1099.

Reverchon, E. et al, 2001, "Supercritical Fluids-Assisted Micronization Techniques. Low Impact Route for Particle Production", Pure and Applied Chemistry, **73(8)**, 1293-1297.

Reverchon, E. G. et al, 2000, "Process Parameters and Morphology in Amoxicillin Micro and Submicro Particles Generation by Supercritical Antisolvent Precipitation", Journal of Supercritical Fluids, **17**, 239-248.

Reverchon, E.G. et al, 1998, Supercritical Antisolvent Precipitation of Nanoparticles of Superconductor Precursors, Industrial & Engineering Chemistry Research, **37**, 952-958.

Reverchon, E.G. et al, 1999, "Biopolymer Micronization by Supercritical Antisolvent Precipitation: The Influence of Some Process Parameters". in 5th Conference on Supercritical Fluids and their Applications., Verona, Italy.

Rezania, A. et al, 1999, Biomimetic peptide surfaces that regulate adhesion, spreading, cytoskeletal organization, and mineralization of the matrix deposited by osteoblast-like cells, Biotechnol. Prog., **15**, 19-32.

Ridy, M.S.E. et al, 1997, Drug. Dev. Ind. Pharm., **23(8)**, 771.

Rihova, B. et al, 1985, Immunogenicity of N-(2-hydroxypropyl) methacrylamide copolymers, Makromol. Chem. 9 (Suppl.), 13– 24.

Rios, M. et al, 2005, Albumin-bound nanoparticle drug nabs FDA approval, Pharm. Technol. **29,** 17.

Robey P. G. et al, 1996, Vertebrate mineralized matrix proteins: structure and function, Connect. Tissue Res., **35,** 131–136.

Ruoslahti, E. et al, 1987, New perspectives in cell adhesion: RGD and integrins, Science, **238**, 491-497.

Ruoslahti, E. et al, 1991, Integrins as receptors for extracellular matrix, in Cell biology of extracellular matrix, Plenum Press: New York, 343-363.

Ruth Duncan et al, 2003, The Dawning Era of Polymer Therapeutics, Nature Reviews Drug Discovery, **2,** 347-360.

Salter, D. M. et al, 1997, Electrophysiological responses of human bone cells to mechanical stimulation: evidence for specific integrin function in mechanotransduction, J. Bone Miner. Res., **12,** 1133–1141.

Schaffner, P. et al, 2003, Structure and function of RGD peptides involved in bone biology, CMLS, Cell. Mol. Life Sci., **60**, 2003.

Schoemaker, N. E. et al, 2002, A phase I and pharmacokinetic study of MAG-CPT, a water soluble polymer conjugate of camptothecin. Brit. J. Cancer, **87**, 608–614.

Schraa, A.J. et al, 2002a, Endothelial cells internalize and degrade RGD-modified proteins developed for tumor vasculature targeting, J. Controlled Release, **83**, 241–251.

Schraa, A.J. et al, 2002b, Targeting of RGD-modified proteins to tumor vasculature: a pharmacokinetic and cellular distribution study, Int. J. Cancer, **102**, 469–475.

Schwendeman, S. et al, 1997, Peptide, protein and vaccine delivery from implantable polymeric systems: Processes and challenges, in Controlled Drug Delivery: Challenges and Strategies K. Park, Editor. American Chemical Society: Washington D.C., 229-267.

Seymour, L. W. et al, 2002, Hepatic drug targeting: Phase I evaluation of polymer-bound doxorubicin., J. Clin. Oncol., **20**, 1668–1676.

Shakesheff, K.M. et al, 1998, Creating biomimetic microenvironments with synthetic polymer-peptide hybrid molecules, in Polymers for tissue engineering, VSP: Utrecht., 113-124.

Sievers, R.E. et al, 1999, "Formation of Aqueous Small Droplet Aerosols Assisted by Supercritical Carbon Dioxide". Aerosol Science and Technology, **30**, 3-15.

Soppimath et al, 2001, Biodegradable polymeric nanoparticles as drug delivery devices, J. Control. Release, **70**, 1-20.

Storm, G. et al, Surface modification of nanoparticles to oppose uptake by the mononuclear phagocyte system, Adv. Drug. Deliv. Rev., **17**, 31-48.

Sukhorukov, G.B. et al, 1998, Layer-by-layer self assembly of polyelectrolytes on colloidal particles. Colloid. Surf. A., **137**, 253-266.

Suryanarayanan, R. et al, 1995, X-Ray Powder Diffractometry in Physical Characterization of Pharmaceutical Solids, H.G. Brittain, editor. Marcel Dekker, Inc.: New York, **10,** 187-221.

Thiering, R. F. et al, 2001, "Current Issues Relating to Anti-Solvent Micronisation Techniques and Their Extension to Industrial Scales". Journal of Supercritical Fluids, **21**, 159-177.

Thote, A.J. et al, 2005, Formation of nanoparticles of a hydrophilic drug using supercritical carbon dioxide and microemulsion for sustained release, Nanomedicine: Nanotech. Biology, **1**, 85-90.

Torchilin, V.P. et al, 2001, p-Nitrophenylcarbonyl-PEG-PE-liposomes: fast and simple attachment of specific ligands, including monoclonal antibodies, to distal ends of PEG chains via p-Nitrophenylcarbonyl carbonyl groups, Biochim Biophys Acta ,**1511**, 391-411.

Torchilin, V.P. et al, 2003, TAT-Liposomes: A Novel Intracellular Drug Carrier, Current Protein and Peptide Science, **4(2),** 133-140.

Ubrich, N. et al, 2004, Preparation and characterization of propranolol hydrochloride nanoparticles: ac omparative study, J. Control. Release, **97(2)**, 291-300.

Vasey, P. et al, 1999, Phase I clinical and pharmacokinetic study of PKI (N-(2-hydroxypropyl)methacrylamide copolymer doxorubicin): first member of a new class of chemotherapeutic agents — drug–polymer conjugates., Clin. Cancer Res., **5**, 83–94.

Vauthier-Holtzscherer, C. et al, 1991, Methodology for the preparation of ultra-dispersed polymer systems. STP Pharma Sciences, **1**, 109-116.

Virji M. et al, 1996, Adhesion receptors in microbial pathogenesis, Mol. Biol. Cell Adhesion Mol., 99–129.

Warwick, B.F. et al, 2000, "Synthesis, Purification, and Micronization of Pharmaceuticals Using the Gas Antisolvent Technique", Industrial & Engineering Chemistry Research, **39(12)**, 4571- 4579.

Winters, M.A. et al, 1996, "Precipitation of Proteins in Supercritical Carbon Dioxide". Journal of Pharmaceutical Sciences, **85(6),** 586-594.

Winters, M.A. et al, 1999, "Protein Purification with Vapor-Phase Carbon Dioxide". Biotechnology and Bioengineering, **62(3)**, 247-258.

Xiao, Y. et al, 1996, Effect of receptor-ligand affinity on the strength of endothelial cell adhesion, Biophys. J., **71**, 2869–2884.

Yeo, S.D. et al, 2000, "Crystal Formation of BaCl2 and NH4Cl Using a Supercritical Fluid Antisolvent". Journal of Supercritical Fluids, **16(3)**, 235- 246.

York, P. et al, 2004, Supercritical Fluid Technology for Drug Product Development, ed. J. Swarbrick. Vol. 138, New York, NY: Marcel Dekker, Inc.

Chapter 3
Analytical Methods

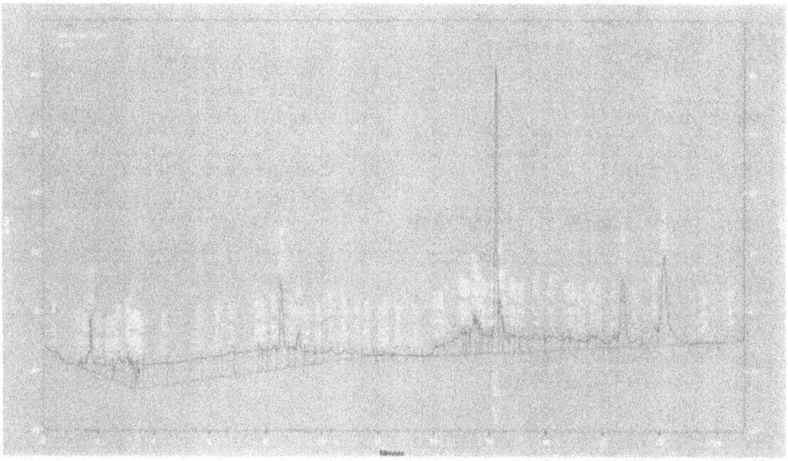

3.1 Introduction

The analytical methods employed in the optimization, preparation and characterization of unconjugated and RGD conjugated nanoparticles of docetaxel are discussed below. The nanoparticles were characterized for particle size, zeta potential, surface morphology, in-vitro drug release, DSC, FTIR, H^1NMR, residual PVA and residual dichloromethane. BT-20 and MDA-MB-231 cells were used to assess the cellular drug levels, in-vitro antiproliferative activity and cellular uptake of the NPs. The stability studies of unconjugated and conjugated NPs were conducted to determine the particle size, zeta potential, % EE, *in- vitro* drug release and the physical changes like caking and discoloration.

3.2 Materials and Equipments

Material	Source
Docetaxel (DC)	Gift samples from Dabur research ltd., Gaziabad, India.
Water (distilled)	Prepared in laboratory by distillation
PLGA (50:50)	Gift samples from gift sample from Boehringer Ingelheim, Germany
Bichinconinic acid (BCA) protein Assay Kit	Banglore Genei, India
6-Coumarin	Gift sample from Neelikon dyes, Mumbai, India
Glacial acetic acid, potassium dihydrogen phosphate, disodium hydrogen phosphate, potassium chloride, potassium hydroxide, sodium chloride, sodium hydroxide.	S.D.Fine chemicals, Mumbai, India
HPLC grade methanol, dichloromethane, acetonitrile	Loba Chemicals, India.
Nuclepore Polycarbonate membrane 2 µm 25mm	Whatman, USA
Polyvinyl alcohol(PVA)	S.D.Fine chemicals, Mumbai, India

Equipments	Source
Calibrated pipettes of 1.0 ml, 5.0 ml and 10.0 ml, volumetric flasks of 10 ml, 25 ml, 50 ml and 100 ml capacity, Funnels (i.d. 5.0 cm), beakers (250 ml) and other requisite glasswares	Schott & Corning (India) Ltd., Mumbai
Analytical balance	Precisa 205A SCS, Switzerland
pH meter	Systronics 335, India
Cyclomixer, three blade stirrer	Remi Scientific Equipments, Mumbai
Cooling Centrifuge	3K 30, Sigma Laboratory centrifuge, Osterode, GmBH.
Lyophilizer, DW1, 0-60E	Heto Drywinner, Denmark
Stability oven	Shree Kailash Industries, Vadodara
UV-Visible Spectrophotometer	Shimadzu UV-1601, Japan
Vacuum Pump F16	Bharat Vacuum pumps, Bangalore
Bath sonicator	INCO, Ambala
Malvern particle size analyser	Malvern Master sizer 2000 SM, U.K.
Scanning electron microscope	JSM-840 SEM, Jeol, Japan
Differential Scanning Calorimeter	Mettler DSC 20, Mettler Toledo, Switzerland
HPLC system	Dionex HPLC with Chromleon 6.5 data processing software

3.3 Chemical analysis

3.3.1 Estimation of Docetaxel

3.3.1.1 Estimation of DC

The drug content was determined using a Dionex HPLC system (Dionex Softron GmbH, Germany). The HPLC system was composed of a pump (P-680, Dionex), a simple 10-µl loop injector (Reodyne 7125) and a UV-visible spectrophotometric detector (UVD 170U, Dionex).The separation was carried out on a 14 cm Kromasil C 18 150-4.6 HPLC column (Merck) having particle size of 5µm. Mobile phase for DC consisted of acetonitrile and water mixture with gradient system. The run time of the assay was 30 min and the retention time of docetaxel was 16.2 min. UV detection wavelength was 227nm and mobile phase flow rate 1 ml/min.

Preparation of standard stock solutions of docetaxel in methanol

50 mg of DC was accurately weighed using single pan electronic balance and transferred to 50 ml volumetric flask. 25 ml of AR grade methanol was accurately measured and transferred to the above volumetric flask, the drug was dissolved properly and then the final volume of the flask was made up to 50 ml with AR grade methanol to produce 1000 µg per ml of DC.

10 ml of the above solution was accurately measured by graduated pipette and transferred to the 100 ml volumetric flask. The final volume was made up to 100 ml with AR grade methanol to prepare stock solution of 100 µg per ml of docetaxel.

Preparation of calibration curve of docetaxel

Suitable aliquots of standard stock solution were accurately measured and transferred to the 10 ml of volumetric flasks. The final volume was made up to 10 ml with HPLC grade methanol to give final concentrations of 0.5, 1, 2, 4, 6, 8 and 10 µg/ml and analyzed in above mentioned HPLC system. The above procedure was repeated three times. Raw data was recorded in Table: 3.1 along with standard deviation and plotted graphically in Figure: 3.1.

Table: 3.1. Calibration for Docetaxel

Concentration (µg / ml)	Mean area(mAU)* ± S.D
0	0
0.5	25336 ±21
1	40538 ±28
2	64861 ±35
6	106573 ±42
10	166045 ±31

Regression equation** Y= 25179x + 12887; Correlation coefficient = 0.9985
*Mean of 3 values

Figure: 3.1. Regressed calibration curve for estimation of Docetaxel

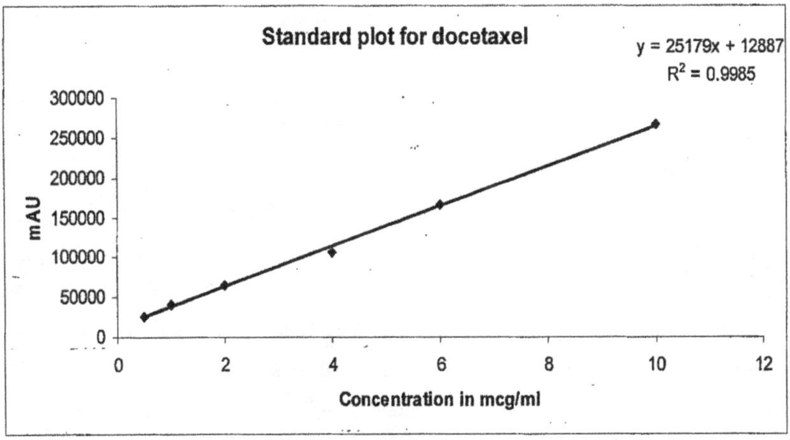

3.3.1.2 Estimation of docetaxel in NPs

To determine the amount of DC entrapped in the NPs, 2mg of NPs were added to 2 ml of acetonitrile and subjected to shaking at room temperature for 4hrs complete dissolution of PLGA. The resulting solution was diluted with mobile phase and centrifuged at 5000rpm for 15mins to remove the precipitated components. The supernatant was analyzed in above explained HPLC system.

3.3.1.3 Estimation of docetaxel for in-vitro release

The release studies for docetaxel nanoparticles in phosphate buffer saline pH 7.4 + 0.1%w/v polysorbate-80. Nanoparticles equivalent to 1mg drug were suspended in 10 ml of release medium in a screw capped tubes, which were placed in a horizontal shaker bath maintained at 37°C and shaken at 60min^{-1}. At specific time intervals following incubation samples were taken out and centrifuged at 25000rpm for 30min. The residue (settled nanoparticles) were collected and dissolved in acetonitrile and analyzed as per the method above. The amount of the drug released was calculated using the following equation:

$$\% \text{ Drug released} = 1 - \frac{\text{Amount of drug in nanoparticles settled}}{\text{Amount of drug initially taken}} \times 100$$

3.4 Estimation of residual PVA

The amount of PVA associated with nanoparticles was determined by a colorimetric method based on the formation of a colored complex between two adjacent hydroxyl groups of PVA and an iodine molecule (Joshi, D.P. et al., 1979). Briefly 10mg of PVA was dissolved in 10ml of distilled water to yield 1000 µg/ml stock solution. From the stock solution, different aliquots were taken and to each sample, 3 ml of a 0.65 M solution of boric acid, 0.5 ml of a solution of I_2/KI (0.05 M/0.15 M), and 1.5 ml of distilled water were added to yield final concentration of 10-250 µg/ml. Finally, the absorbance of the samples was measured vs. water treated in same manner at 690 nm after 15 min incubation. The above procedure was repeated three times and the mean absorbance was determined. The data was recorded in Table: 3.8 along with standard deviation. Figures: 3.7 show calibration curve of PVA in water.

Table: 3.2. Calibration Curve of PVA (λmax= 690nm)

Concentration (µg/ml)	Mean Absorbance ± SD (n=3)
5	0.035 ± 0.006
10	0.051 ± 0.005
20	0.098 ± 0.004
30	0.146 ± 0.02
40	0.195 ± 0.04
50	0.236 ± 0.05
100	0.474 ± 0.04
250	1.242 ± 0.12

Regression equation** Y= 0.0049X-0.0025; Correlation coefficient R^2= 0.9994
*Mean of 3 values

Figure: 3.2. Calibration plot for PVA

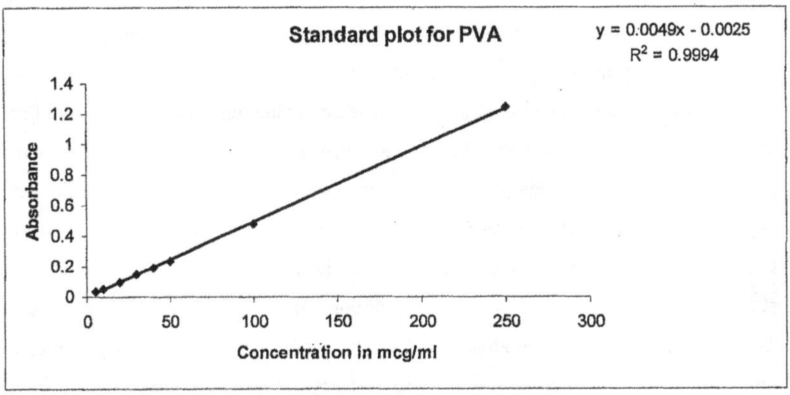

3.5 Determination of residual dichloromethane in NPs

As per USP, residual solvents are tested under General Chapter <467> "Organic Volatile Impurities." Dichloro methane (DCM)s belongs to class 2 solvents. Class 2 solvents are non-genotoxic animal carcinogens. Solvents of this class should be limited in pharmaceutical products because of their inherent toxicity. Limit for DCM is 600 ppm and permissible daily exposure is 6 mg/day. DCM was analyzed by Gas chromatography coupled with static head space sampling, the operating parameters of which are listed in Table: 3.3.

Table: 3.3. Headspace Operating Parameters

	Headspace Operating Parameter Sets		
	1	2	3
Equilibration temperature °C	80	105	80
Equilibration time (min.)	60	45	45
Transfer-line temperature °C	85	110	105
Carrier gas: nitrogen or helium at an appropriate pressure			
Pressurization time (s)	30	30	30
Injection volume (mL)	1	1	1

3.6 Determination of peptide (RGD) by BCA method

Protein Assay based on bicinchoninic acid (BCA) is a most sensitive and detergent compatible method for the colorimetric detection and quantitation of total protein. This method is a combination of the well-known biuret reaction, the reduction of Cu^{2+} to Cu^{1+} by protein in an alkaline medium and the highly sensitive and selective colorimetric detection of the cuprous cation (Cu^{2+}) with reagent containing Bichinconinic acid (Smith et al). The macromolecular structure of protein, the number of peptide bonds and the presence of four amino acids (cysteine, cystine, tryptophan and tyrosine) (Wiechelman et al., 1988). The purple-colored reaction product of this assay is formed by the chelation of two molecules of BCA with one cuprous ion. This water-soluble complex exhibits a strong absorbance at 562 nm. A series of dilutions of known concentration are prepared from the protein and assayed alongside the unknown(s) before the concentration of each unknown is determined based on the standard curve. The BCA reagent does not reach a true end point, color development continues even after cooling to RT, but because the color development is slow at room temperature, no significant error is introduced if readings of all the test tubes are done within 10 min.

BCA-Protein Reaction

1. protein (peptide bonds) + Cu^{2+} tetradentate- $Cu1^{+}$ complex
2. $Cu1^{+}$ + 2 Bichinchoninic Acid BCA- Cu^{1+} complex (purple colored, read at 562nm)

Materials:

Genei's BCA Protein Assay kit KT-31

Distilled water containing 0.05-0.1 % sodium azide.

UV-Visible spectrophotometer

Methods:

1. The powder in the standard vial of the Genei's BCA Protein Assay kit KT-31 was dissolved in distilled water containing 0.05 % sodium azide to yield 5 mg/ml of Transferrin stock solution.
2. A fresh set of standard solutions was prepared from this stock solution by diluting it according to Table: 3.4.
3. To prepare BCA working Reagent (BWR), 50 parts of Reagent A was mixed with 1 parts of Reagent B. Upon addition of reagent A to reagent B, initially turbidity is observed that quickly disappears upon mixing to yield a clear green BWR. This BWR is stable for at least 24 hours when stored in a closed container at room temperature.
4. 0.2 ml of each standard or unknown sample was taken into labeled test tubes. 0.2 ml of the diluent (distilled water) was taken for blank reading.
5. 2 ml of the BWR was added to each test tube and mixed well.
6. All the test tubes were incubated at 60°C for 30 min.
7. The test tubes were then cooled down to room temperature and the absorbance measured at 562 nm Vs a water reference used as a blank and recorded in Table: 3.5.
8. A standard curve was prepared by plotting the average absorbance reading for each RGD standard vs. its concentration in µg/ml and plotted as shown in Figure: 3.3.
9. Using this standard curve, the protein concentration for each unknown sample was determined.

Table: 3.4. Preparation of diluted RGD standards

Volume of the RGD solution	Volume of Diluent	Final RGD concentration
300 µl of stock	1200 µl	1000 µg/ml **(A)**
375 µl of (A)	125 µl	750 µg/ml **(B)**
250 µl of (A)	250 µl	500 µg/ml **(C)**
125 µl of (A)	375 µl	250 µg/ml **(D)**
75 µl of (A)	425 µl	150 µg/ml **(E)**
50 µl of (A)	450 µl	100 µg/ml **(F)**
25 µl of (A)	475 µl	50 µg/ml **(G)**
12.5 µl of (A)	487.5 µl	25 µg/ml **(H)**
6.25 µl of (A)	493.75 µl	12.5 µg/ml **(I)**

Table: 3.5. Calibration of RGD by BCA method

Sample	Concentration µg/ml	Mean Absorbance* ± S.D at 562nm
A	1000	0.972 ± 0.21
B	750	0.824 ± 0.18
C	500	0.563 ± 0.06
D	250	0.315 ± 0.04
E	150	0.283 ± 0.05
F	100	0.227 ± 0.06
G	50	0.166 ± 0.03
H	25	0.135 ± 0.03
I	12.5	0.110 ± 0.02

*Mean of 3 values;

Regression equation; $Y = 0.0009x + 0.1218$ Correlation coefficient; $R^2 = 0.9935$

Figure: 3.3. Calibration plot for RGD

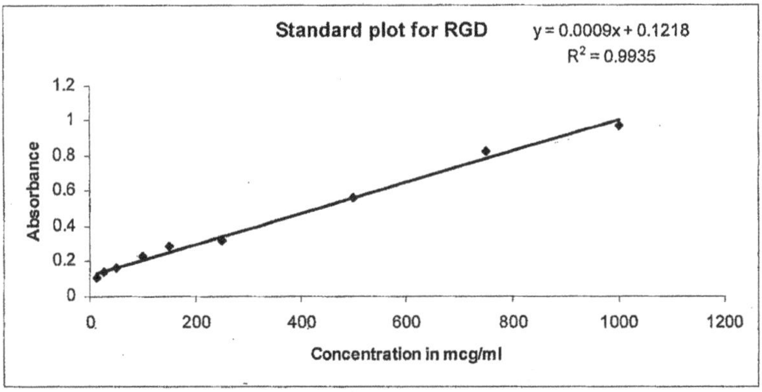

3.6.1 Estimation of Phosphatidyl Choline

The Stewart assay (Stewart et al., 1980) was used for estimating phosphatidyl choline in liposomes. This method utilizes the ability of phospholipids to form a complex with ammonium ferrothiocyanate in organic solution.

3.6.1.1 Solutions

1. Ammonium ferrothiocyanate solution (0.1M) was prepared by dissolving 27.03g of ferric chloride hexahydrate and 30.4g of ammonium thiocyanate in double distilled water and making up the volume of the resulting solution to 1 litre.
2. Stock solution of phosphatidyl choline in chloroform (0.1mg/ml) was prepared by dissolving 50mg of phosphatidyl choline in 10ml of chloroform. 2ml of this solution was diluted 100 times to yield a solution of the required concentration.
3. Saturated sodium chloride solution: Sodium chloride was dissolved in distilled water with heating to form a supersaturated solution. This solution was then cooled to room temperature and filtered to give the required saturated solution.

3.6.1.2 Procedure for calibration curve

Suitable aliquots (0.1 – 1.5 ml) of the stock solution of phosphatidyl choline were transferred to 10ml centrifuge tubes. Appropriate quantities of chloroform were then added such that the total volume of the contents of the tubes was 3ml. To each tube, 2ml of ammonium ferrothiocyanate solution (0.1M) was then added. The contents of each tube were mixed by vigorous vortexing on a cyclomixer for 15sec. The tubes were then spun for 5min at 1800 rpm in a tabletop centrifuge. The lower, organic colored layer was then removed using a syringe and long needle (18 gauge) and transferred to a test tube. The absorbance of these solutions was measured at 485 nm on a Shimadzu 1601 UV-Visible spectrophotometer with glass cells of 10mm path length using a blank prepared in the same manner omitting the phospholipids.

The above procedure was repeated six times. Mean absorbance values along with the regressed values and the regression equation obtained are shown in Table: 3.6.

3.6.1.3 Stability and selectivity

Stability of the colored solutions, prepared above for the calibration curve of phosphatidyl choline, was ascertained by observing the changes in absorbance of the solutions over a period of 4 h. The selectivity of the method for phosphatidyl choline was investigated by carrying out the procedure detailed above in the presence of potential interferences such as cholesterol, Sucrose, etc., at the levels at which these materials were included in the liposomes.

Table: 3.6. Calibration for estimation of phosphatidyl choline (Stewart assay)

Concentration (μg/3ml)	Mean Absorbance* ± S.E.M	Regressed value
10	0.026 ± 0.004	0.031
20	0.055 ± 0.002	0.056
40	0.103 ± 0.004	0.106
60	0.160 ± 0.002	0.156
80	0.211 ± 0.007	0.206
100	0.263 ± 0.003	0.256
150	0.373 ± 0.004	0.381

Regression equation** Y= 0.0025 X + 0.0057
Correlation coefficient = 0.9979
*Mean of 6 values

3.6.1.4 Estimation of phosphatidyl choline from liposomes/ supernatant

The Bligh-Dyer two-phase extraction method (New et al., 1990) was modified for estimating phosphatidyl choline from liposomes. Briefly, 0.1ml of liposomal dispersion or 0.5ml of the supernatant was taken in a centrifuge tube and to this 1ml of saturated sodium chloride solution was added. 2ml of chloroform was then added to the contents followed by vigorous vortexing on a cyclomixer for 30 sec and centrifugation at 1800 rpm for 5 min in a tabletop centrifuge. The lower chloroform layer was separated using a syringe and needle (18 gauge) and passed over a bed of anhydrous sodium sulfate into a 10ml volumetric flask. The process was repeated with a further 2ml and 1ml of chloroform. The chloroform layers were then pooled and the volume made up to 10ml with chloroform. To 0.5ml of this chloroform extract in a centrifuge tube, 2.5ml of chloroform and 2ml of 0.1M ammonium ferrothiocyanate solution was added. The contents were then subjected to the same procedure as detailed above for the standards (Section 3.6.1.2). Duplicate estimations were performed and the mean absorbance was used to determine the amount of phosphatidyl choline in the liposomes or supernatant using the regression equation.

3.6.2 Estimation of cholesterol

The Zlatkis, Zak and Boyle's method was used for cholesterol estimation. This method utilizes the ability of cholesterol in acetic acid to form a complex with ferric chloride and sulphuric acid (Zlatkis et. al., 1953).

3.6.2.1 Solutions

1. Ferric chloride solution: A 0.05% w/v solution of ferric chloride hexahydrate in glacial acetic acid was prepared by dissolving 50mg of ferric chloride hexahydrate in 100ml glacial acetic acid.
2. Stock solution of cholesterol: A 0.5mg/ml solution of cholesterol in glacial acetic acid was prepared by dissolving 25mg of cholesterol in 50ml of glacial acetic acid.
3. Saturated sodium chloride solution: It was prepared in the same manner as for the estimation of phosphatidyl choline from liposomes (Section 3.6.1.1)

3.6.2.2. Procedure for calibration curve

Suitable aliquots of the stock solution of cholesterol (0.1 to 1ml) were transferred accurately into 10ml volumetric flasks. To each flask, 4ml of ferric chloride solution and 4ml of concentrated sulphuric acid was added. The contents were mixed, made up to the volume with glacial acetic acid and allowed to stand for 30 min. The absorbance of the resulting coloured solutions of the complex, formed between cholesterol, ferric chloride and sulphuric acid was measured at 550nm using Shimadzu 1601 UV-Visible spectrophotometer with glass cells of 10mm path length, against a blank prepared in the same manner as the standard solutions except cholesterol. The above procedure was repeated six times. The experimental data along with the results of the statistical evaluation of the data are shown in Table: 3.4.

3.6.2.3 Stability and selectivity

Stability of the solutions of the complex, prepared for obtaining the calibration curve of cholesterol, was ascertained by observing the changes in their absorbance over a period of 24 h. Cholesterol was estimated in the presence of phosphatidyl choline, Sucrose, etc., at the same concentrations at which these materials were included in the liposomes to ascertain the selectivity of the method.

3.6.2.4. Estimation of cholesterol from liposomes/ supernatant

1ml of the chloroform extract, obtained as described before in the estimation of phosphatidyl choline form liposomes or supernatant (Section 3.6.1.4) was taken in a 10ml volumetric flask and evaporated to dryness by heating at 90°C in a thermostatically controlled, electrically heated water bath. The dried contents were then subjected to the same procedure as discussed previously (Section 3.6.2.2). The amount of cholesterol in the liposomes or supernatant was then obtained using the regression equation of the calibration curve.

Table: 3.7. Calibration for estimation of cholesterol (Zlatkis, Zak and Boyle's method)

Concentration (μg/ml)	Mean Absorbance* ± S.E.M	Regressed value
5	0.065 ± 0.001	0.069
10	0.154 ± 0.0021	0.155
20	0.344 ± 0.003	0.327
30	0.475 ± 0.004	0.499
40	0.695 ± 0.003	0.671
50	0.836 ± 0.004	0.843

Regression equation** Y= 0.0172X –0.0173
Correlation coefficient = 0.9966
*Mean of 6 values

3.7 Determination of Particle Size, Polydispersity and Zeta potential

The particle size was measured with Malvern zetasizer NanoZS. The instrument is based on the principle of dynamic light scattering (DLS), also sometimes referred to as photon correlation spectroscopy (PCS) or quasi elastic light scattering. DLS is a technique of measuring the size of particles typically in the sub-micron region and is usually applied to the measurement of particle suspended within a liquid. The technique measures particle diffusion due to Brownian motion and relates this to the size of the particles. Brownian motion is the random movement of particles due to the bombardment by the solvent molecules that surround them. The parameter calculated is defined as the translational diffusion coefficient. The particle size is then calculated from the translational diffusion coefficient using the Strokes-Einstein equation.

Malvern zetasizer NanoZS was used to measure the zeta potential of the particles based on the electrophoresis and electrical conductivity of the formed nanoparticle dispersion. The electrophoretic mobility (μm/s) of the particles was converted to the zeta potential by in-built software based on Helmholtz- Smoluchowski equation.

A 2.0 mg sample of nanoparticles was suspended in distilled water, and the particle size, polydispersity index and zeta potential were measured using the principle of laser light scattering with zeta sizer (Nano-ZS, Malvern Instruments, UK).

3.8 Morphological characterization

The morphology of the nanoparticles was analyzed using EDAX (Energy dispersion analysis by X-ray) Scanning Electron Microscopy (SEM) and TEM (Transmission Electron Microscopy). Aqueous nanoparticle suspensions were layered on the SEM stubs, and they were allowed to dry at room temperature. Samples were then observed with Phillips SEM 51S set at 10 kV.

Aqueous liposomal suspension was negatively stained with phosphotungstic acid (0.5%) while nanoparticles were analyzed without any staining. Samples were then observed with Morgagni, Philips, Eindhoven, Netherlands

3.9 Differential scanning calorimetry

The DSC of samples was carried out by scanning the samples using differential scanning colorimeter (Mettler). Thermograms were analyzed using Mettler Toledo star SW 7.01. An empty aluminium pan was used as the reference for all measurements. During each scan, 2 to 3 mg of sample was heated, in a hermetically sealed aluminium pan, at a heating rate of 10° C/min, from 35° C to 300° C, under a nitrogen atmosphere.

3.10. Discussions

DC in nanoparticles, liposomes and in-vitro release medium was estimated by HPLC method. RGD was estimated by BCA protein assay and amino acid analysis. The estimation in the nanoparticles, liposomes and *in vitro* release studies for DC was performed by HPLC method. The calibration curve of DC was established in acetonitrile: water gradient system by HPLC at 227nm. The linearity of DC was found to be 0.5-10µg/ml (R^2=0.9985). To determine the amount of drug entrapped nanoparticles were dissolved in acetonitrile. The resulting system was centrifuged to remove the precipitated components and the supernant was diluted with the solvent system and subjected to analysis.

The invitro release study was performed using the tube shaking method. At different time intervals, the samples were removed and centrifuged at 25000 rpm and the settled nanoparticles were dissolved in acetonitrile and analyzed for the drug remaining in the nanoparticles as the same method for entrapment efficiency. The drug released was calculated by taking the difference of the drug taken initially and the drug remaining in the nanoparticles.

The estimation of RGD conjugation was carried out using BCA protein estimation. The calibration curve was established at 12.5-1000 μg/ml (R^2=0.9935). The amount of PVA associated with nanoparticles was determined by a colorimetric method based on the formation of a colored complex between two adjacent hydroxyl groups of PVA and an iodine molecule. A standard plot for known concentrations of PVA was established at 5-250 μg/ml. (R^2=0.9994). Residual solvents in pharmaceuticals, commonly known as organic volatile impurities (OVIs), are chemicals that are either used or produced during the manufacture of active pharmaceutical ingredients (APIs), excipients and drug products. OVIs are classified into three classes on the basis of their toxicity level and the degree to which they can be considered an environmental hazard. DCM belongs to class 2 solvents which are non-genotoxic animal carcinogens. Solvents of this class should be limited in pharmaceutical products because of their inherent toxicity. Limit for DCM is 600 ppm and recommended daily exposure is 6 mg/day.

The Stewart assay was used for estimating phosphatidyl choline in liposomes (Stewart, 1980). This method is based on complex formation between ammonium ferrothiocyanate and phospholipids in organic solution. The complex in chloroform exhibits maximum absorbance at 485nm. The advantage of this method is that the presence of inorganic phosphate does not interfere with the assay. A disadvantage, however, is that this method is not applicable to samples where mixtures of unknown phospholipids may be present (New et al., 1990a). A correlation coefficient of 0.9979 indicated a linear relationship between absorbance and concentration of phosphatidyl choline taken for complex formation. Beer's law was found to be obeyed between 10 – 150 μg/3ml.

The Zlatkis, Zak and Boyle method (Zlatkis et. al., 1953) was used for estimating cholesterol in liposomes. Here, cholesterol in acetic acid forms a colored complex with ferric chloride and sulphuric acid, which exhibits maximum absorbance at 550nm. Linearity of the method was observed from a correlation coefficient of 0.9966. Beer's law was found to be obeyed between 5 – 50 μg/ml. The regression equation obtained was $Y = 0.0172 X + 0.0146$. Monitoring of the absorbance of the solutions, used for preparing the calibration curve revealed that the color of the complex was retained as its original intensity for only 2h.

3.11. Rreferences

Ferrothiocyanate, Anal. Biochem., **104**, 10-14.

ICH Harmonized Tripartite Guideline for Residual Solvents, 1997, Step 4, 17 July.

Joshi, D.P. et al., 1979, Determination of poly (vinyl alcohol) via its complex with boric acid and iodine, Anal. Chim. Acta., **104,** 153–160.

Smith, P. K. et al., 1985, Measurement of protein using bicinchoninic acid, Anal. Biochem., **150**, 76-85.

Stewart J.C.M. et al, 1980, Colorimetric determination of phospholipids with ammonium ferrothiocyanate, Anal.Biochem., **104**, 10-14.

Uday B. et al., 2003, Nano- and Microparticles Sustain Retinal Delivery of Budesonide, a Corticosteroid Capable of Inhibiting VEGF Expression, IOVS, **44**, (3).

USP 25-NF20 (US Pharmacopeia, 12601 Twinbrook Parkway, Rockville, Maryland 20852, USA, 2002).

Wiechelman K. et al., 1988, Investigation of the bicinchoninic acid protein assay: Identification of the groups responsible for color formation, Anal. Biochem., **175**, 231-237.

Zlatkis A. et al., 1953, A new method for the direct determination of serum cholesterol, J. Lab. Clin Med., **41**, 486-492.

Chapter 4

Preparation and RGD Conjugation of Nanoconstructs

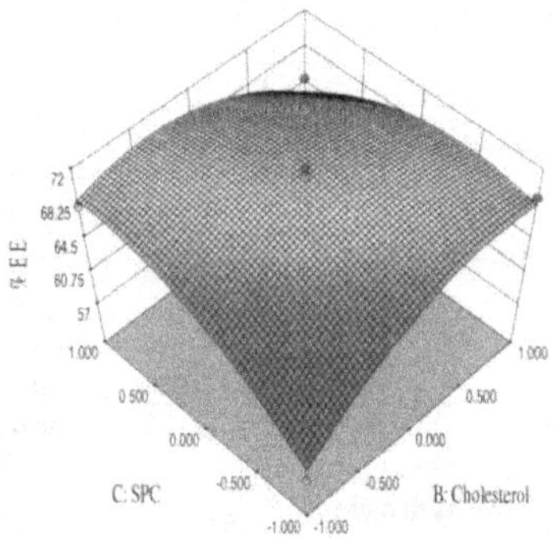

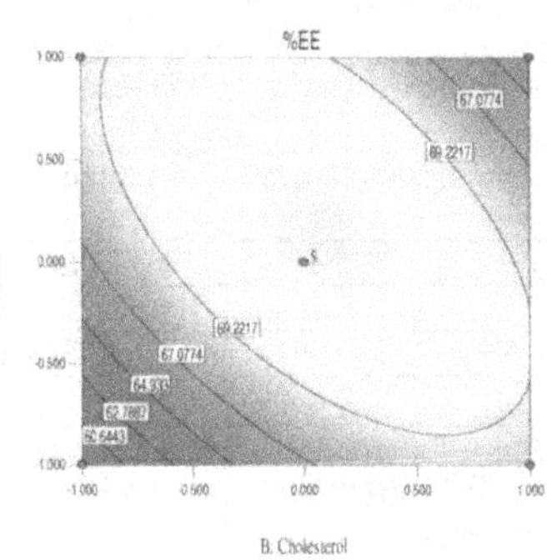

4.1. Introduction

Design and fabrication of pharmaceutical particulate systems is still largely an art as opposed to a fundamental science. However, a more systematic design and manufacture of particulate systems including nanoparticles is being enabled by the application of novel technologies, such as supercritical fluid (SCF) technology. A fluid is supercritical when it is compressed beyond its critical pressure (Pc) and heated beyond its critical temperature (Tc). SCF technology has emerged as an important technique for particle manufacturing. (Ram Gupta et al., 2006)

Liposomes are prepared using several methods such as thin film hydration method, reverse phase evaporation, double emulsification, pH gradient method, solvent dispersion, detergent removal method. However, all these methods are used for preparation of multilamellar vesicles as the final product. To convert multilamellar vesicles into large unilamellar vesicles/small unilamellar vesicles techniques like sonication, extrusions etc. are used (Castor et al., 1996).

Table: 4.1. Materials and Equipments

Material	Source
Water (distilled)	Prepared in laboratory by distillation
PLGA (50:50)	Gift samples from Boehringer Ingelheim, Germany
Bichinconinic acid (BCA) protein Assay Kit	Banglore Genei, India
6-Coumarin	Gift sample from Neelikon dyes, Mumbai, India
Glacial acetic acid, potassium dihydrogen phosphate, disodium hydrogen phosphate, potassium chloride, potassium hydroxide, sodium chloride, sodium hydroxide, hydrochloric acid	S.D. Fine chemicals, Mumbai, India
HPLC grade methanol, acetonitrile acetic acid	S.D. Fine chemicals, India.
Nuclepore Polycarbonate membrane 2 µm 25mm	Whatman, USA
RGD Peptide	USV Limited, Mumbai
Polyvinyl alcohol	Sigma chemicals, USA
DSPE PEG 2000, HSPC, SPC	Lipoid, Germany
Equipments	**Make**
Calibrated pipettes of 1.0 ml, 5.0 ml and 10.0 ml, volumetric flasks of 10 ml, 25 ml, 50 ml and 100 ml capacity, Funnels (i.d. 5.0 cm), beakers (250 ml) and other requisite glasswares	Schott & Corning (India) Ltd., Mumbai

Analytical balance	AX 120, EL 8300, Shimadzu Corp., Japan
pH meter	Pico$^+$ Labindia, Mumbai, India
Cyclomixer, magnetic stirrer	Remi Scientific Equipments, Mumbai
Cooling Centrifuge	3K 30, Sigma Laboratory centrifuge, Osterode, GmBH.
Supercritical Antisolvent instrument	SAS-50,Thar incorporation ltd.
Lyophilizer	DW1, 0-60E, Heto Drywinner, Denmark
UV-Visible Spectrophotometer	Shimadzu UV-1601, Japan
Spectrofluorimeter	Rf540, Shimadzu Corp., Japan
Particle and Zeta size Analyzer	Malvern zeta sizer NanoZS, U.K.
Transmission electron microscopy	Morgagni, Philips, Netherlands
^{1}H-NMR	av300, Bruker, UK
HPLC system	Dionex HPLC with Chromleon 6.5 data processing software

4.2. Methods

4.2.1. Preparation of Liposomes by Supercritical Carbon dioxide (SC-CO_2)

Docetaxel, HSPC, SPC and cholesterol in different molar ratios were dissolved in Chloroform: Methanol (2:1). The different molar ratios of aforesaid lipids and cholesterol with respect to drug are mentioned in Table: 4.6a & 4.6b. along with different operation conditions. This solution of mix lipids and drug were sprayed through solvent pump into the high pressure vessel. The pressure and temperature of the vessel was achieved and maintained through Automated Back Pressure Regulator (ABPR) and temperature control panel, respectively. The Liquefied CO_2 was converted to supercritical CO_2 in high pressure vessel at preset temp and pressure above critical point of CO_2 and was continuously pumped into the vessel by a high pressure pump through out the process. Once the system reached steady state (temperature and pressure), the solution of mix lipids and drug were introduced through a solvent pump into the stream of SC-CO_2 in high pressure vessel at the flow rate of 0.15ml/min. This allows mixing of the SC-CO_2 with the organic solvent and results in the precipitation of the drug encapsulated Proliposomes (lipid particles) in the vessel. The SC- CO_2 was allowed to flow continuously through the high pressure vessel after the completion of the solvent spraying process to achieve complete removal of the residual solvent from the precipitates. The precipitated proliposomes form liposomes on hydration with 10 ml of PBS pH 7.4 at 50°C. The DSPE-PEG was added in 2-8 mole% ratios to the prior optimized mix lipid ratio from aforesaid method and same process was repeated with optimized process parameters to prepare PEGylated liposomes.

4.2.2. Apparatus

An apparatus for making liposomes is schematically described in Figure: 4.1 which comprised of the following elements: CO_2 storage take 1, Heat exchanger 2, CO_2 flow pump 3, Heat exchanger 4, a high pressure vessel or chamber 5, Co-solvent container 6, Co solvent pump 7, a second vessel 8, Automated Back pressure regulator 9, solvent collection valve 10 and Co-solvent spraying nozzle 11.

Figure: 4.1. Schematic diagram of Supercritical fluid particle former.

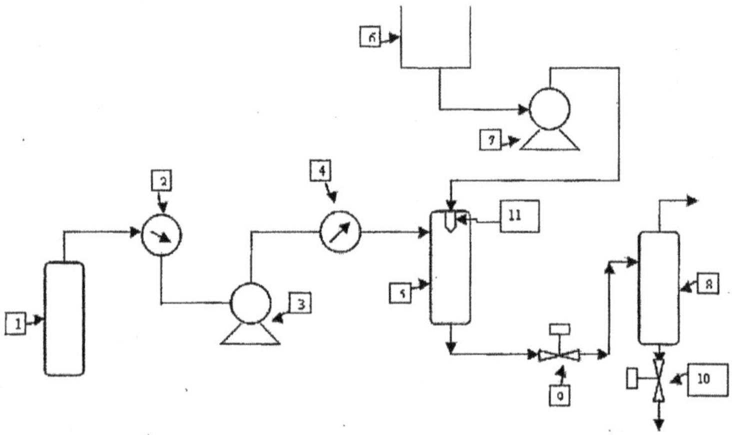

For optimizing the liposomal formulation here two basic parameters were taken in to consideration:

1] Process parameters: CO_2 flow rate, Processing Temperature and CO2 pressure.

2] Formulation parameters: Drug to lipid ratio, transition temperature.

4.3. Optimization of Process Parameters

Quantitative aspects of the effects and relationships among various process parameters of high therapeutics payload Liposomes produced by Supercritical Fluid Antisolvent technique are investigated using Response Surface Methodology (RSM).

To study this, we performed, "Box-Behnken" design (BBD) on three critical process factors known to affect their results. The BBD is a popular template for RSM because it requires only three-levels of each process factor and only a fraction of all the possible combinations. In this design, the experimental region is assumed to be a cube, and experiments are performed at points corresponding to midpoint of each edge and replicated experiments at the center of this multidimensional cube.

This design is suitable for exploring quadratic response surfaces and constructing second-order polynomial models. The complete design consisted of 15 experimental points that included twelve factor points and three replications at the centre point. The non-linear quadratic model generated by the design is as follow:

$$Y= \beta_0+ \beta_1A+ \beta_2B+ \beta_3C+ \beta_{12}\, AB+ \beta_{13}AC+ \beta_{23}BC+ \beta_{11}A^2+ \beta_{22}B^2+ \beta_{33}C^2$$

------ Equation [4.1]

Where, Y is the measured response (dependant variable) associated with each factor-level combination; expressed in terms of size of the liposomes, β_0 is an intercept, β_1, β_2, β_3, β_{12}, β_{13}, β_{23}, β_{11}, β_{22} and β_{33} are the regression coefficients. A, B and C are the (independent factors studied) Temperature (°C), Pressure (Bar), and CO_2 flow rate (Gm/Min) respectively. The independent factors and the dependent variable used in the design are listed in Table 1. The Design Expert (Version 7.1, State Ease Inc, USA) program was used for design of experiment and analysis of this second-order model and for drawing of three dimensional response surface and contour plots.

Table: 4.2.Variables in Box Behnken Design

X_i	Independent variables	Units	Coded values			Response	Response
			-1	0	1		
A	Temperature	°C	34	40	46	Particle size in nm	Yield %w/w
B	Pressure	Bar	100	160	220		
C	CO_2 Flow	Gm/Min	30	75	120		

Table: 4.3. Matrix of Box Behnken Design and Particle size response of each experimental run

Std	Run	Factor: A	Factor: B	Factor C	Particle size (nm)	Predicted particle size (nm)
12	1	40	220	120	255.2±10.5	303.75
4	2	44	220	75	650.3±8.4	768.125
3	3	36	220	75	740.1±11.4	553.125
13	4	40	160	75	800.2±9.7	850
11	5	40	100	120	780.4±6.9	760
8	6	44	160	120	460.3±8.9	508.125
10	7	40	220	30	1780.2±8.4	1800
14	8	40	160	75	970.4±10.5	850
7	9	36	160	120	560.2±8.9	483.125
15	10	40	160	75	780.3±10.5	850
1	11	36	100	75	860.4±6.8	956.875
2	12	44	100	75	800.2±12.4	771.875
5	13	36	160	30	2000.4±20.7	1951.875
9	14	40	100	30	1800.2±16.5	1751.25
6	15	44	160	30	1450.3±14.2	1526.875

Table: 4.4. Matrix of Box Behnken Design and yield as response of each experimental run

Std	Run	Factor: A	Factor: B	Factor C	Yield %	Predicted yield %
12	1	40	220	120	67.5±3.2	64.5
4	2	44	220	75	23.6±2.7	24.5
3	3	36	220	75	53.5±3.5	54.5
13	4	40	160	75	55.1±2.8	53.33333
11	5	40	100	120	51.2±2.4	51.5
8	6	44	160	120	36.1±3.3	37
10	7	40	220	30	44.1±4.2	43.5
14	8	40	160	75	53.2±4.5	53.33333
7	9	36	160	120	57.5±3.4	58
15	10	40	160	75	52.2±2.8	53.33333
1	11	36	100	75	38.1±3.2	36.5
2	12	44	100	75	31.2±2.6	29.5
5	13	36	160	30	42.3±3.4	41
9	14	40	100	30	41.4±4.2	43.5
6	15	44	160	30	26.1±2.4	25

Data Processing:

Liposomes were prepared by supercritical fluid Antisolvent (SAS) technique using SPC/drug/HSPC. Process parameters, such as operating temperature, pressure and flow rate of the SCF were found to have significant influence on preparation of liposome (SCF-LP). Hence, process parameters were optimized and kept unaltered in subsequent experiments. In order to optimize process parameters, a Box Behnken Design (BBD) of RSM was used. Fifteen batches of SCF-LP were prepared by SAS process using a 3-factor, 3-level BBD varying three independent variables (Temperature (A), Pressure (B) and CO_2 flow rate (C) of the formulation according to Table: 4.2. The influence of these variables on observed response (Y, particle size and yield) is recorded in Table: 4.3 and Table: 4.4. Each batch of SCF-LP was prepared three times and was evaluated for particle size and yield. The maximum response as particle size was 2000nn and minimum response was 255nm. The mathematical relationship for the same in terms of a polynomial equation relating the response Y and independent variables was: $Y= +850.00 -100.00* A -101.88* B -621.88 * C -7.50* A * B +112.50 *A * C -126.25 *B *C -61.87 *A^2 -25.62 * B^2+329.37 * C^2$ and $Y = +53.33-9.25 * A+3.25 * B+7.25 * C-5.75 * A * B -1.25 * A* C +3.25 * B * C-13.79 * A^2-3.29 * B^2+0.71* C^2$ for particle size and yield respectively. ······· Equation [4.2] & [4.3]

Equation expresses the quantitative effect of the individual formulation components (A, B, and C) and combination thereof on the response (Y) in terms of interaction coefficients. The values of the coefficients A to C are related to the effect of these variables on the response (Y). Coefficients with more than one factor term and those with higher order terms represent interaction terms and quadratic relationships respectively. A positive and negative signs suggest a positive and negative effect on response respectively. The theoretical (predicted) values and the observed values were in reasonably good agreement as seen from Table: 4.3 and Table: 4.4. The significance of the ratio of mean square variation due to regression and residual error was tested using analysis of variance (ANOVA). The ANOVA indicated a significant ($P < 0.05$) effect of factors on response. Lack of fit was not significant (p = 0.4636, p = 0.2193) and regression was strongly significant (p =0.01, R^2= 0.9834 and p =0.01, R^2= 0.9856). Also the predicted R^2 is 0.81 and 0.80 for particle size and yield respectively, which is very good for chosen factorial model. So it was concluded that the second-order model adequately approximated the true surface. After optimizing process parameters, formulation parameters were optimized for % Entrapment Efficiency (%EE).

4.4. Optimization of Formulation Parameters

In order to optimize different phosphatidyl choline (PC) to cholesterol ratio, liposomes were formulated using PC to cholesterol in molar ratio [9:1, 8:2 and 7:3] and the drug concentration was kept constant. The initial trials were carried out with synthetic saturated phosphatidyl cholines. The natural phospholipids were excluded from the initial trials on the basis of unsaturation in their structure and these lipids are prone to oxidation and hydrolysis and less stable compare to saturated lipids. Again these PCs can not form rigid bilayer and hence rapid release of encapsulated materials from the vesicles has been observed.

The synthetic phospholipids and cholesterol system with different molar ratios were applied as enumerated in Table: 4.5.

Table: 4.5. Percent Entrapment Efficiency and Particles size of DC liposomes using various lipids

Types of Lipids	Lipid composition
HSPC:Chol	9:1
	8:2
	7:3
DMPC:Chol	9:1
	8:2
	7:3
DPPC:Chol	9:1
	8:2
	7:3

Use of mixture of lipids:

The second attempt was carried out by using mixture of lipids containing both unsaturated and saturated lipid in one liposomal system to improve hydration and encapsulation.

The unsaturated and saturated lipids were SPC and HSPC respectively along with cholesterol to design conventional liposomes. The ratio of drug to total lipid was taken as 1:15, 1:20 and 1:25 mole %. The liposomes were characterized for particle size, percent entrapment, vesicle morphology and zeta potential. The formation of two distinct regions by the use of mix lipids accounts for higher percent entrapment of free drug in the mix lipid liposomal system. It also helps in restricting the interaction of hydrophobic chain of drugs to each other and hence stabilized the system. The marvelous work was carried out by *Korlach et al 1999* on mix lipid bilayer in the same system. They revealed that the existence of the two distinct phase in the same system, exemplified the liposomes made from mixture of two phospholipids, unsaturated and saturated. The studies were supported by evaluating the liposomal system with confocal fluorescence microscopy and simultaneous measurement of diffusion properties by fluorescence correlation spectroscopy. They further explained that liquid crystalline phase and gel phase was existed in the same system at specific ratio of the phospholipids and at specific transition temperature. In detail the saturated lipid, generally having higher transition temperature exists as gel phase while the unsaturated lipid, low transition temperature forms liquid crystal phase and these both phases were existed while the liposomes were prepared from mixture of lipid. *Semmler et al., 2000* in his paper supported the study that both the phases existed in the same system and form stabilized liposomes. At last the stability could be attained in a way that the bilayer of discontinuous phase limited boundaries which ultimately lessen the later moment of the chains and contact between the drug molecules.

The work carried out by *Needham and Beech et al* disclosed the use of secondary lipid as surface active agent or lysolipid. The work concentrates on the site specific release of the active materials from the liposomes in a condition like hyperthermia, generally seen in cancer like disorders where inflammation is predominant. So, in the mixed lipid system, one lipid acts as lysolipid and once the carrier reaches to the disease site it will release its content easily as natural lipid release the content faster than the synthetic lipid. Here in case of hyperthermia natural lipids release the drug faster as temperature plays a critical role. The advantage of mix phospholipids system is that it has both unsaturated and saturated phospholipids components. The unsaturated phospholipids alone lead to easy formation of liposomes but suffer from low stability as it easily degraded by oxidation or hydrolysis. The saturated lipids alone are unable to entrap high percent drug load and the essential presence of cholesterol leads to increase in hydrophobicity and hence difficulty in hydration of lipids which results in formation of precipitates. Hydration can be improved by addition of unsaturated lipids which have polar heads and so it can help in hydration. Hence in this study we used mix phospholipids which proved to be better than liposomes prepared from single phospholipid Table: 4.5.

The optimized process parameters were kept constant and the formulation parameters were further optimized by the BBD of Response surface methodology. This design is suitable for exploring quadratic response surfaces and constructing second-order polynomial models. The complete design consisted of 17 experimental points that included twelve factor points and five replications at the centre point. The non-linear quadratic model generated by the design is as follow:

$$Y = \beta_0 + \beta_1 A + \beta_2 B + \beta_3 C + \beta_{12} AB + \beta_{13} AC + \beta_{23} BC + \beta_{11} A^2 + \beta_{22} B^2 + \beta_{33} C^2$$

...... Equation [4.4]

Where, Y is the measured response (dependant variable) associated with each factor-level combination; expressed in terms of % entrapment efficiency of the liposomes, β_0 is an intercept, β_1, β_2, β_3, β_{12}, β_{13}, β_{23}, β_{11}, β_{22} and β_{33} are the regression coefficients. A, B and C are the (independent factors studied) mole % of HSPC, mole % of cholesterol, and mole % of SPC respectively. The independent factors and the dependent variable used in the design are listed in Table: 4.6a & Table: 4.6b, respectively. The Design Expert (Version 7.1, State Ease Inc, USA) program was used for design of experiment and analysis of this second-order model and for drawing of three dimensional response surface and contour plots.

Table: 4.6a. Variables in Box Behnken Design for formulation parameters

X_i	Independent variables	Units	Coded values			Response (Y)
			-1	0	1	
A	HSPC	% Mole	4	7	10	% Entrapment efficiency
B	cholesterol	% Mole	0.5	1	1.5	
C	SPC	% Mole	2	3	4	

Table: 4.6b. Matrix of Box Behnken Design for optimizing formulation parameters

Std	Run	Factor A HSPC	Factor B Cholesterol	Factor C SPC	%EE	Predicted %EE
9	1	7	0.5	2	57.1±2.4	58.5
1	2	4	0.5	3	50.2±3.1	48.625
2	3	10	0.5	3	70.2±2.5	69.125
13	4	7	1	3	71.1±3.6	71.2
10	5	7	1.5	2	69.2±1.8	68.25
14	6	7	1	3	70.3±4.2	71.2
5	7	4	1	2	50.1±4.1	49.875
7	8	4	1	4	53.2±3.7	53.625
17	9	7	1	3	72.1±2.8	71.2
6	10	10	1	2	69.1±3.2	68.375
8	11	10	1	4	70.2±2.4	70.125
11	12	7	0.5	4	68.3±4.7	68.75
3	13	4	1.5	3	53.4±3.6	53.875
12	14	7	1.5	4	65.1±4.1	63.5
16	15	7	1	3	72.1±2.8	71.2
4	16	10	1.5	3	67.3±1.5	68.375
15	17	7	1	3	71.1±3.8	71.2

- Drug to total lipid ratio was 1:15 mole %

Figure: 4.2. **Response surface plots of a) the effects of Temperature (A) and Pressure (B), b) effects of Temperature(A) and CO_2 flow rate(C) and c) effects of Pressure (B) and CO_2 flow rate(C) on the particle size of the SC-LP**

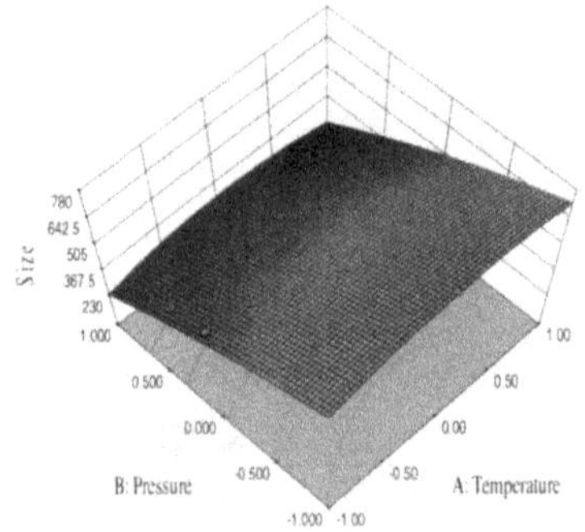

(a)

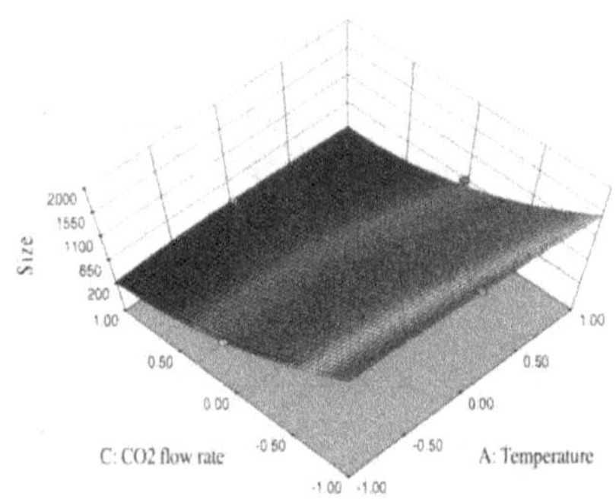

(b)

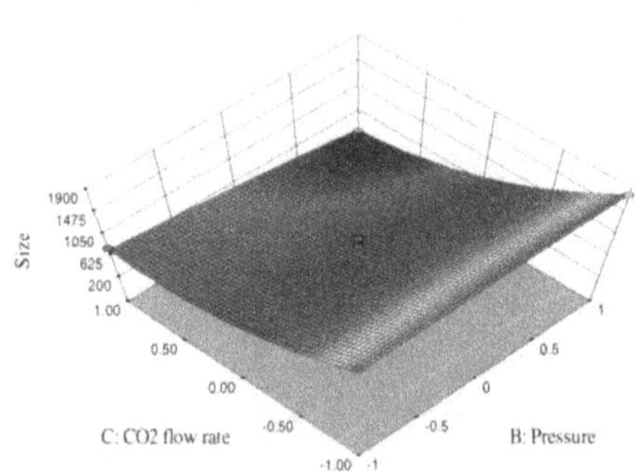

(c)

Figure:4.3. **Contour plots of a) the effects of Temperature (A) and Pressure (B), b) effects of Temperature(A) and CO_2 flow rate(C) and c) effects of Pressure (B) and CO_2 flow rate(C) on the particle size of the SC-LP**

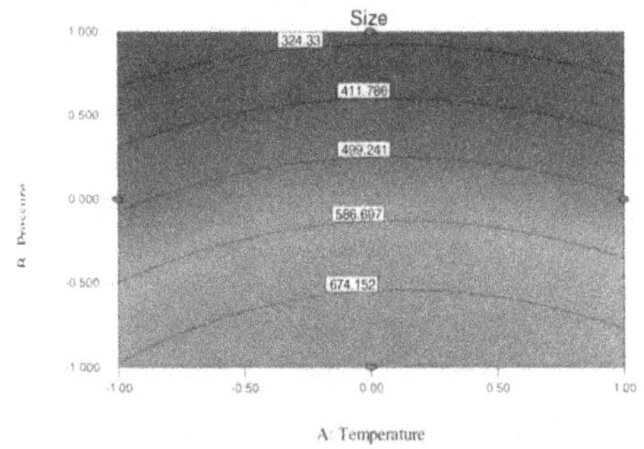

(a)

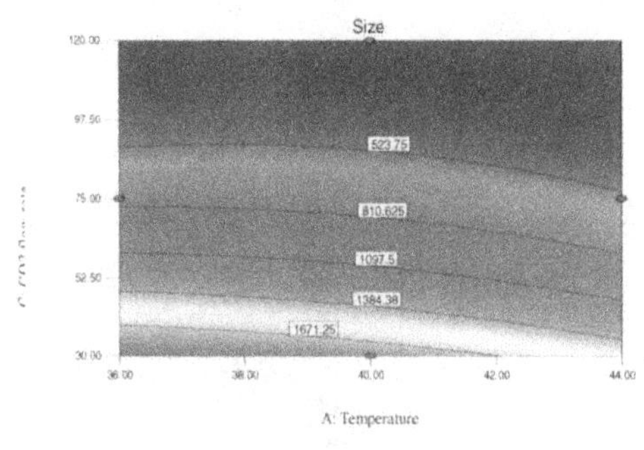

(b)

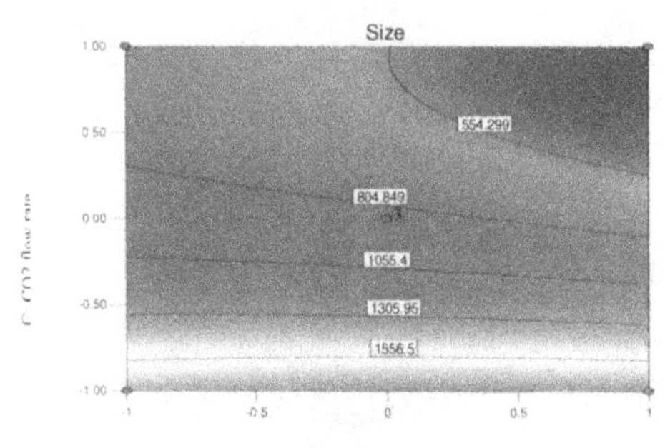

(c)

Figure: 4.4. **Response surface plots of a) the effects of Temperature (A) and Pressure (B), b) effects of Temperature(A) and CO_2 flow rate(C) and c) effects of Pressure (B) and CO_2 flow rate(C) on the yield of the SC-LP**

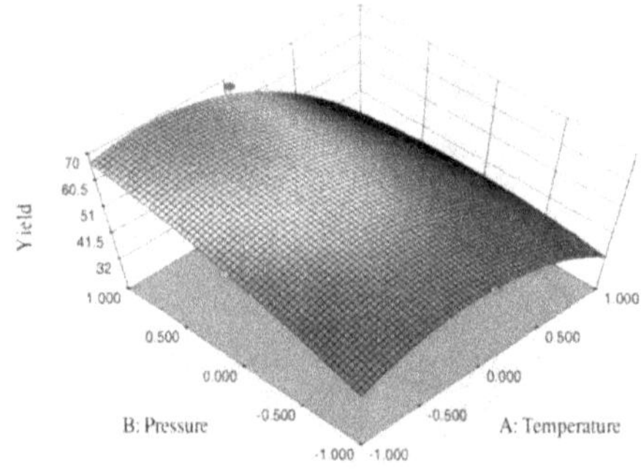

(a)

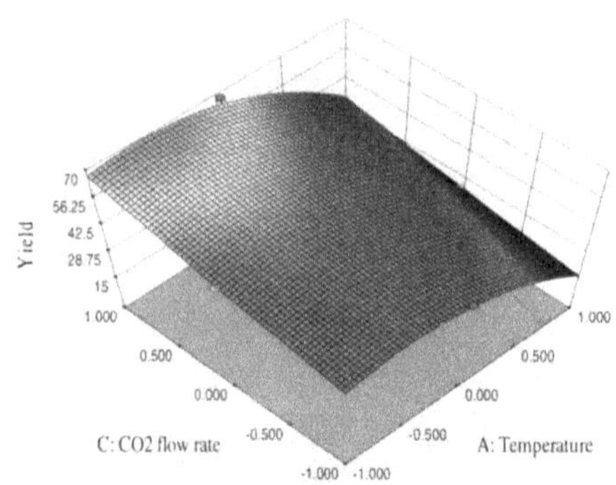

(b)

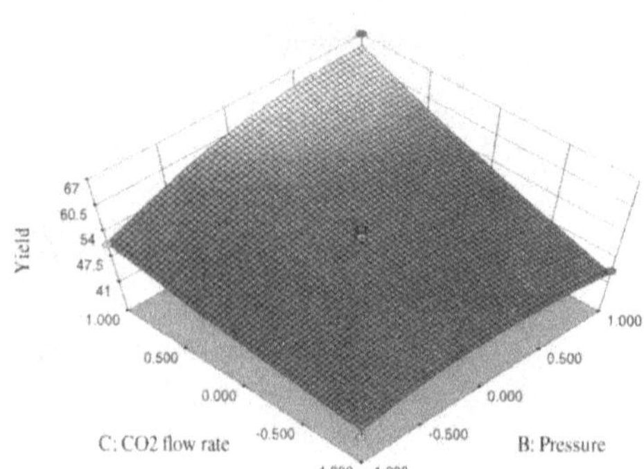

(c)

Figure: 4.5. **Contour plots of a) the effects of Temperature (A) and Pressure (B), b) effects of Temperature(A) and CO_2 flow rate(C) and c) effects of Pressure (B) and CO_2 flow rate(C) on the Yield of the SC-LP**

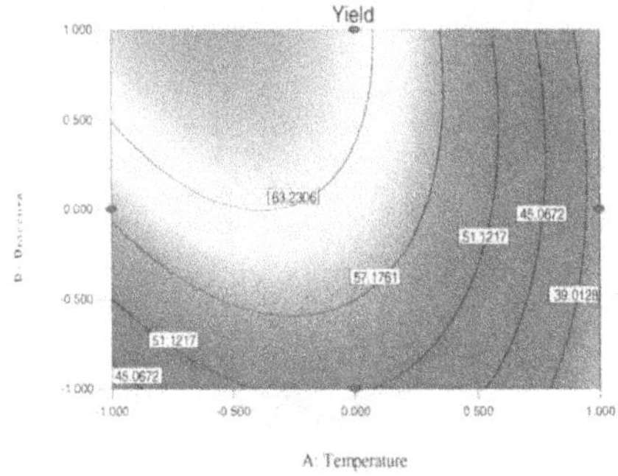

(a)

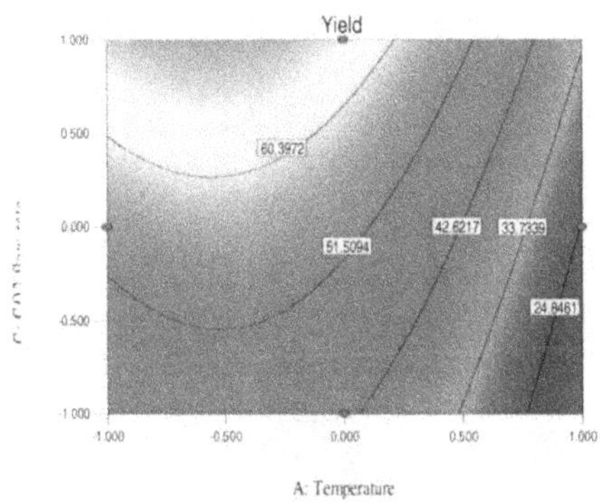

(b)

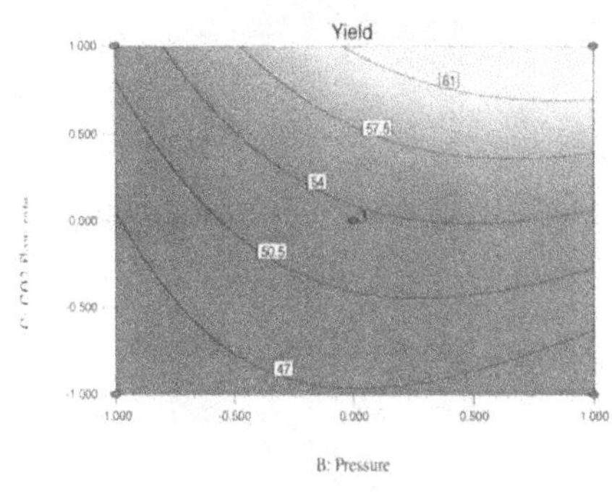

(c)

Figure: 4.6. **Response surface plots of a) the effects of the amount of HSPC (A) and the amount of Cholesterol (B), b) effects of the amount of HSPC (A) and the amount of SPC(C) and c) effects of the amount of Cholesterol (B) and the amount of SPC(C) on the %EE of the SC-LP**

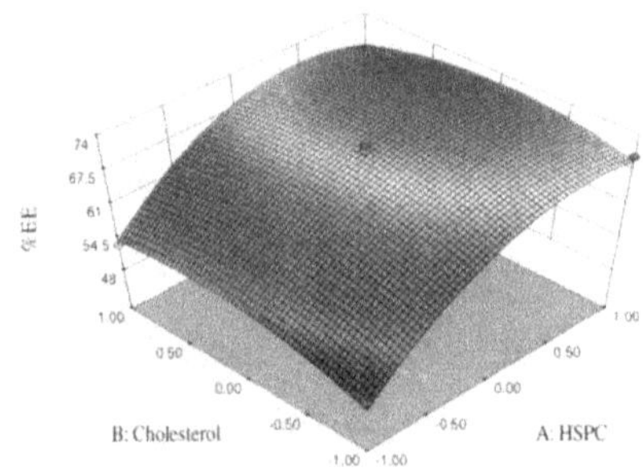

(a)

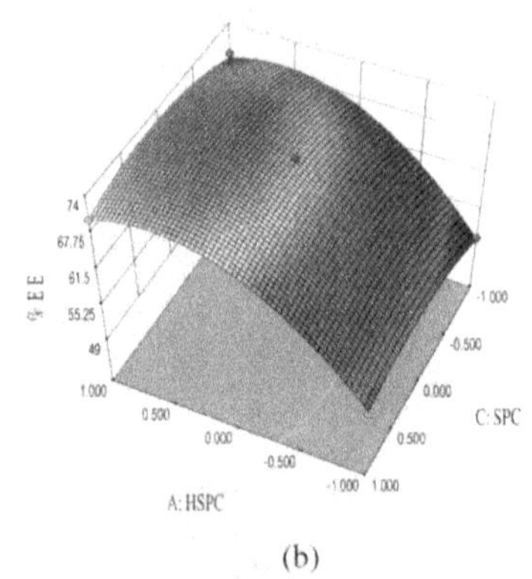

(b)

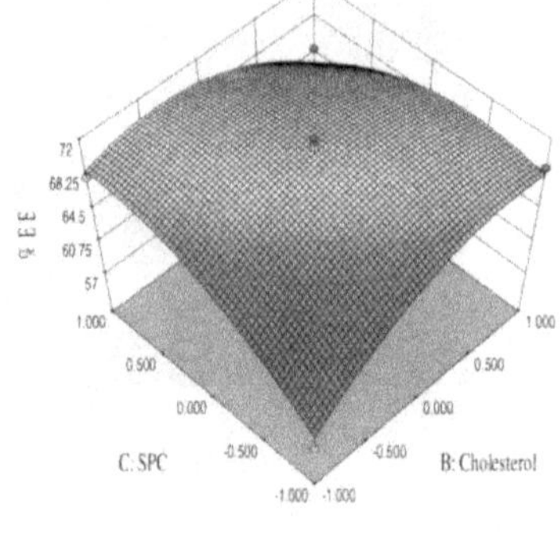

(c)

Figure: 4.7. Contour plots of a) the effects of the amount of HSPC (A) and the amount of Cholesterol (B), b) effects of the amount of HSPC (A) and the amount of SPC(C) and c) effects of the amount of Cholesterol (B) and the amount of SPC(C) on the %EE of the SC-LP

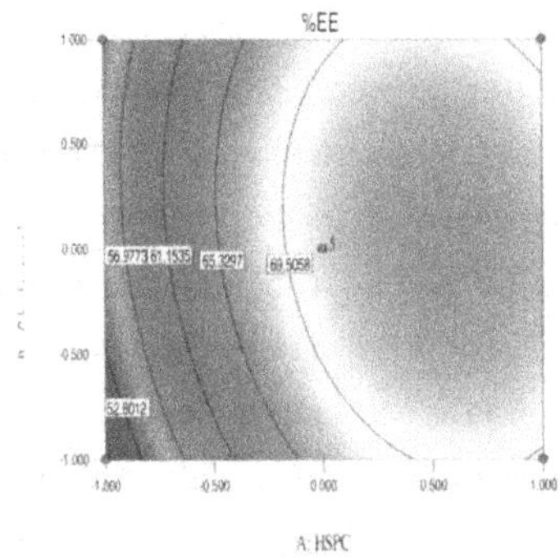

(a)

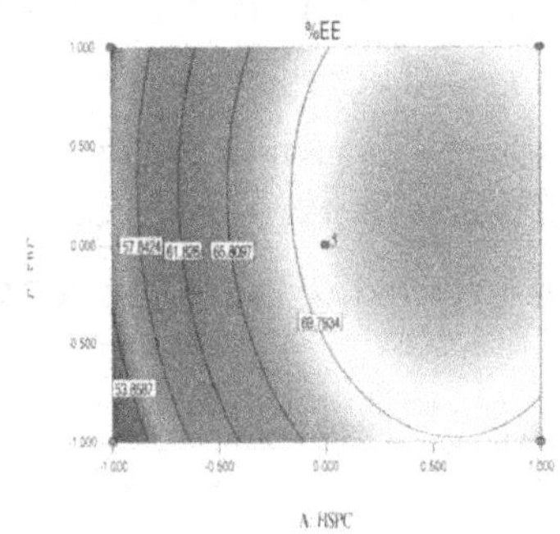

(b)

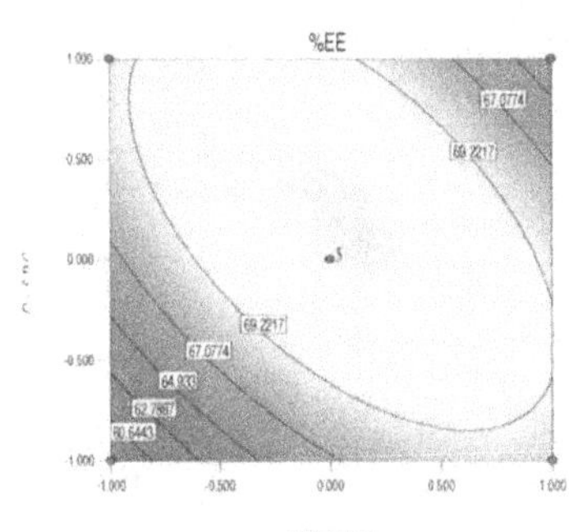

(c)

ANOVA

The three factors with lower and upper design points in coded and uncoded values are shown in Table: 4.1 and Table: 4.3. All the responses observed for fifteen runs were fitted to various models using Design- Expert software in RSM. It was observed that the best-fitted models were quadratic. The values of R^2, adjusted R^2, predicted R^2, Degree of freedom (Df), Sum of squares(SS) and Mean square(MS) are given in Table: 4.7 & Table: 4.8, along with the regression equation generated for each response. The results of ANOVA in Table: 4.7 & Table: 4.8 for the dependent variables demonstrate that the model was significant for both the response variables. It was observed that all the three independent variables *viz* A (Temperature), B (Pressure) and C (CO_2 Flow rate) had a negative effect on particle size (Y1), but, a mix effect on yield (Y2). The mathematical relationship for the same in terms of a polynomial equation relating the response Y and independent variables was: $Y= +850.00 -100.00*A -101.88* B -621.88*C -7.50*A* B +112.50*A* C -126.25*B*C -61.87*A^2-25.62*B^2+329.37*C^2$ and $Y = +53.33-9.25*A+3.25*B+7.25*C-5.75*A*B -1.25*A*C+3.25*B*C-13.79*A^2-3.29*B^2+0.71*C^2$ ......Equation [4.5] & Equation [4.6] for particle size and yield respectively.

The similar equation for formulation parameter was $Y=+71.20+8.75*A+1.13*B+1.38*C-1.50*A* B-0.50*A*C-3.75*B*C-7.73*A^2-3.48* B^2-2.97*C^2$ Where Y is the % EE

......Equation [4.7]

Table: 4.7. Analysis of Variance for BBD Model of Process parameters

Parameters		Df	SS	MS	R^2	AdjR^2	PredR^2	F	Lack of fit
Particle size	Model	9	3.808E+006	4.231E+005	0.9834	0.9536	0.8123	0.0006	0.4636
	Residual	5	64156.25	12831.25	-	-	-	-	-
Yield	Model	9	2104.93	233.88	0.9856	0.9598	0.8003	0.0004	0.2193
	Residual	5	30.67	6.13	-	-	-	-	-

*Df- Degree of freedom
SS- Sum of squares
MS-Mean square
F- Significance

Table: 4.8. Analysis of Variance for BBD Model of formulation parameters

Parameters		Df	SS	MS	R^2	AdjR^2	PredR^2	F	Lack of fit
%EE	Model	9	1073.69	119.30	0.9866	0.9694	0.8232	0.0001	0.0648
	Residual	7	14.55	2.08	-	-	-	-	-

A key obstacle to liposome and other colloidal delivery using phospholipids frequently is limited by their rapid detection and removal from blood by layer and basement membrane of blood vessels to the Mononuclear Phagocytic System (MPS) (Lasic, et al., 1993, Senior et al., 1992 & Strom et al., 1993). In late 1980s, some feedback comes on the in vivo fate of liposomes by work from two independent teams, *Allen et al, 1989 and Gabizon et al 1988.* In their work, inclusion of small proportion of glycolipids in bilayer had a remarkable effect in lengthening the blood residence time. This long circulation time of the liposomes was correlated with the accumulation of the same in the tumor implanted in the suitable model. Initially the term *"Stealth®"* was coined on the basis of avoidance of rapid detection and uptake by MPS. Later on the term *"Stearically stabilized"* become popular due to their enhanced stability and reduced reactivity to plasma proteins and cell surface receptor. In early stages, neutral phospholipids and high concentration of cholesterol along with small portion of acidic phospholipids were used to avoid their in vivo recognition. High content of cholesterol provided stability in presence of plasma proteins and negative charge of acidic phospholipids helps to render aggregation and at the same time increase encapsulation of drug in the liposomes.

Individual work by Papahadjopoulos and coworkers first reported the ability of specific glycolipids such as ganglioside [GM1], cerebroside sulfate or phosphatidylinositol [PI] to increase the half life of vesicles in blood, since all the molecule have negative charge and are shielded by large carbohydrate residue which possibly provided stearic stabilization. The mechanism accounting for the long circulation of the pegylated liposomes is supposed to be that the bulky polyethylene glycol (PEG) head group served as a barrier preventing interactions with plasma opsonins as a result of its concentration of highly hydrated groups that sterically inhibit hydrophobic and electrostatic interactions of a variety of blood components at the liposome surface, as described by *Ceh et al. 1997*. The main questions for construction of such a platform are how to get high encapsulation efficiency for many drugs. DSPE- PEG 2000 was used as polymer to provide stearic layer on the surface of vesicles. Different mol % of DSPE- PEG 2000 was incorporated in the bilayer and effect on percent encapsulation efficiency of DC liposomes was studied (Table: 4.18).

4.5. Preparation of Nanoparticles

Nanoparticles are defined as particulate dispersions or solid particles with a size in the range of 10-1000nm. The drug is dissolved, entrapped, encapsulated or attached to a nanoparticle matrix. Depending upon the method of preparation, nanoparticles, nanospheres or nanocapsules can be obtained. Nanocapsules are systems in which the drug is confined to a cavity surrounded by a unique polymer membrane, while nanospheres are matrix systems in which the drug is physically and uniformly dispersed. In recent years, biodegradable polymeric nanoparticles, particularly those coated with hydrophilic polymer such as poly(ethylene glycol) (PEG) known as long-circulating particles, have been used as potential drug delivery devices because of their ability to circulate for a prolonged period time target a particular organ, as carriers of DNA in gene therapy, and their ability to deliver proteins, peptides and genes (Mohanraj, V.J. et al., 2006). There are a variety of nanoparticles systems currently being explored for cancer therapeutics (Haley, et. al., 2008). There is an increased interest in developing biodegradable nanoparticles since they offer a suitable means of delivering small molecular weight drugs, proteins or genes by either localized or targeted delivery to the tissue of interest (Moghimi, S.M. et al., 2001) The types of nanoparticles currently used in research for cancer therapeutic applications include dendrimers, liposomes, polymeric nanoparticles, micelles, protein nanoparticles, ceramic nanoparticles, viral nanoparticles, metallic nanoparticles, and carbon nanotubes. (Byrne, J.D. et al., 2008). Amongst these nanoparticulate delivery systems polymeric nanoparticles have shown promising properties for targeted drug delivery and for sustained action. Nanoparticles are colloidal systems that range in size typically from 10 to 1000 nm in diameter, and are formulated from a biodegradable polymer in which the therapeutic agent is entrapped in, adsorbed or chemically coupled onto the polymer matrix (Labhasetwar, V. et al., 1997). Biodegradable polymers are unique tools for the preparation of nanoparticles, owing to their low toxicity profiles. (Si shen feng et al., 2004) Despite the potential promise of cyanoacrylate polymers for brain targeting, the clinical safety of cyanoacrylates has not yet been established. Although a number of different polymers have been investigated for formulating biodegradable nanoparticles, polyepsilon caprolactone (PCL), poly (lactide-co-glycolide) (PLGA) and poly lactic acid (PLA), FDA approved biocompatible and biodegradable polymers, have been the most extensively studied (Langer, R. et al., 1997 and. Jain, R.A. et al., 2000).

Nanoparticles can be prepared by polymerization of monomers entrapping the drug molecules leading to *in situ* polymerization or from preformed polymers. Several techniques have been suggested to prepare the biodegradable polymeric nanoparticles from preformed polymers such as poly (D, L-lactide) {PLA}, poly (D, L-glycolide) {PGA} and poly (D,L-lactide-co-glycolide) {PLGA}. Various methods proposed for the preparation of PLGA nanoparticles include emulsification/solvent evaporation, solvent displacement/diffusion (nanoprecipitation), emulsification/solvent diffusion and salting out using synthetic polymers. Solvent diffusion (nanoprecipitation method) leads to the nanoparticles of uniform size and narrow size distribution. *Fessi et al 1989* PVA is used as stabilizer to form particles of relatively small size and uniform size distribution (Sahoo et al., 2002 and. Scholes, P.D. et al., 1993).

4.5.1. Method of Preparation

DC encapsulated PLGA nanoparticles were prepared by using emulsion-solvent evaporation technique (Kompella, U.B. et al., 2001). Briefly, the drug and polymer (different drug: polymer ratios) were added to dichloromethane, and the contents were allowed to stand at room temperature for 30 to 45 min with occasional stirring to allow complete solubilization of the drug and the polymer. This solution was poured into an aqueous PVA solution (0.5%-1.5%) and the resulting mixture was stirred with the help of high speed homogenizer (Ultra-turaxx, T-25, Ultrapure Scientific, Mumbai) to get a primary O/W emulsion. The primary emulsion was passed through high pressure homogenizer (Emulsiflex, C5, Avestin, Canada). The homogenized O/W emulsion was allowed to stir overnight with a magnetic stirrer (Remi Equipments, Mumbai) to evaporate the methylene chloride. Nanoparticles were recovered by centrifugation for 30 min at 25000 rpm, washed two times with distilled water to remove unentrapped drug and PVA, and then lyophilized for 24 hrs using different types and concentrations of cryoprotectants.

4.5.2. Optimization of process variables:

Based on the results obtained in preliminary experiments, number of homogenization cycles and homogenizing pressure were found to be the major variables in determining the particle size and entrapment efficiency. Hence, the primary emulsion as described in 4.5.1 was subjected to different number of cycles and different pressures to find the optimized process parameters for lowest particle size and highest % EE. The results are recorded in Table: 4.9.

Table: 4.9. Optimization of process variables

Batch No.	No of cycles	Homogenizing pressure (MPa)	DC-NPs	
			Particle size (nm)	% EE
1	1	45	4000±10	60±2.0
2	2	45	2200±15	53±2.5
3	3	45	1150±9	35±2.1
4	1	70	2500 ± 10	62±2.1
5	2	70	1100 ± 8	54±1.8
6	3	70	850 ± 8	37±2.0
7	1	105	950 ± 15	61±1.5
8	2	105	460 ± 10	54±2.4
9	3	105	280 ± 7	34±2.0
10	1	125	410 ± 12	62±2.2
11	**2**	**125**	**220 ± 5**	**53±2.3**
12	3	125	180 ± 2	36±1.8

The optimized process parameters were kept constant and the formulation parameters were further optimized by the BBD of Response surface methodology.

Table: 4.10. Variables in Box Behnken Design

X_i	Independent variables	Units	Coded values			Response (Y1)
			-1	0	1	
A	Drug	% w/w	1	1.5	2	% Entrapment efficiency
B	Polymer	% w/w	2	6	10	
C	PVA	% w/v	1	1.5	2	

Table: 4.11. Matrix of Box Behnken Design for optimizing formulation parameters

Std	Run	Factor A Drug concentration	Factor B Polymer concentration	Factor C PVA concentration	%EE	P%EE	run
11	1	1.5	2	2	20.2±1.3	32.125	11
4	2	2	10	1.5	53.1±1.5	8.125	14
15	3	1.5	6	1.5	45.2±2.1	73.875	6
10	4	1.5	10	1	66.3±2.6	49.875	2
7	5	1	6	2	57.3±1.2	60.375	15
3	6	1	10	1.5	72.4±2.3	33.375	16
14	7	1.5	6	1.5	42.1±1.9	53.625	5
16	8	1.5	6	1.5	41.3±2.2	32.625	12
17	9	1.5	6	1.5	45.2±1.8	12.5	10
9	10	1.5	2	1	14.3±0.9	65.75	4
1	11	1	2	1.5	29.4±1.4	20.25	1
8	12	2	6	2	31.3±1.5	50.5	13
12	13	1.5	10	2	49.2±1.2	43.2	17
2	14	2	2	1.5	10.3±0.3	43.2	7
5	15	1	6	1	62.4±1.4	43.2	3
6	16	2	6	1	30.3±2.1	43.2	8
13	17	1.5	6	1.5	43.2±1.4	43.2	9

4.5.3. Method of Preparation using solvent diffusion technique

The nanoparticles of the drugs Docetaxel (DC) was also prepared by using the solvent diffusion (nanoprecipitation) technique (Fessi et. al, 1989). The method was optimized for process parameters followed by formulation parameters. The basic process parameters standardized were the speed of the magnetic stirrer and rate of addition of organic phase to aqueous phase. The rate of addition of organic phase was kept at 0.5ml/min throughout the entire optimization process as per the literature. The speed of the stirrer was standardized using qualitative examination of nanoparticle dispersion. The process parameters were standardized using placebo batches without drug. The standardization of stirrer speed is enumerated in Table: 4.12.

Table: 4.12 Influence of Stirring Speed

Sr. No.	Stirrer speed	Observation
1	Low	Non uniform dispersion
2	Moderate	Uniform dispersion
3	High	Aggregation in the dispersion

The critical formulation parameters considered for optimization were drug: polymer ratio, % PVA concentration and organic: aqueous phase ratio. Briefly, 5mg DC and PLGA (25mg, 50mg and 100mg corresponding to different drug: polymer ratio of 1:05, 1:10 and 1:20) were added to acetone to make organic: aqueous phase ratio of 01:04, 01:03 and 01:02 equating to 0.25, 0.33 and 0.5 respectively in decimal values). The organic phase containing drug and polymer was injected at 0.5mL/min into vortex 10ml of aqueous phase containing PVA (0.5, 1 and 1.5%w/v) as stabilizer on a magnetic stirrer (Remi Equipments, Mumbai). With the diffusion of solvent in to the aqueous phase, the polymer precipitates while encapsulation of DC also occur leading to formation PLGA-DC-NP. The resulting nanoparticle dispersion was further stirred to evaporate the organic phase. NPs were recovered by centrifugation for 30 min at 25000 rpm, washed thrice with distilled water to remove unentrapped drug and excess PVA.

4.5.4. Optimization of formulation parameters

Table: 4.13. Variables in Box Behnken Design

X_i	Independent variables	Units	Coded values			
			-1	0	1	Response
A	Polymer concentration*	mg	1	2	3	% Entrapment efficiency
B	PVA concentration	%w/v	1	1.5	2	
C	Organic to Aqueous phase ratio	-	0.2	0.35	0.5	

*Polymer concentration 1, 2 & 3 denotes 25, 50 & 100 mg, respectively

Table: 4.14. Matrix of Box Behnken Design for optimizing formulation parameters

Std	Run	Factor A: Polymer concentration mg	Factor B: PVA concentration %w/w	Factor C: Organic to Aqueous phase ratio	Particle size	%EE	Predicted particle size	Run	Predicted %EE	Run
14	1	2	1.5	0.35	165.2±3.1	47.2±1.8	159	14	39.125	14
5	2	1	1.5	0.2	150.3±1.8	33.3±1.6	172	5	56.625	5
7	3	1	1.5	0.5	140.2±1.4	29.2±2.1	143	9	37.375	9
15	4	2	1.5	0.35	164.5±3.2	45.3±1.8	166	10	58.875	10
2	5	3	1	0.35	170.6±3.3	55.4±1.5	151.25	2	33.875	2
8	6	3	1.5	0.5	157.3±3.1	49.5±2.2	173.25	12	54.375	12
16	7	2	1.5	0.35	164.2±1.9	46.4±1.9	141.75	3	29.625	3
13	8	2	1.5	0.35	162.4±2.1	46.2±3.1	155.75	6	48.125	6
3	9	1	2	0.35	145.3±2.2	39.4±1.2	169.75	17	60	17
4	10	3	2	0.35	165.2±1.8	59.5±2.1	156.75	11	56.75	11
10	11	2	2	0.2	156.4±2.2	56.6±3.2	154.25	15	51.25	15
6	12	3	1.5	0.2	175.6±2.1	55.2±1.5	145.25	16	55	16
17	13	2	1.5	0.35	162.4±2.4	45.3±1.6	163.4	8	45.8	8
1	14	1	1	0.35	160.3±1.9	39.4±2.3	163.4	1	45.8	1
11	15	2	1	0.5	155.3±2.5	52.2±1.4	163.4	4	45.8	4
12	16	2	2	0.5	145.5±2.2	54.3±2.1	163.4	7	45.8	7
9	17	2	1	0.2	170.6±4.1	61.4±1.8	163.4	13	45.8	13

4.5.5. Response surface and countour plots for Solvent evaporation method

Figure: 4.8. **3D-Response surface plot (a) and Contour plot (b) showing the effect of the amount of Drug (A) and Polymer (B) on the response Y (%EE) of NPs.**

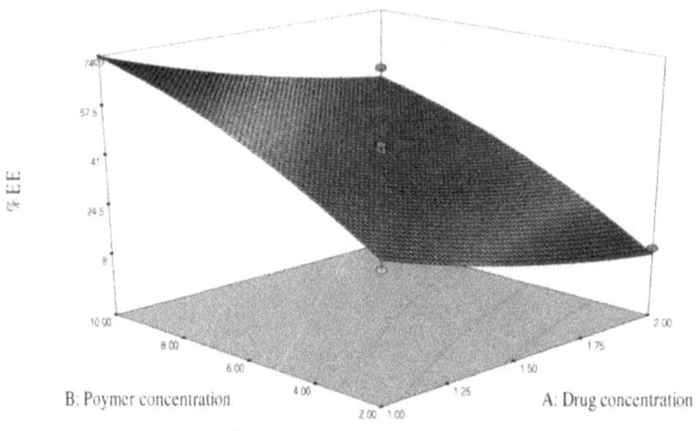

(a)

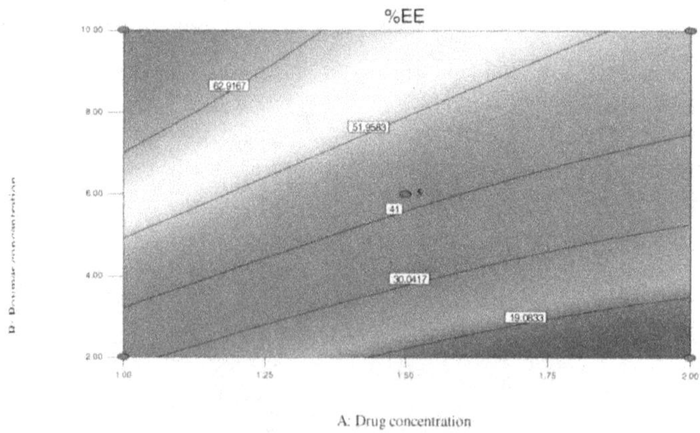

(b)

Figure: 4.9. **3D-Response surface plot (a) and Contour plot (b) showing the effect of the amount of Drug (A) and PVA (C) on the response Y (%EE) of NPs**

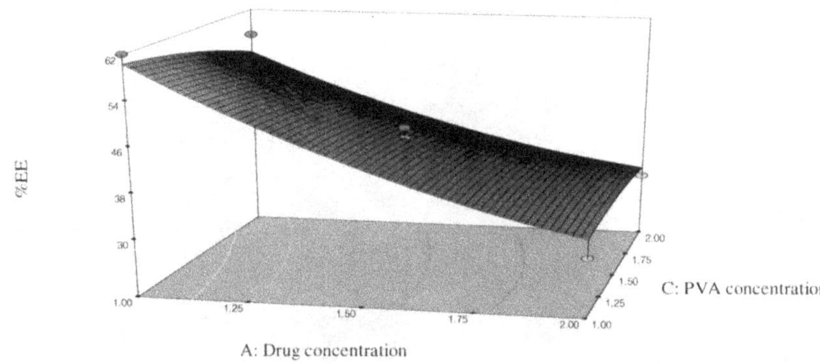

(a)

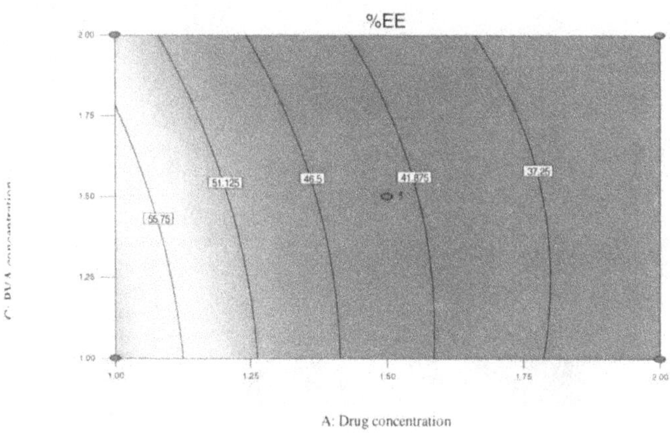

(b)

Figure: 4.10. **3D-Response surface plot (a) and Contour plot (b) showing the effect of the amount of Polymer (B) and PVA (C) on the response Y (%EE) of NPs.**

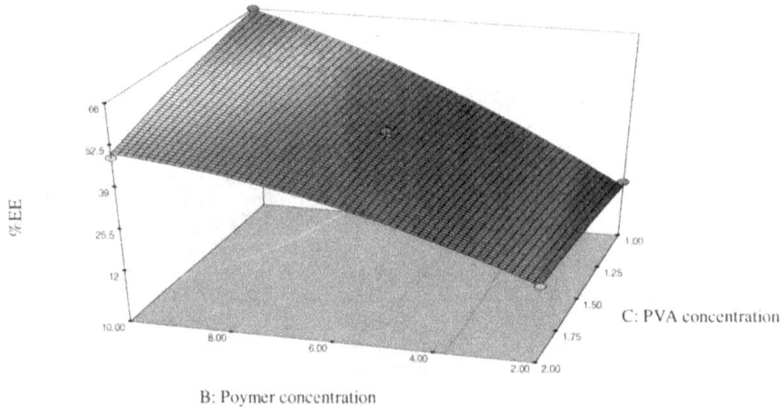

(a)

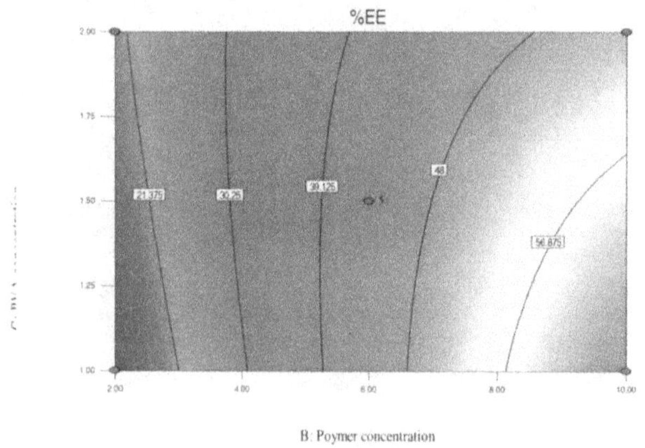

(b)

4.5.6. Response surface and countour plots for nanoprecipitation method

Figure: 4.11. **3D-Response surface plot (a) and Contour plot (b) showing the effect of the amount of Polymer (A) and PVA (B) on the response Y (particle size) of NPs**

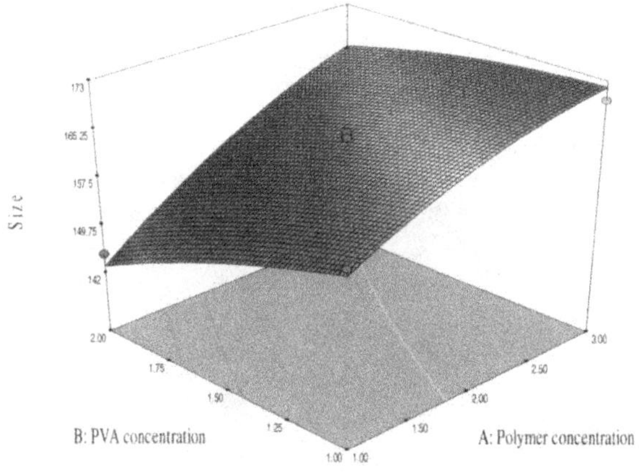

(a)

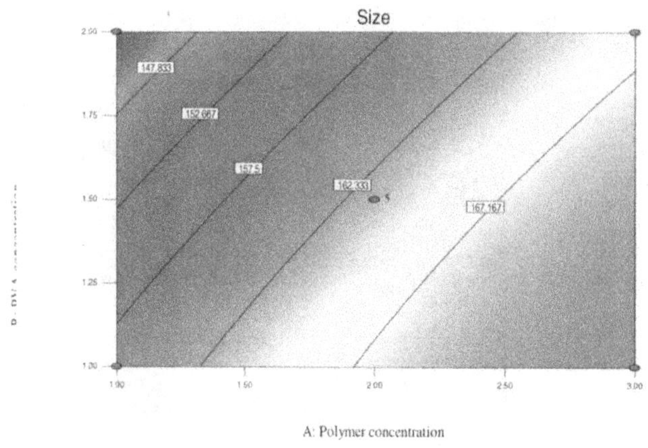

(b)

Figure: 4.12. **3D-Response surface plot (a) and Contour plot (b) showing the effect of the amount of Polymer (A) and Organic to Aq. Phase ratio (C) on the response Y (particle size) of NPs**

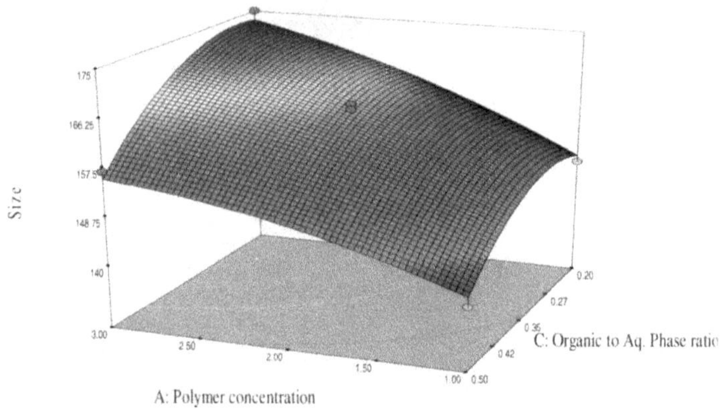

(a)

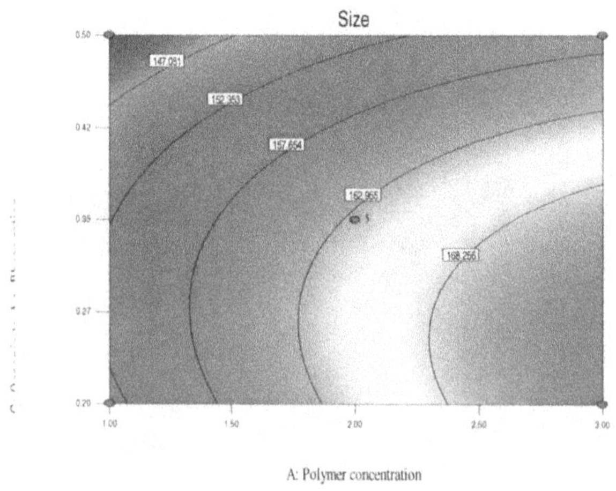

(b)

Figure: 4.13. **3D-Response surface plot (a) and Contour plot (b) showing the effect of the amount of PVA (B) and Organic to Aq. Phase ratio (C) on the response Y (particle size) of NPs**

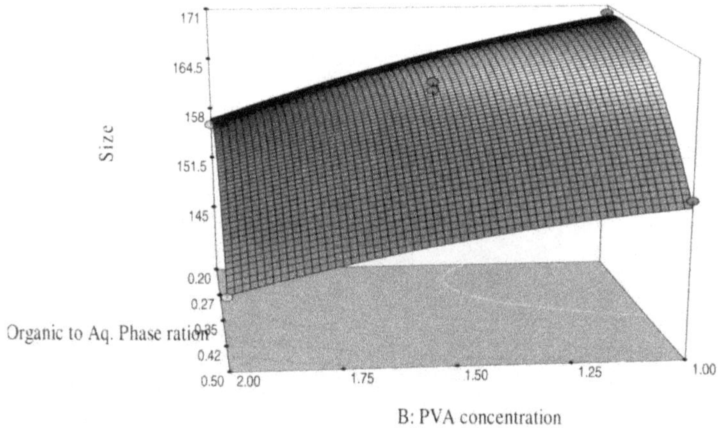

(a)

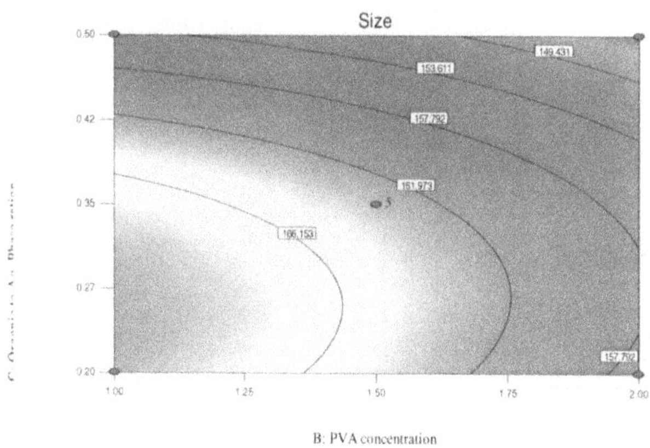

(b)

Figure: 4. 14. **3D-Response surface plot (a) and Contour plot (b) showing the effect of the amount of Polymer (A) and PVA (B) on the response Y (%EE) of NPs**

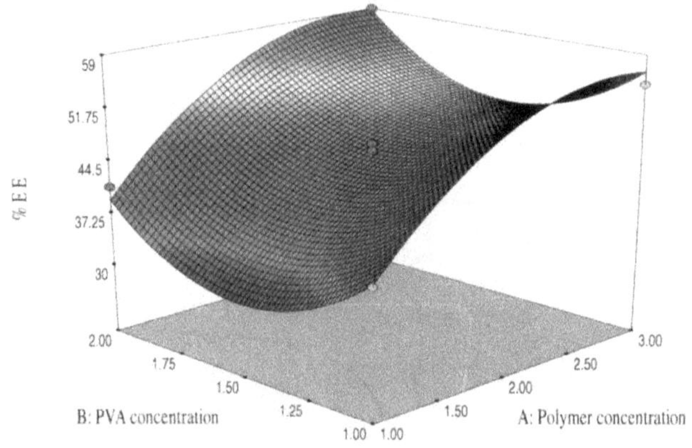

(a)

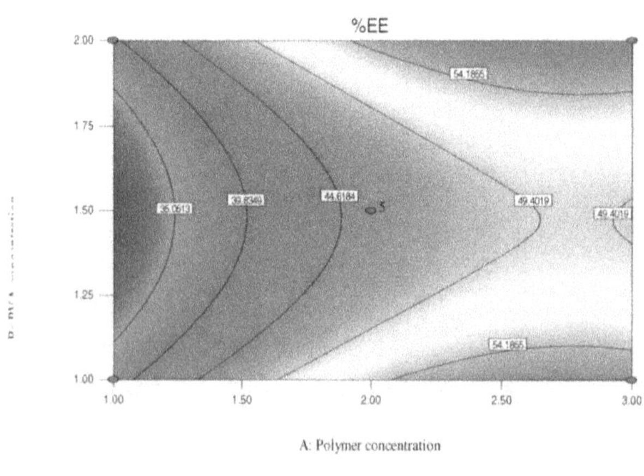

(b)

Figure: 4.15. **3D-Response surface plot (a) and Contour plot (b) showing the effect of the amount of Polymer (A) and Organic to Aq. Phase ratio (C) on the response Y (%EE) of NPs**

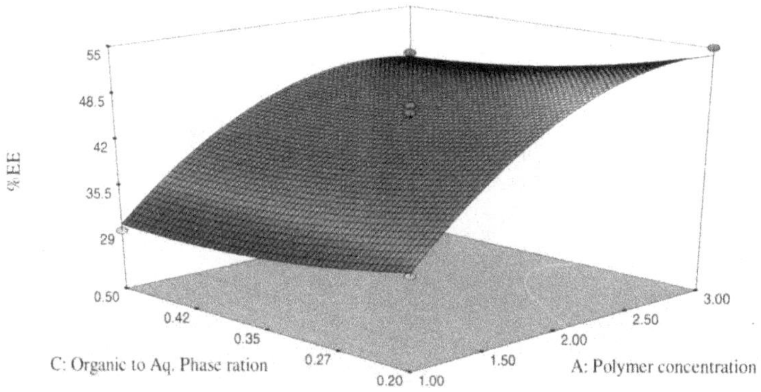

(a)

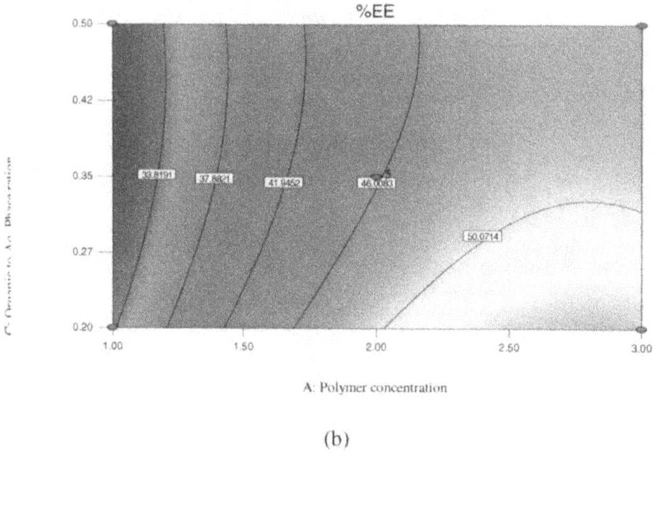

(b)

Figure: 4.16. **3D-Response surface plot (a) and Contour plot (b) showing the effect of the amount of PVA (B) and Organic to Aq. Phase ratio (C) on the response Y (%EE) of NPs**

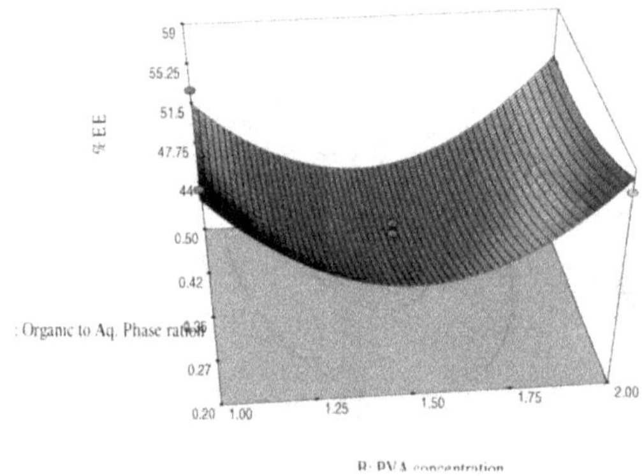

(a)

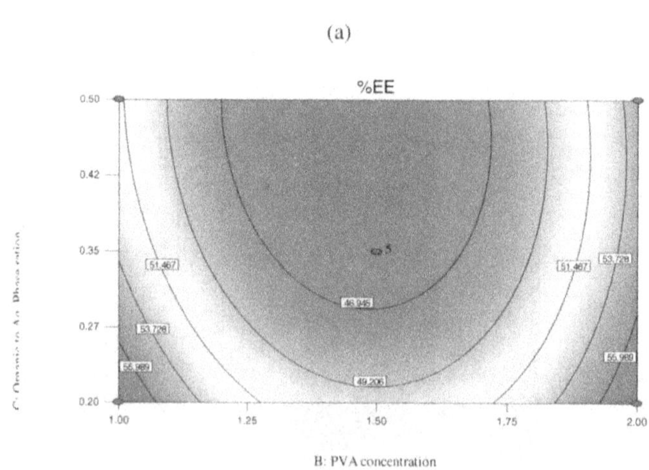

(b)

Table: 4.15. Analysis of Variance for BBD Model of formulation parameters for solvent evaporation method

Parameters		Df	SS	MS	R^2	AdjR^2	PredR^2	F	Lack of fit
%EE	Model	9	4943.48	549.28	0.9856	0.9672	0.8070	0.0001	0.0555
	Residual	7	72.05	10.29	-	-	-	-	-

*Df- Degree of freedom
SS- Sum of squares
MS-Mean square
F- Significance

Table: 4.16. Analysis of Variance for BBD Model of formulation parameters for nanoprecipitation method

Parameters		Df	SS	MS	R^2	AdjR^2	PredR^2	F	Lack of fit
Particle size	Model	9	1474.6	163.78	0.9816	0.9578	0.7741	0.0001	0.1151
	Residual	7	27.70	3.96		-	-	-	-
%EE	Model	9	1226.08	136.23	0.9873	0.9709	0.8290	0.0001	0.0553
	Residual	7	15.80	2.26	-	-	-	-	-

4.6. Lyophilization and optimization of cryoprotectant concentration

The nanoparticle & liposomal dispersions have thermodynamic instability upon storage and lead to the formation of aggregates. Freeze drying/lyophilization is one of the known methods to recover the nanoparticles & liposomes in the dried form and suitably redisperse it at the time of administration. To the suspension of the nanoparticles different cryoprotectants like sucrose, mannitol and trehalose were added in different concentrations at nanoparticle (NP): cryoprotectant (CP) ratio of 1:1, 1:2 and 1:3 before freeze-drying. The effect these cryoprotectants on the redispersibility of the freeze-dried formulations and the size of the nanoparticles & liposomes after freeze-drying was investigated and recorded in Table 4.19 & Table: 4. 20, respectively.

4.7. RGD attachment to PLGA nanoparticles

The Cyclic RGD peptide was conjugated to the surface of the PLGA nanoparticles by using a two step process as described by (Zhang et al., 2008). In the first step, the nanoparticles were activated using a sulfo NHS/EDC and in the second step the NH_2-

PEG-COOH was attached to the activated nanoparticles. The RGD was attached to pegylated nanoparticles by the same process with repetition of conjugation steps.

Step 1: Attachment of PLGA nanoparticle with bifunctional PEG

$$\text{i)}\quad \text{PLGA-COOH} + \text{NH2-PEG-COOH} \xrightarrow[\text{pH 5.5}]{\text{EDC/sulfo NHS}} \text{PLGA- PEG-COOH} \quad \text{.....Equation [4.8]}$$

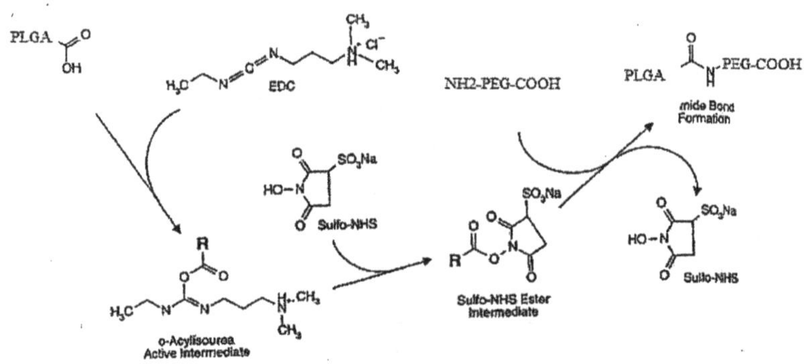

Step 2: Attachment of RGD peptide

$$\text{ii) PLGA- -PEG-COOH} + \text{RGD4c} \xrightarrow[\text{pH 5.5}]{\text{EDC/NHS}} \text{PLGA-PEG-RGD} \quad \text{.....Equation [4.9]}$$

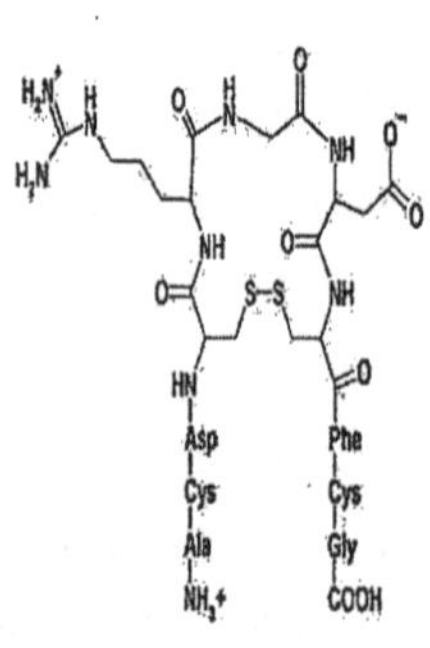

RGD 4C

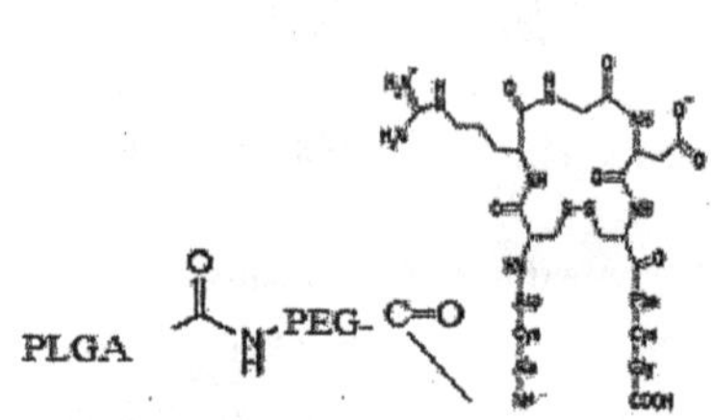

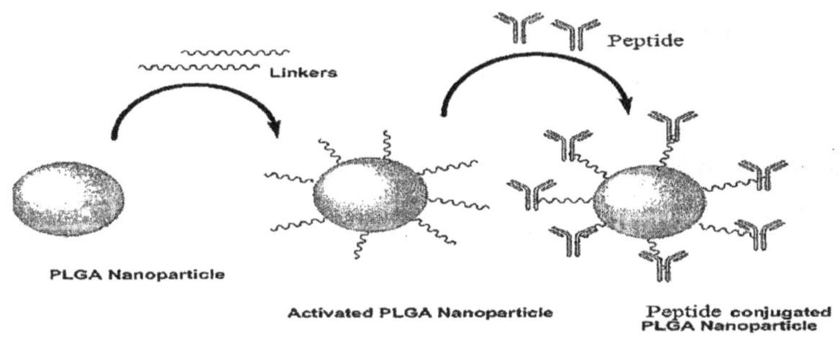

Briefly, 0.3, 0.7, 1.5 and 3mmol solution of NHS and 0.5, 1, 2 and 4 mmol of EDC in 20mM HEPES/NaOH buffer, pH 7.0, were added to a suspension of 5 mg nanoparticles in the same buffer and incubated for 2 hr at room temperature with gentle stirring. The activated nanoparticles were used to conjugate 10mg of NH_2-PEG-COOH. The resulting PLGA-PEG-COOH nanoparticles were washed twice with buffer used for conjugation of RGD. The same process of carboxyl group activation was repeated and 0.5,1 and 2 and 4 mg of RGD was used to achieve optimum conjugation with Pegylated nanoparticles. The NPs were centrifuged at 25,000 rpm for 30mins at 4°C, to remove the unreacted RGD. Finally, the particles were washed with 20mM HEPES/NaOH buffer, pH 7.0 and lyophilized for 24 hrs.

Deprotection of amine group

Deprotection of the amine of Fmoc-PEG_8-COOH was accomplished by stirring Fmoc-PEG_8-COOH in 1.5 mL of 20% piperidine in DMF for 2 h at room temperature. The solution was further subjected to extensive dialysis in 500 MWCO to ensure a complete removal of Fmoc before being lyophilized to dryness.

Influence of amount of activating agents

To check the influence of amount of activating agents on surface RGD conjugated by keeping the weight of nanoparticles (5 mg) and RGD taken for conjugation (200 μg) constant, different concentrations of activating agents were used and results were recorded in Table: 4.21 and Figure: 4.17 for docetaxel nanoparticles.

Influence of amount of RGD

To check the influence of amount of RGD taken for conjugation on surface RGD conjugated and conjugation efficiency, to 5 mg of activated nanoparticles, different concentrations of RGD was added and results recorded in Table: 4.22 & Figure: 4.18 for docetaxel nanoparticles.

Estimation of surface RGD density

To estimate the amount of RGD conjugated to the surface of PLGA-DC-NPs, the amount of RGD in the supernatant and the washings was subtracted from the amount of RGD taken for conjugation. The % conjugation efficiency (CE) was calculated using the following expression.

% CE = (Amount of RGD conjugated/RGD added for conjugation) * 100

RGD attachment to docetaxel encapsulated pegylated liposomes:

Cyclic RGD peptide was conjugated to the surface of the pegylated liposomes by the same method adopted for RGD conjugation to PLGA nanoparticles in the same section of 4.7.

4.8. Preparation of 6-coumarin loaded nanoparticles

Nanoparticles containing fluorescent containing dye 6-coumarin were formulated using the solvent evaporation and supercritical Antisolvent method. The dye acts as a fluorescent probe for NPs & LPs and offers a sensitive method to quantitatively determine their intracellular uptake (Panyam et al., 2003). A solution of 6-coumarin and PLGA in chloroform was emulsified into aqueous PVA solution. This primary emulsion was passed through high pressure homogenizer (Emulsiflex, C5, Avestin, Canada) for 2 cycles at 125 MPa pressure. The homogenized O/W emulsion was immediately added drop-wise to an aqueous PVA solution and the contents were stirred overnight with a magnetic stirrer (Remi Equipments, Mumbai) to evaporate the methylene chloride. Nanoparticles were recovered by centrifugation for 30 min at 25000 rpm, washed and lyophilized for 24 hrs. Results of characterization of 6-coumarin nanoparticles is tabulated and discussed in chapter 5. Similarly the process for liposomes were repeated by replacing the drug with 6-coumarina and keeping all the optimized process and formulation parameters same. Results of characterization of 6-coumarin nanoparticles are tabulated and discussed in chapter 5.

4.9. Results and discussion

4.9.1. Preparation of liposomes by supercritical fluid technology

The supercritical fluid technology with CO_2 as an Antisolvent provides easy and reproducible method for preparation of liposomes.

Optimization of process parameters

The effects of process variables like solute concentration and solvent flow rate were well studied and reported in literature (Magnan, C. et al., 2000 & Reverchon, E. et al., 1999) and our preliminary experiments also support these data. Hence, in ongoing section we have discussed the influence of temperature, pressure and CO_2 flow rate in detail. Three dimensional response surface plots generated by the Design Expert software are presented in Figures: 4.2, 4.4 & 4.6, while two dimensional contour plots are presented in Figures: 4.3, 4.5 & 4.7 for the studied responses, i.e. particle size and yield. The relationship between the dependent and independent variables were elucidated using contour and response surface plots by keeping the third factor at a same level.

The effect of A (temperature) and B (pressure) and their interaction on Y at a fixed level of C are given in contour plot shown in Figure: 4.2: (a) & Figure: 4.3 (a) and response surface shown in Figure: 4.4 (a) & Figure: 4.5 (a). As shown in figures, at mean level of A (Temp at 40°C), particle size decreases from 780nm to 255nm and yield increases from 51 to 67%w/w when the amount of Pressure (B) Increases from 100 to 220bar. Similarly, at higher level of A (at 46 °C), particle size and yield decrease from 460nm to 324nm and from 36 to 23%w/w respectively when B increases from 160 to 200bar. The effect of A and C and their interaction on Y at a fixed level of B are given in Figure: 4.2: (b) & Figure: 4.3 (b) and Figure: 4.4 (b) & Figure: 4.5 (b), shows that at mean level of A (at 40 °C), particle size decreases from 1800nm to 780nm and yield increases from 44 to 67%w/w when the C increases from 30 to 120gm/min. The effect of B and C and their interaction on Y at a fixed level of A are given in Figure: 4.2: (c) & Figure: 4.3 (c) and Figure: 4.3 (c) & Figure: 4.4 (c), shows that at lower level of B(at 100 bar), particle decreases from 1800nm to 780nm and yield increases from 41 to 51 %w/w when the C increases from 30 to 120gm/min. Similarly, at higher levels of B (at 220 bar), particle size decreases from 1780 to 255nm while yield increases from 44 to 67%w/w when C increases from 30 to 120gm/min.

The influence of CO_2 flow rate, temperature and pressure on the particle size and yield of Liposomes:

It has been observed that the increase in CO2 flow rate results in decrease in particle size and increase in the yield of the SC-LP. The possible explanation for this is the high mixing energy and fine atomization of solvent droplets in the stream of SC-CO2 at high flow rate. Generally, a higher mixing energy leads to smaller particles of spherical morphology. Due to the high flow rate, the incoming solvent droplet converts in to fine form and the supercritical fluid removes the organic solvent and leaves behind the small particles in the vessel. As a result of the rapid removal of organic solvent from each droplet, the solute precipitates faster in the high pressure vessel and it is a factor responsible for high yield. It has been found that, as the pressure increases at high temperature the particle size and yield decreases. While at the pressure increases at moderate temperature the particle size decreases but yield increases. The pressure of the SC-CO_2 in the high pressure vessels depicts its quantity. This means at high pressure, more amount of CO_2 is available in the vessel. The proportion of CO_2 directly affects the process of supersaturation for the particle production. The high amount of CO_2 hastens the supersaturation process and results in the precipitation of small particles with spherical morphology. The temperature has significant ($p<0.05$) influence on the yield but non-significant ($p>0.05$) influence on particle size. With increase in temperature along with high pressure, yield decreases might be because of the low T_g (49°C) of the mix lipid system. It is known from the literature that the SC-Co_2 lowers the T_g of the polymers (Conway, S.E. et al., 2001, Sparacio, D. et al., 1998 & Mandel, F.S. et al., 2002). We are anticipating the similar effect responsible for low yield of the final product. The process variables with minimum particle size and maximum yield were considered as optimum and kept constant for further processing.

Table: 4.17. Percent Entrapment Efficiency and Particles size of DC liposomes using various lipids

Types of Lipids	Lipid composition	%EE	Particle size (nm)
HSPC:Chol	9:1	68.5±3.2	255.2±3.2
	8:2	Flocculation	
	7:3	Flocculation	
DMPC:Chol	9:1	69.5±6.5	265.4±3.6
	8:2	63.6±3.4	257.3±4.2
	7:3	Flocculation	
DPPC:Chol	9:1	61.5±4.1	272.2±3.9
	8:2	64.7±5.3	258.5±2.8
	7:3	Flocculation	

In case of Hydrogenated Soya Phosphatidyl Choline [HSPC], in molar ratio of 9:1 with cholesterol the percent entrapment was found to be 68.5±3.2 % and particle size 255.2±3.2 nm. Increase in cholesterol ratio to 8:2 and 7:3 leads to flocculation and formation of free drug crystals. To improve encapsulation of DC in the liposomal bilayer, other synthetic saturated lipids used were Dimyristoyl phosphatidyl choline [DMPC] and Dipalmitoyl phosphatidyl choline [DPPC]. The maximum entrapment was observed 69.55±6.5 % with DMPC and 64.7±5.3 %with DPPC. The results are listed in Table: 4.17.

The three components of the liposomal bilayer i.e. lipids, cholesterol and DC increase the hydrophobicity and this leading to partial hydration and ultimate results in flocculation. *Bernsdorff et al 1999* in the different experiments observed that paclitaxel loaded liposomes remains stable only for 2 days in a drug/lipid ratio of 4 mole%, further increases concentration of paclitaxel up to 8 mole% it precipitate out as needle shaped crystal and similar problem has occurred at the time of hydration. Also this study reveals that paclitaxel, a hydrophobic drug, incorporated in liposomes is thermodynamically prone to self aggregation, then precipitating from liposomes. The stability of the bilayer was observed with low drug to lipid ratio but this ratio is unsuitable for clinical applications as higher lipid may exhibit some level of toxicity and also increase the cost of production. It becomes necessary to design a liposomal system which encapsulate higher amount of drug in minimum possible lipid to avoid above mentioned drawbacks.

The use of mix lipid systems:

Optimization of formulation parameters:

Liposomes were prepared by supercritical fluid Antisolvent (SAS) technique using SPC/drug/HSPC. Process parameters, such as operating temperature, pressure and flow rate of the SCF were optimized and kept unaltered in subsequent experiments. In order to optimize formulation parameters, a Box Behnken Design (BBD) of RSM was used. Seventeen batches of SCF-LP were prepared by SAS process using a 3-factor, 3-level BBD varying three independent variables (mole % of HSPC, mole % of cholesterol, and mole % of SPC) of the formulation according to Table: 4.6a & Table: 4.6b. The influence of these variables on observed response (Y, %EE) is recorded in Table: 4.6b. Each batch of SCF-LP was prepared three times and was evaluated for %EE. The maximum response as %EE was 72 and minimum response was 50. The mathematical relationship for the same in terms of a polynomial equation relating the response Y and independent variables was: $Y= Y=+71.20+8.75*A+1.13*B+1.38*C-1.50*A*B-0.50*A*C-3.75*B*C-7.73*A^2-3.48*B^2-2.97*C^2$ for %EE. ......Equation [4.10]

Equation expresses the quantitative effect of the individual formulation components (A, B, and C) and combination thereof on the response (Y) in terms of interaction coefficients. The values of the coefficients A to C are related to the effect of these variables on the response (Y). Coefficients with more than one factor term and those with higher order terms represent interaction terms and quadratic relationships respectively. A positive and negative signs suggest a positive and negative effect on response respectively. The theoretical (predicted) values and the observed values were in reasonably good agreement as seen from Table: 4.6b. The significance of the ratio of mean square variation due to regression and residual error was tested using analysis of variance (ANOVA). The ANOVA indicated a significant ($P < 0.05$) effect of factors on response. Lack of fit was not significant ($p = 0.0648$) and regression was strongly significant ($p = 0.01$, $R^2 = 0.9866$). Also the predicted R^2 is 0.82 %EE, which is very good for chosen factorial model. So it was concluded that the second-order model adequately approximated the true surface.

The effect of A (amount of HSPC) and B(amount of cholesterol) and their interaction on Y at a fixed level of C(amount of SPC) are given in Figure: 4.6a & Figure: 4.7a shows that at lower levels of A, %EE increases from 50 to 53% when the amount of Cholesterol

(B) Increases from 0.5 to 1.5 %. Similarly, at higher levels of A, %EE decreases from 70 to 67% when B increases from 0.5 to 1.5%. The effect of A and C and their interaction on Y at a fixed level of B are given in Figure: 4.6b & Figure: 4.7b shows that at lower level of A, % EE increases from 50 to 53% when the C increases from 2 to 4% and at higher level of A, %EE increases from 69 to 70% when the C increases from 2 to 4%. The effect of B and C and their interaction on Y at a fixed level of A are given in Figure: 4.6c & Figure: 4.7c shows that at lower level of B, %EE increases from 57 to 68 % when the C increases from 2 to 4%. Similarly, at higher levels of B, % EE decreases from 69 to 65% when C increases from 2 to 4%. The formulation variables with maximum %EE were considered as optimum for further processing.

In our initial trials, we found difficulty in hydration during the preparation of liposomes for docetaxel with saturated lipid (HSPC). Hence, we applied a mix lipid system containing unsaturated lipid (SPC) and saturated lipid with cholesterol. In mix lipid system, the saturated phospholipids and cholesterol provide the rigidity to the membrane and hence improve the stability while unsaturated phospholipid improves the hydration through its polar head groups. The drug entrapment was found to be increase from 72.82±2.18% to 81.4±4.6% with decrease in drug to total lipid ratio from 1:15 to 1:20 mole % in an optimized batch. However, further decrease in drug to total lipid ratio from 1:20 to 1:25mole% did not have any significant effect on %EE. Hence, 1:20 mole % was considered as an optimum drug to total lipid ratio for maximum drug entrapment.

Effect of DSPE-PEG$_{2000}$-COOH on particle size and % EE

The Different mol % of DSPE- PEG 2000 was incorporated in the bilayer and effect on percent encapsulation efficiency of DC liposomes was studied (Table: 4.18). It was found that 6 mol % of DSPE-PEG$_{2000}$-COOH incorporated in liposomes gave optimum entrapment i.e. 79.2±4.4 % among the other molar percentage tried. The percent entrapment was found from 81±4.6 and %, 75.8±2.2%, to their respective molar percent 2 and 8 mole % of DSPE-PEG$_{2000}$-COOH. Entrapment was decreases to 75.8±2.2% when 8 mol % of the polymer was incorporated in the liposome composition. Fall in the percent entrapment was supported by theory that the hydrophobic chain of DSPE-PEG$_{2000}$-COOH would align with the hydrophobic chain of lipids in bilayer and therefore competes with the DC to accommodate in bilayer. There was no significant effect on the particle size observed when the ratio of polymer increased up to 8 mole%. The particle size was found in the range of 260 to 274 nm.

Table: 4.18. Effects of PEGylation on %EE and Particle Size

Composition	%EE	Particle Size [nm].
SPC: HSPC: Cholesterol	81.4±4.6	260.3± 2.4
$DSPE-PEG_{2000}-COOH$ in Mol%		
2	81.4±1.4	265.4± 2.8
4	80.2±2.8	267.2 ± 3.6
6	79.2±4.4	269.2 ± 2.6
8	75.8±2.2	274± 3.2

(Mean ± S.D., *n* = 3)

***Drug to lipid ratio was 1:20 mole %**

4.9.2. Preparation of Nanoparticles by SOLVENT EVAPORATION

Several techniques have been reported to prepare the biodegradable polymeric nanoparticles from preformed polymers such as poly (D,L-lactide) (PLA), poly (D,L-glycolide) (PLG) and poly (D,L-lactide-co-glycolide) (PLGA). Some of the commonly used preparation methods are emulsion-evaporation, double solvent evaporation, salting out, emulsification/diffusion, solvent displacement and nanoprecipitation. Emulsion-evaporation is one of the most frequently used methods yielding spherical nanoparticles with smooth surfaces and hence was used to prepare nanoparticles

Optimization of Process variables

The process parameters *viz.* homogenization pressure and no. of cycles were optimized for maximum %EE and minimum particle size <250nm. The homogenization pressures along with no. of cycle in respect of particle size were found to be inversely proposal. As we increased the pressure and no. of cycle, the particle size was decreasing. However, the % EE was also decreasing with increase in no. of cycles. Hence, the 125MPa pressure and 2 no. of cycles were optimized to get particle size of 220 ± 5nm and % EE of 53±2.3

Optimization of formulation variables

The mathematical relationship for the same in terms of a polynomial equation relating the response Y and independent variables was:

$$\%EE = +43.20-12.00*A+20.88*B-1.88*C+0.000*A*B +1.50*A*C-5.75*B*C+2.77*A^2-4.98*B^2 \quad \text{Equation [4.11]}$$

Equation expresses the quantitative effect of the individual formulation components (A, B, and C) and combination thereof on the response (Y) in terms of interaction coefficients. The values of the coefficients A to C are related to the effect of these variables on the response (Y).

The relationship between the dependent and independent variables was further elucidated using contour and response surface plots. The effect of A and B and their interaction on Y at a fixed level of C are given in Figure: 4.8a & Figure: 4.8b. As shown in Figure: 4.8a, at lower levels of A, %EE increases from 29 to 72% when the amount of Polymer (B) Increases from 2 to10 %. Similarly, at higher levels of A, %EE increases from 10 to 53% when B increases from 2 to 10%. Figure: 4.9a & Figure: 4.9b shows that at lower level of A, % EE decreases from 62 to 57% when the C increases from 1 to 2% and at higher level of A, %EE increases from 30 to 31% when the C increases from 1 to 2%. Figure: 4.10a & Figure: 4.10b shows that at lower level of C, %EE increases from 14 to 66 % when the B increases from 2 to 10%. Similarly, at higher level of C, %EE increases from 20 to 49 % when the B increases from 2 to 10%

The highest %EE achieved was 72.4 ± 4.6 % with particle size of 240 ± 3 nm for DC-NPs. This was at low level of A (1%), high level of B (10%) and at medium level of C (1.5%). The drop in the particle size and higher % EE with the increase in PVA concentration is probably due to the differences in the stability of the emulsions formulated with different concentrations of PVA. Further, the viscosity of PVA solution increases with increasing PVA concentrations. This could result in the formation of a stable emulsion with smaller and uniform droplet size, leading to the formation of smaller sized nanoparticles. There was not much reduction in particle size or increase in %EE when the PVA was increased from 1.5 to 2%. Hence, drug: polymer ratio 1: 10 and 1.5% w/v PVA as an emulsifier were taken as optimized parameters for the preparation of NPs for further studies.

The nanoparticles were negatively charged, which is attributed to the presence of ionized carboxyl groups on the surface of the nanoparticles. (Stolnik, S. et al., 1995). But, the zeta potential values were higher for nanoparticles prepared with 0.5% PVA compared to those prepared with 2% PVA. In several other studies, a clear differentiation in the zeta potential values of coated and non-coated nanoparticles has been reported, with high negative zeta potential values for non-coated nanoparticles and less negative zeta potential values for coated nanoparticles. It has been reported that the zeta potential of PLGA nanoparticles without any PVA in neutral buffer is about −45 mV (Stolnik, S. et al., 1995). This high negative charge is attributed to the presence of uncapped end carboxyl groups of the polymer at the particle surface. Coating of nanoparticles with some amphiphilic polymers normally decreases the zeta potential because the coating layers shield the surface charge and move the shear plane outwards from the particle surface (Hawley, A.E. et al., 1997 & Tobio, M. et al., 1998). Redhead et al. have reported a similar reduction in the zeta potential of PLGA nanoparticles after coating with amphilphilic polymers like poloxamer 407 and poloxamine 908 (Redhead, H.M. et al., 2001). Thus, the PVA layer at the surface of the nanoparticles also probably shielded the surface charge of PLGA. Since the amount of residual PVA is relatively lower in case of nanoparticles prepared with 0.5% PVA, less shielding and therefore higher zeta potential was observed in these nanoparticles.

To optimize the process parameters for lowest particle size and highest % entrapment efficiency, the primary emulsion was subjected to different number of homogenization cycles and pressures. The results recorded in Table: 4.9 show that when the pressure was kept constant, the particle size and the % entrapment efficiency decreased with the increase in number of homogenization cycles from one to three. Increase in the pressure from 45 to 125MPa also decreased the particle size as well as the entrapment efficiency. With the decrease in particle size, the total surface area of the particles increases resulting in diffusion of drug from the particles. This may be the reason for decreased entrapment with decrease in particle size. Two cycles at 125MPa was found to be the optimized process parameter. Further increase in the number of cycles resulted in lower particle size which was also accompanied by decreased entrapment efficiency.

4.9.3. Preparation of Nanoparticles by Nanoprecipitation

Optimization of process parameters

The process parameters such as the stirrer speed and rate of addition of organic phase affect the formation of the nanoparticles. As commonly reported in the literature (Fessi et al., 1989 & Derakhshandeh et al., 2007) the rate of addition of the organic phase to the aqueous phase was kept constant at 0.5ml/min. The speed of stirring was evaluated for the formation of nanoparticles. The process was executed at slow, moderate and high speed of the stirrer and the observations are tabulated in Table: 4.14. At moderate speed of the stirrer there was uniform nanoparticle dispersion with no particle aggregation. However, at slow speed the vortex formation was inadequate and hence leads to the deposition of the solids at the surface of the aqueous phase. At high stirrer speed there was aggregation of the nanoparticles. This may be due to the high shear causing insufficient stabilization of nanoparticles and causing particle aggregation. Hence the all the batches further were prepared at the moderate speed of the stirrer.

Optimization of formulation parameters

The mathematical modeling equation for size and %EE are as below:

Size =+163.40+9.00*A-5.50*B-6.75*C+2.50*A*B-2.00*A*C+1.00*B*C-2.20*A^2-1.20*B^2-5.70* C^2.......Equation [4.12]

R^2=0.9816, lack of fit=0.1156, Pred. R^2=0.7741

%EE=+45.80+9.50*A+0.75*B-2.50*C+0.25*A*B-0.75*A*C+0.75*B*C-6.02*A^2+8.47*B^2+1.48*C^2.......Equation [4.13]

R^2=0.9873, lack of fit=0.0553, Pred. R^2=0.8290

The relationship between the dependent and independent variables was further elucidated using contour and response surface plots. The effect of A and B and their interaction on Y at a fixed level of C are given in Figure: 4.11a & Figure: 4.11b and Figure: 4.14a & Figure: 4.14b. As shown in Figure: 4.11a & Figure: 4.14a at lower levels of A , particle size decreases from 162nm to 145nm and %EE decreases from 41 to 38%w/w when the amount of PVA decreases from 2 to 1%. Similarly, at higher levels of A, particle size decreases from 170 to 165nm and %EE increases from 55 to 59%w/w when B increases from 1 to 2%. Figure: 4.12a & Figure: 4.12b and Figure: 4.15a & Figure: 4.15b shows that at lower level of A, particle size decreases from 150 to 140nm and %EE decreases from 33 to 29%w/w when the C increases from 0.20 to 0.50. Similarly at higher level of A particle size decrease from 175 to 157 nm and %EE decreases from 55 to 48% when the C increases from 0.20 to 0.50. Figure: 4.13a & Figure: 4.13b and Figure: 4.16a & Figure: 4.16b shows that at lower level of B, particle decreases from 170 to 155nm and %EE decreases from 59 to 53 %w/w when the C increases from 0.2 to 0.5. Similarly, at higher levels of B, particle size decreases from 156 to 145nm while %EE decreases from 57 to 54%w/w when C increases from 0.2 to 0.5..

In this study, the main parameters affecting the nanoparticle formulation were found to be polymer concentration (keeping the amount of the drug constant), %w/v PVA concentration in aqueous phase and the ratio of the organic: aqueous phase (represented in decimal form). Hence, polymer concentration, %w/v PVA concentration and organic: aqueous phase ratio were selected as independent variables to find the optimized condition for small particle size (PS) and highest % drug entrapment efficiency (%EE) using a BBD of Response Surface Methodology (RSM)

Influence of the Polymer (PLGA) Concentration

For DC nanoparticles, the increase in the concentration of PLGA resulted in the increase in the particle size of the nanoparticles. The viscosity of the organic phase in which the PLGA is dissolved appears to affecting the nanoparticles size due to hindrance in rapid dispersion of PLGA solution into the aqueous phase and resulted increase in the droplet and nanoparticle size. (Chorny, et al., 2002) Availability of PVA on the surface of nanoparticles prevents the aggregation of nanoparticles during solvent evaporation but due to higher PLGA concentration, deposition of PVA on the particle surface may not be uniform and sufficient leading to aggregation. Increase in concentration of PLGA increases the drug entrapment efficiency for DC. It may be due to increase in drug entrapping polymer and due to the decrease in the diffusion of the drug towards the aqueous phase (Song et al., 2008 a & b).

Influence of PVA concentration

The increase in the PVA concentration leads to increase of particle size of nanoparticles. This increase in the nanoparticles size may be due to increase in the viscosity of the aqueous phase thereby increasing the resistance to the diffusion rate of the organic phase. The miscibility of organic phase (acetone) with aqueous phase results in orientation of PVA at the interface of PLGA solution in acetone present as droplets in the system (Sahoo et al., 2002). The increase in the PVA concentration leads to enhanced orientation of PVA towards PLGA and hence increases in the particle size. The drug entrapment efficiency was also found to increase with increase in the PVA concentration. This increase in the drug entrapment efficiency may be probably due to reduction in diffusion rate of the organic phase in the aqueous phase.

4.9.4. Lyophilization of Nanoconstructs

The results for lyophilization of nanoparticles and liposomes are shown in Table: 4.19 and Table: 4.20, respectively.

Table 4.19: Effect of different cryoprotectants on the particle size and redispersion of Nanoparticles

Type of cryoprotectant	NP: CP	Particle size (nm)		S_f/S_i	Redispersion
		Before lyophilization S_i	After lyophilization S_f		
Initial	1:0	230.7 ± 2.3	NA	NA	NA
Sucrose	1: 1	--	--	--	Poor redispersibility
Sucrose	1:2	--	570.4 ± 14.6	2.47	Poor redispersibility
Sucrose	1:3	--	431.5 ± 13.8	1.87	Poor redispersibility
Mannitol	1: 1	--	451.3 ± 16.8	1.95	Difficult redispersibility
Mannitol	1:2	--	372.4 ±12.7	1.61	Difficult redispersibility
Mannitol	1:3	--	325.6 ± 14.7	1.41	Difficult redispersibility
Trehalose	1: 1	--	283.5 ± 12.6	1.22	Easy redispersibility
Trehalose	1:2	--	262.4 ± 15.4	1.13	Easy redispersibility
Trehalose	1:3	--	237.8 ± 7.9	1.03	Easy redispersibility

(Mean ± S.D., n = 3)
NA: Not Applicable

Table 4.20: Effect of different cryoprotectants on the particle size and redispersion of liposomes

Type of cryoprotectant	LP: CP	Particle size (nm)		S_f/S_i	Redispersion
		Before lyophilization S_i	After lyophilization S_f		
Initial	1:0	278.4±5.2	NA	NA	NA
Sucrose	1: 1	--	--	--	Poor redispersibility
Sucrose	1:2	--	711.5 ± 21.5	2.55	Poor redispersibility
Sucrose	1:3	--	615.4 ± 12.5	2.21	Poor redispersibility
Mannitol	1: 1	--	427.6 ± 15.9	1.53	Difficult redispersibility
Mannitol	1:2	--	452.6 ±15.8	1.62	Difficult redispersibility
Mannitol	1:3	--	386.5± 16.8	1.38	Difficult redispersibility
Trehalose	1: 1	--	326.5± 11.7	1.17	Easy redispersibility
Trehalose	1:2	--	308.9 ± 14.3	1.10	Easy redispersibility
Trehalose	1:3	--	291.4 ± 12.5	1.04	Easy redispersibility

(Mean ± S.D., n = 3)
NA: Not Applicable

In aqueous suspensions, the chemical and physical stability of nanoparticles has been reported to be poor (Saez, A. et al., 2000 & Konan, Y.N. et al., 2002).Freeze-drying has been the most utilized drying method of nanoparticle suspensions. Because the freeze-drying process is highly stressful for nanoparticles, addition of cryoprotectants becomes essential. For nanoparticles carbohydrates have been perceived to be suitable freeze-drying protectants. There are considerable differences in the cryoprotective abilities of different carbohydrates. It has been proposed in case of liposomes that sugars preserve membrane structure (cryoprotection) by hydrogen bonding to the phospholipid head group and effectively replacing the bound water.

The optimized batch of nanoconstructs was lyophilized using sucrose, mannitol and trehalose (at 1:1, 1:2 and 1:3 nanoconstructs: cryoprotectant) to select suitable cryoprotectant and its concentration. The redispersibility of the freeze-dried formulations and particle size of the nanoconstructs before and after freeze-drying were evaluated and recorded in Table: 4.19 and Table: 4.20.

When sucrose was used as a cryoprotectant, at all concentrations studied, the redispersion of freeze-dried NPs was difficult due to the formation of flakes or aggregates and also there was substantial increase in particle size after lyophilization. The Sf/Si values were 2.47 and 1.87 with 1:2 and 1:3 NPs: sucrose, respectively. For liposomes, the Sf/Si values were 2.55 and 2.21 with 1:2 and 1:3 LPs: sucrose, respectively. The increase in the particle size could have been due to the cohesive nature of the sucrose. Further, it was observed that the lyophilized nanoparticles with sucrose had tendency to absorb moisture very quickly.

With mannitol, the nanoparticle formulation showed free flowing ability, however the redispersion was difficult and possible only after vigorous shaking. The Sf/Si values were 1.95, 1.61 and 1.41 with 1:1, 1:2 and 1:3 NPs:Mannitol respectively. For liposomes, the Sf/Si values were 1.95, 1.61 and 1.41 with 1:1, 1:2 and 1:3 LPs: Mannitol, respectively.

With trehalose as cryoprotectant, the lyophilized nanoparticles were redispersed easily and the increase in particle size was not significant as indicated by S_f/S_i values which were 1.22, 1.13, and 1.03 for 1:1, 1:2 and 1:3 NPs: trehalose respectively recorded in table 4.13. For liposomes, the Sf/Si values were 1.17, 1.10 and 1.04 with 1:1, 1:2 and 1:3 LPs:trehalose respectively. The redispersion of the nanoparticles depends on the hydrophilicity of the surface. The easy redispersibility is probably due to the higher solubility of trehalose in water i.e. 0.7 parts in 1 part of water. The cryoprotective effect may be attributed to the ability of trehalose to form a glassy amorphous matrix around the particles, preventing the particles from sticking together during removal of water (Konan et al 2002). Furthermore, trehalose, a non-reducing disaccharide of glucose, has previously exhibited satisfactory cryoprotective effects for pharmaceutical and biological materials.

4.9.5. RGD conjugation of nanoparticles and Liposomes

Several strategies have been employed for surface modifications of PLGA-NPs & DC-LPs. RGD-modified PLGA-NPs & LPs have been employed to provide cytoadhesive/cytoinvasive character to NPs & LPs. The surface modification of PLGA-NPs with RGD was achieved in two steps using carbodiimide coupling method. This active ester method yields stable amide bonds. As a prerequisite, the polymer has to contain free carboxyl groups at the surface as represented by the H-type of PLGA which are activated by carbodiimide/N-hydroxysuccinimide. In contrast to the activation of carboxyls with only carbodiimide, the presence of N-hydroxysuccinimide yields N-hydroxysuccinimide esters as stable intermediates which rather acylate amino groups of proteins than to be subject of hydrolysis in aqueous medium (Grabarek, Z. et al., 1990). The amounts of activating agents (EDAC/NHS) and RGD were optimized to achieve minimum particle size and maximum RGD density on the surface of NPs.

Table: 4.21. Influence of amount of RGD

Amt of RGD added (mg)	RGD Density (µg/mg) PLGA-DC-NP
0.5	6.2 ± 1.7
1	11.9±2.5
2	26.4±3.5
4	30.2 ± 4.5

Table: 4.22. Influence of Concentration of Activating Agents

Batch no	Activating agents	RGD density (µg/mg)
	EDC/SulfoNHS (mmol/mmol)	
1	0.5/0.3	5.3±1.8
2	1/0.7	14.2 ± 3.7
3	2/1.5	26.4 ± 3.5
4	4.0/3.0	28.2 ±4.7

Figure: 4.17. Influence of Concentration of Activating Agents

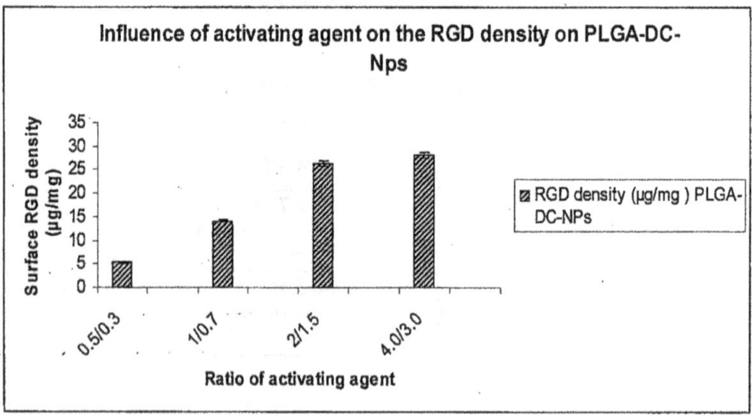

Figure: 4.18. Influence of amount of RGD

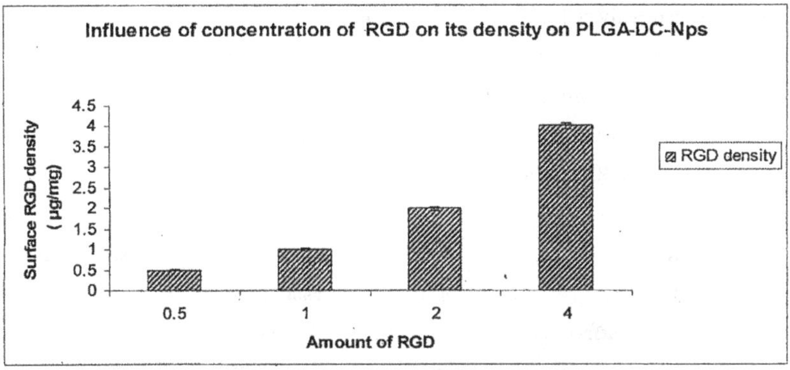

Figure: 4.19. Influence of Concentration of Activating Agents

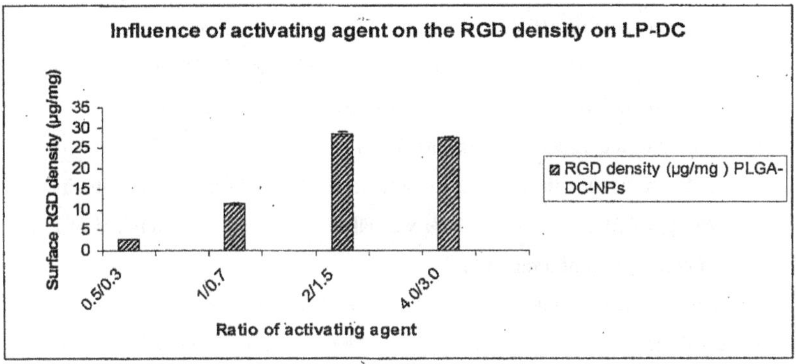

Figure: 4.20. Influence of amount of RGD

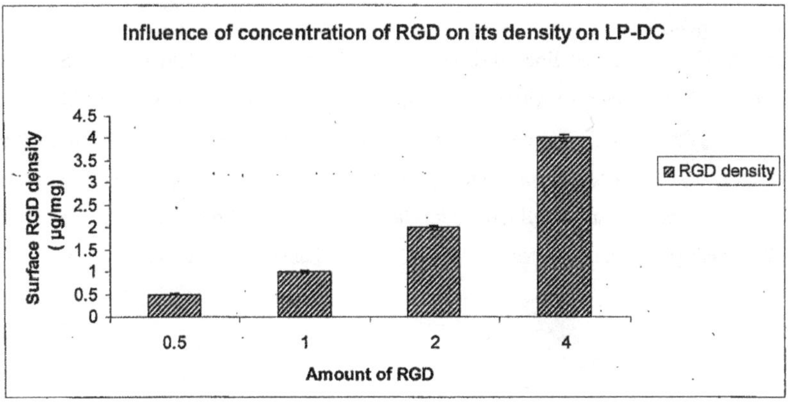

To check the influence of concentration of activating agents on density of surface RGD, 5 mg of NPs were activated with different concentrations of EDAC/NHS, and the density of surface RGD and particle size of conjugated NPs were measured (Table: 4.19). It was found that at 0.5/0.3 mmol EDAC/NHS, the surface bound RGD was detectable for conjugated NPs of DC. Increase of EDAC/NHS concentration from 1/0.7 mmol to 2/1.5 mmol increased the RGD density of PLGA-DC-NPs from 14.2 ± 3.7 to 26.4 ± 3.5 µg/mg of nanoparticle surface and further increase in the concentration of EDAC/NHS did not increase the RGD density significantly. The presence of the protein on the surface, as well as the loss of the fine particles during processing caused the NPs to increase in mean particle size after surface modification. Therefore 2/1.5 mmol EDAC/NHS was taken as the optimized concentration for the activation of PLGA-DC-NPs for the conjugation process.

To maximize conjugation efficiency, different amounts of RGD solution were added to 5 mg of activated PLGA-DC-NPs and the density of conjugated RGD was measured (Table 4.20). For PLGA-DC-NPs as the amount of RGD was increased from 0.5 to 4 mg, the density of conjugated RGD /NPs increased from 6.2 ± 1.7µg/mg to 30.2 ± 4.5 µg/mg. However, the % conjugation efficiency was found to be insignificant with increased amounts (4mg) of RGD. Therefore, 2mg was taken as the optimized amount of RGD to be used for conjugation of 5 mg of PLGA-DC-NPs.

The influences of concentrations of activating agents and amount of RGD on its density on docetaxel encapsulated liposomes have been demonstrated in Figure: 4.19 and Figure: 4.20 respectively.

4.10. Conclusions

Docetaxel encapsulated liposomes comprising of mix lipid system (HSPC, SPC and DSPE-PEG) and Nanoparticles of PLGA were successfully prepared by supercritical fluid technology with CO_2 as an anti-solvent method and solvent evaporation method respectively. The nanoparticles and liposomes were surface conjugated with RGD for preferential breast cancer cell targeting. The particle observed for both unconjugated and RGD conjugated nanoparticles was below 300nm suitable for intravenous administration.

4.11. References

Allen, T.M. et al., 1989, Liposomes with prolonged circulation times: factors affecting uptake by reticuloendothelial and other tissues, Biochim Biophys Acta, **19; 981(1)**, 27-35.

Bernsdorff, C. et al, 1999, Interaction of the anticancer agent Taxol (paclitaxel) with phospholipid bilayers, J. Biomed. Mater. Res., **46(2)**, 141-149.

Byrne, J.D. et al, 2008, Advanced Drug Delivery Reviews, **60**, 1615–1626.

Castor, et al., 1996, Method and Apparatus for making Liposomes, **5**,554, 382 9.

Ceh B et al., 1997, A Rigorous Theory of Remote Loading of Drugs into Liposomes: Transmembrane Potential and Induced pH-Gradient Loading and Leakage of Liposomes, J. Colloid. Interface. Sci., **1;185 (1)**, 9-18.

Chorny M. et al, 2002, Lipophilic drug loaded nanospheres prepared by nanoprecipitation: effect of formulation variables on size, drug recovery and release kinetics, Journal of Controlled Release, **83**, 389–400.

Conway, S.E.et al, 2001, Poly (lactide-co-glycolide) solution behavior in supercritical CO_2, CHF3, and $CHClF_2$, J. Appl. Polym. Sci., **80**, 1155-1161.

Derakhshandeh K. et al, 2007, Encapsulation of 9-nitrocamptothecin, a novel anticancer drug, in biodegradable nanoparticles: Factorial design, characterization and release kinetics, European Journal of Pharmaceutics and Biopharmaceutics, **66**, 34–41.

Fessi, H. et al, 1989, Nanocapsule formation by interfacial polymer deposition following solvent displacement, Int. J. Pharm., **55**, R1-R4.

Gabizon, A. Liposome formulations with prolonged circulation time in blood and enhanced uptake by tumors, Proc Natl Acad Sci U S A., **85(18)**, 6949-53.

Grabarek, Z. et al, 1990, Zero-length cross-linking procedure with the use of active esters, Anal. Biochem., **185**, 131– 135.

Haley, E. et al, 2008, Nanoparticles for drug delivery in cancer treatment, Urol. Oncol. **26 (1)**, 57–64.

Hawley, A.E. et al, 1997, Preparation of biodegradable, surface engineered PLGA nanospheres with enhanced lymphatic drainage and lymph node uptake, Pharm. Res., **14 (5)**, 657–661.

Jain, R.A et al, 2000, The manufacturing techniques of various drug loaded biodegradable poly(lactide-co-glycolide) devices. Biomaterials, **21**, 2475–2490.

Kompella, U.B. et al, 2001, Poly (lactic acid) Nanoparticles for Sustained Release of Budesonide, Drug Delivery Technology, **1**, 29–35.

Konan, Y.N. et al., 2002, Preparation and characterization of sterile and freeze-dried sub-200nm nanoparticles, Int. J. Pharm., **233**, 239–52.

Labhasetwar, V. et al, 1997, Nanoparticles for drug delivery, Pharm. News, **4**, 28–31.

Langer, R. et al, 1997, Tissue engineering: a new field and its challenges, Pharm. Res., **14** 7, 840–841.

Magnan, C. et al, 2000, Soya lecithin micronization by precipitation with a compressed fluid antisolvent influence of process parameters, J. Supercrit. Fluids., **19**, 69–77.

Mandel, F.S. et al, 2002, Prolong release of drug prepare by treatment of supercritical fluid techniques, PCT. Int. Appl., WO0220624.

Moghimi, S.M. et al, 2001, Long-circulating and target specific nanoparticles: theory to practice, Pharmacol. Rev., **53** 2, 283–318.

Mohanraj, V.J. et al, 2006, Nanoparticles – A Review, Trop. J. Pharm. Res, **5 (1)**, 561-573.

Needham and Beech et al, Identification of Lysolipid Receptors Involved In Inflammatory Response, WO patent **99065466.**

Ram Gupta et al., 2006, Nanoparticle Technology For Drug Delivery, Taylor & Francis, Pharmaceutical Science, 336.

Redhead, H.M. et al, 2001, Drug delivery in poly (lactide-co-glycolide) nanoparticles surface modified with poloxamer 407 and poloxamine 908: in vitro characterization and in vivo evaluation, J. Controlled Release, **70** (3), 353–363.

Reverchon, E. et al, 1999, Biopolymers micronization by supercritical Antisolvent precipitation: influence of some process parameters, Proceedings of the Fifth Conference on Supercritical Fluids and their Applications, 473.

Saez, M. et al., 2000, Eur. J. Pharm.Biopharm, **50**, 379.

Sahoo, S.K. et al, 2005, Enhanced Antiproliferative Activity of Transferrin-Conjugated Paclitaxel-Loaded Nanoparticles Is Mediated via Sustained Intracellular Drug Retention Molecular Pharmaceutics, **2(5)**, 373-383.

Scholes, P.D. et al, 1993, The preparation of sub-200 nm poly(lactide-co-glycolide) microspheres for site-specific drug delivery, J. Controlled Release, **25**, 145–153.

Semmler, K. et al, 2000, The structure and thermotropic phase behaviour of dipalmitoylphosphatidylcholine codispersed with a branched-chain phosphatidylcholine, Biochim. Biophys. Acta., **20;1509(1-2)**, 385-396.

Si Shen Feng et al, 2004, Nanoparticles of biodegradable polymers for new-concept chemotherapy, Expert Reviews Medical Devices, **1 (1)**, 115-125.

Song, X. et al, 2008a, Dual agents loaded PLGA nanoparticles: systematic study of particle size and drug entrapment efficiency, European Journal of pharmaceutics and biopharmaceutics, **69**, 445-453.

Song, X. et al, 2008b, PLGA nanoparticles simultaneously loaded with vincristine sulfate and verapamil hydrochloride: Systematic study of particle size and drug entrapment efficiency, International Journal of Pharmaceutics, **350**, 320–329.

Sparacio, D. et al, 1998, Generation of microcellular biodegradable polymers using supercritical carbon dioxide, ACS Symposium Series 713. In: Solvent-Free Polymerization and Processes. Washington, DC: American Chemical Society, 181-193.

Stolnik, S. 1995, The colloidal properties of surfactant-free biodegradable nanospheres from poly (malic acid-co-benzyl malate)s and poly (lactic acid-co-glycolide). Coll. Surf., **97**, 235–245.

Tobio, M. et al, 1998, Stealth PLA–PEG nanoparticles as protein carriers for nasal administration, Pharm. Res., **15 (2)**, 270–275.

Chapter 5
Characterizations of Nanoconstructs

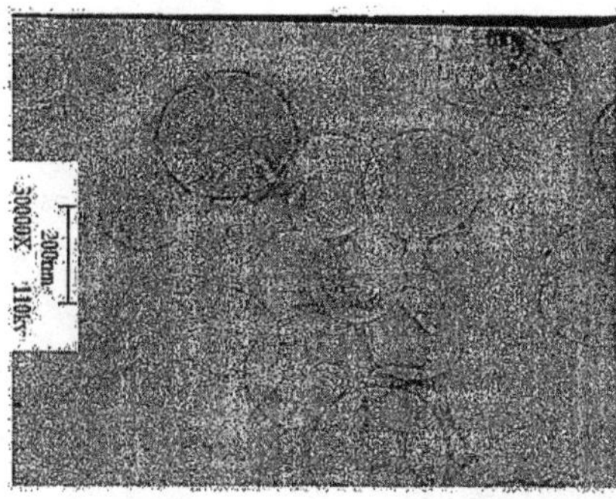

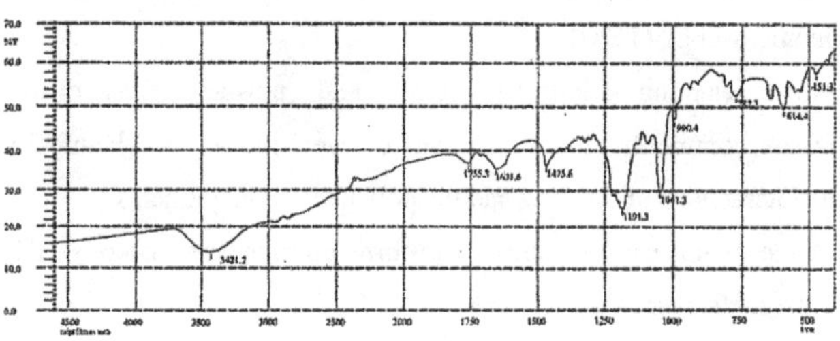

5.1. Introduction

Colloidal systems like nanoparticles and liposomes differ from macroscopic objects because of sub-micron properties such as high surface area and energy, and movement of the particles by diffusion (Brownian motion). The different behavior of nanoparticles and liposomes leads, to some extent, to the use of a different pattern of characterization methods. Extensive characterization of a nanoparticles system is essential for understanding and prediction of the performance of the system in the body. As the field of pharmaceutical nanoconstructs is evolving constantly; the need for more thorough characterization and comprehensive understanding of the systems increases.

Size, morphology and physical state of the encapsulated drug as well as MW and crystallinity of the polymer influence drug release and degradation of the nanoparticles. Meanwhile, size, surface charge and hydrophobicity/hydrophilicity are parameters that affect the body distribution and interactions with the biological environment. Stability of nanoconstructs are also a general issue governing the above mentioned properties.

Various techniques for characterization of nanoparticles include:

- Photon correlation spectroscopy (PCS), a technique based on dynamic (laser) light scattering, is widely used in size determinations of nanoconstructs.
- The surface charge of the particle was determined by Zeta(ζ) Potential measurement
- The determination of drug entrapment efficiency by techniques of spectrophotometry and chromatography gives the amount of drug present in the nanoconstructs.
- The surface morphology by scanning electron microscopy (SEM), transmission electron microscopy (TEM).
- Differential scanning calorimetry (DSC) and (powder) x-ray diffractometry (XRPD) are commonly used techniques to reveal the physicochemical state and possible interactions of the drug and the polymer in nanoparticles
- The surface chemistry by Fourier transform infrared spectroscopy (FTIR), and nuclear magnetic resonance spectroscopy (NMR).
- The surface hydrophilicity of the nanoparticles influences the cellular uptake and also the invivo pharmacokinetic behavior of the nanoparticles. (Sahoo, et. al., 2002) The PVA is estimated using the colorimetric iodine reaction estimated spectrophotometrically. (Joshi, D.P. et al., 1979)

Table: 5.1. Materials and Equipments

Material	Source
Water (distilled)	Prepared in laboratory by distillation
Bichinconinic acid (BCA) protein Assay Kit	Banglore Genei, India
Glacial acetic acid, potassium dihydrogen phosphate, disodium hydrogen phosphate, potassium chloride, potassium hydroxide, sodium chloride, sodium hydroxide.	S.D.Fine chemicals, Mumbai, India
HPLC grade methanol, glacial acetic acid, acetonitrile	S.D.Fine chemicals, Mumbai, India
Nuclepore Polycarbonate membrane 2 μm 25mm	Whatman, USA
Polyvinyl alcohol	Sigma Chemicals, USA
Equipments	**Make**
Calibrated pipettes of 1.0 ml, 5.0 ml and 10.0 ml, volumetric flasks of 10 ml, 25 ml, 50 ml and 100 ml capacity, Funnels (i.d. 5.0 cm), beakers (250 ml) and other requisite glasswares	Schott & Corning (India) Ltd., Mumbai
Analytical balance	AX 120, EL 8300, Shimadzu Corp., Japan
pH meter	$Pico^+$ Labindia, Mumbai, India
Cyclomixer, three blade stirrer	Remi Scientific Equipments, Mumbai
Cooling Centrifuge	3K 30, Sigma Laboratory centrifuge, Osterode, GmBH.
Lyophilizer	DW1, 0-60E, Heto Drywinner, Denmark
UV-Visible Spectrophotometer	Shimadzu UV-1601, Japan
Spectrofluorimeter	RF-540, Shimadzu corporation, Japan
Particle size and zeta potential analyzer	NanoZS, Malvern Instruments, U.K.
Transmission electron microscope	Morgagni, Philips, Netherlands
Differential Scanning Calorimeter	Mettler DSC 20, Mettler Toledo, Switzerland
HPLC system	Dionex HPLC with Chromleon 6.5 data processing software

5.2. Methods

5.2.1. Particle size and zeta potential: A 2.0 mg sample of nanoconstructs was suspended in distilled water, and the particle size and zeta potential were measured using the principle of laser light scattering with zeta sizer (Nano-ZS, Malvern Instruments, UK). The observations are tabulated in Table: 5.2 and Figures: 5.1 to Figure: 5.4.

5.2.2. Entrapment efficiency: To determine the amount of Docetaxel entrapped in the NPs, 2mg of NPs were added to 5 ml of methylene chloride and subjected to shaking at room temperature for 5 hrs to ensure complete dissolution of the particles. The resulting solution was evaporated to dryness, and the dried residue was reconstituted with 1 ml of mobile phase. The reconstituted solution was centrifuged and the supernatant was injected into the HPLC column. The % entrapment efficiency (EE) was calculated using the following expression.

% EE = (Amount of drug in the NPs/drug added in the formulation) * 100

The same process was repeated with liposomes with 5 ml of chloroform.

The results are recorded in Table: 5.2 & Table: 5.3 for nanoparticles and liposomes respectively

5.2.3. In-vitro drug release

The *in vitro* drug releases of the nanoconstructs of docetaxel were performed in phosphate buffer saline pH 7.4 + 0.1%w/v polysorbate-80 (Puglisi G., et al., 2006). Nanoconstructs equivalent to 1mg drug were suspended in 10 ml of release media in a screw capped tubes, which were placed in a horizontal shaker bath maintained at 37°C and shaken at 60min^{-1}. At fixed time intervals the tubes were taken out from the bath and centrifuged at 25,000 rpm for 30 min. The pellets were resuspended in 10ml of fresh PBS 7.4 + 0.1%w/v polysorbate-80 and placed back into the bath to continue release measurement (Feng et al., 2003b). For in vitro drug release study in serum the same process was repeated as above with the change of release media as 10ml of fetal bovine serum.

Results for In vitro release profile of DC encapsulated plain, and peptide tagged pegylated liposomes are tabulated in Table: 5.4 and Figure: 5.5. Results for In vitro release profile of DC encapsulated plain, and peptide tagged nanoparticles are tabulated in Table: 5.5

and Figure: 5.6. Results of in vitro serum study for nanoconstructs are shown in Figure: 5.7.

5.2.3. Transmission electron microscopy

Nanoconstructs were dispersed in de-ionized water at a concentration of 500μg/ml. To measure the morphology and size distribution of nanoparticles, a drop of sample was placed onto a 300-mesh copper grid coated with carbon. The grid was air-dried overnight to remove surface water. The images were taken for Nanoparticles without negative staining. While in case of liposomes, negative staining was performed using a droplet of 0.5% w/v phosphotungstic acid. Transmisssion electron microscopy was performed using Morgagni 268, Philips (Netherlands) transmission electron microscope. The TEM RGD conjugated nanoparticles and liposomes for docetaxel are shown in Figure: 5.8 and Figure: 5.9, respectively.

5.2.4. Surface morphology

The morphology was examined by scanning electron microscopy (SEM) (JSM-5610LV, JEOL, Japan). Samples were attached to sample stubs using double sided tape, and then viewed using an accelerating voltage of 15 kilovolt at the magnification of 250X to 20000X. Results are recorded in Figure: 5.10 and Figure: 5.11 for DC encapsulated nanoparticles and liposomes, respectively.

5.2.5 X- ray diffraction studies (XRD)

Powder X-ray diffraction patterns were obtained using an X-ray diffractometer (Philips PW 1710) with Cu Kα radiation generated at 30 mA and 40 kV. The source of X - ray was copper anode with a wavelength of 1.54060 Å. The XRD patterns were recorded for DC, PLGA, PLGA-DC NPs, PLGA-DC-RGD NPs, HSPC-SPC-DC LPs and HSPC-SPC-DC-RGD LPs. Results are recorded in Figure: 5.12 and Figure: 5.13 for nanoparticles and liposomes, respectively.

5.2.6. Differential Scanning Colorimetry:

The DSC of DC, PLGA, PLGA-DC NPs, PLGA-DC-RGD NPs, HSPC-SPC-DC LPs and HSPC-SPC-DC-RGD LPs was carried out by scanning the samples using differential scanning colorimeter (Mettler). Thermograms were analyzed using Mettler Toledo star SW 7.01. An empty aluminium pan was used as the reference for all measurements. During each scan, 2 to 3 mg of sample was heated, in a hermetically sealed aluminium pan, at a heating rate of 10° C/min, from 25° C to 300° C, under a nitrogen atmosphere.

Figures: 5.14 and Figure: 5.15 show the differential scanning colorimetric grams for nanoparticles and liposomes, respectively.

5.2.7. Determination of residual PVA

The amount of PVA associated with nanoparticles was determined by a colorimetric method based on the formation of a colored complex between two adjacent hydroxyl groups of PVA and an iodine molecule (Joshi, D.P. et al., 1979). Briefly, 2 mg of lyophilized nanoparticles sample was treated with 2 ml of 0.5 M NaOH for 15 min at 60 °C. Each sample was neutralized with 900 ml of 1 N HCl and the volume was adjusted to 5 ml with distilled water. To each sample, 3 ml of a 0.65 M solution of boric acid, 0.5 ml of a solution of I_2/KI (0.05 M/0.15 M), and 1.5 ml of distilled water were added. Finally, the absorbance of the samples was measured at 690 nm after 15 min incubation. A standard plot of PVA was prepared under identical conditions.

5.2.8. [1H]NMR of the RGD conjugated nanoconstructs

^{1}H-NMR spectroscopy was used to ascertain the conjugation of RGD to the nanoconstructs. The ^{1}H-NMR spectra of PLGA, PLGA-DC-RGD NPs, LPs and RGD-DC-LPs are shown in Figure: 5.16 a, b, c and d, respectively.

5.2.9 Infrared spectra of nanoparticles

Infrared spectra of the drug loaded unconjugated and the RGD conjugated nanoparticles and liposomes were obtained (Figure: 5.17a, b, c and d) and analyzed for confirmation of the RGD conjugation.

5.3. Results and Discussion:

5.3.1. Particle size, zeta potential and drug entrapment efficiency

The particle size, zeta potential and drug entrapment efficiency (%EE) for PLGA-DC-NP and PLGA-DC-RGD-NP are recorded in Table: 5.2. The particle size and zeta potential are shown in Figure: 5.1 and Figure: 5.2, respectively.

Table: 5.2. Characterization of optimized RGD conjugated and unconjugated PLGA nanoparticles of Docetaxel

Parameter	* PLGA-DC-NP	# PLGA-DC-PEG-NP	** PLGA-DC-PEG-RGD-NP
Mean particle size (nm)	210.3 ± 2.7	221.4 ± 1.6	230.7 ± 2.3
Zeta potential (mV)	-38.4 ± 2.6	-11.3±1.8	-10.2 ± 2.8
Entrapment efficiency (%)	71.6 ± 2.4 %	59.7 ± 3.3	58.4 ± 1.6

(Mean ± S.D., n = 3)
* PLGA-DC-NP- Docetaxel loaded PLGA nanoparticles
# PLGA-DC-PEG-NP –pegylated Docetaxel loaded PLGA nanoparticles
** PLGA-DC-PEG-RGD-NP- RGD conjugated docetaxel loaded PLGA nanoparticles

Figure: 5.1. Particle size distribution plots of docetaxel loaded PLGA nanoparticles, before and after RGD conjugation.

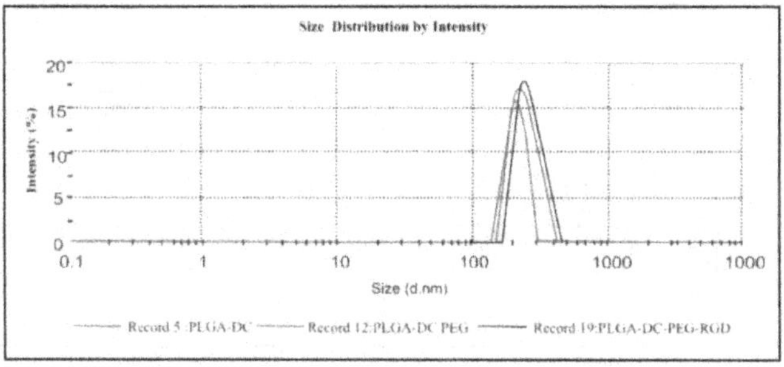

Figure: 5.2. Zeta Potential plots of docetaxel loaded PLGA nanoparticles, before and after RGD conjugation.

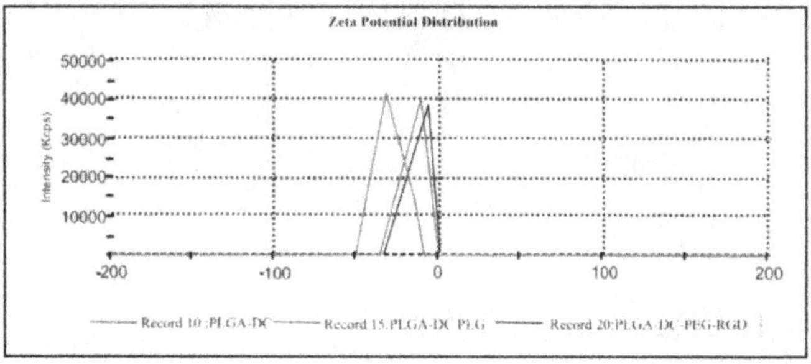

Figure: 5.3. Particle size distribution plots of docetaxel loaded Liposomes, before and after RGD conjugation.

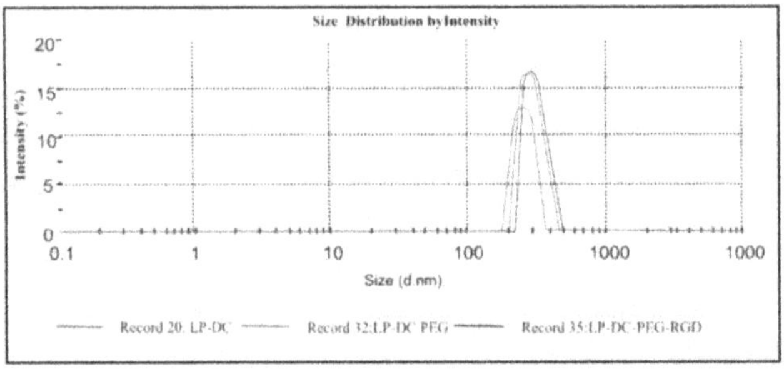

Figure: 5.4. Zeta Potential plots of docetaxel loaded liposomes before and after RGD conjugation.

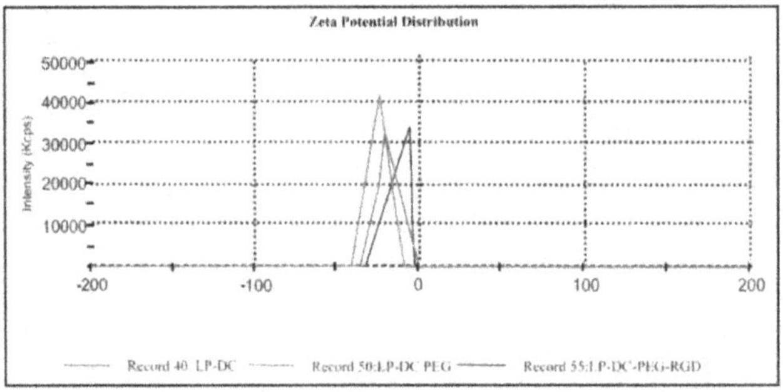

Table: 5.3.Characterization of optimized RGD conjugated and unconjugated Liposomes of Docetaxel

Parameter	*** LP-DC**	**# LP-DC-PEG**	****LP-DC-PEG-RGD**
Mean particle size (nm)	260.4 ± 4.6	269.2 ± 2.8	278.6±3.4
Zeta potential (mV)	-28.7 ± 1.3	-27.2±1.8	-11.6±0.4
Entrapment efficiency (%)	72.8 ± 2.2 %	69.2±5.8	64.5±1.5

(Mean ± S.D., *n* = 3)
* **LP-DC** Docetaxel loaded Liposomes
\# LP-DC-PEG Docetaxel loaded pegylated liposomes
****LP-DC-PEG-RGD** – RGD conjugated Docetaxel loaded Liposomes

Mean particle size and zeta potential of PLGA-DC-NP and PLGA-DC-RGD-NP were found to be 210.3 ± 2.7nm and -38.4 ± 2.6mV and 230.7 ± 2.3nm and -10.2 ± 2.8mV respectively. Increase in the particle size after RGD conjugation was due to RGD conjugated. The %EE for PLGA-DC-NP and PLGA-DC-RGD-NP was found to be 71.6 ± 2.4 % and 58.4 ± 1.6% respectively. The reduced drug entrapment efficiency for PLGA-DC-RGD-NP may be due to dissociation of the drug on the surface of PLGA-DC-NP during the RGD conjugation process.

Similarly, the particle size and zeta potential for LP-DC, LP-DC-PEG and LP-DC-RGD are recorded in Table: 5.3. The particle size and zeta potential are shown in Figure: 5.3 and Figure: 5.4, respectively. Mean particle size and zeta potential of LP-DC & LP-DC-PEG were found to be 260.4 ± 4.6nm& 269.2 ± 2.8nm and -28.7 ± 1.3 & -27.2±1.8mV respectively. While the LP-DC-PEG-RGD demonstrated 278.6±3.4nm particle size and -11.6±0.4mV zeta potential. The %EE for LP-DC, LP-DC-PEG and LP-DC-PEG-RGD was determined to be 72.8 ± 2.2 %, 67.9 ± 3.1% and 64.5±1.5%, respectively.

5.3.2. In-vitro Drug Release

Release of the entrapped therapeutic agent from PLGA matrix has been found to occur through diffusion-cum-degradation-mediated processes (Crotts, G. et al., 1998). It has been demonstrated that during the early phases, the release of the entrapped therapeutic agent occurs mainly through its diffusion in the polymer matrix while during the later phases, the release is mediated through both diffusion of the therapeutic agent and the degradation of the polymer-matrix itself. Thus, degradation rate of the polymer matrix is an important determinant of the in vitro release of the therapeutic agent from PLGA matrices (Anderson, J.M. et al., 1997). The acidic (lactic acid and glycolic acid) monomers and oligomers formed catalyze the further degradation of the parent polymer. Thus, any factor that influences the formation and/or retention of the acidic monomers in the particles could affect the polymer degradation rate and the in vitro release of the entrapped therapeutic agent (Panyam, J. et al., 2003).

Figure: 5.5. In-vitro release of Docetaxel from PLGA NPs before and after conjugation with RGD

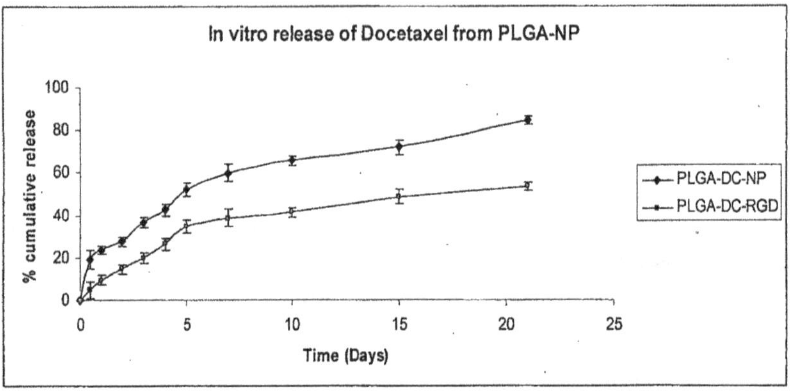

(Mean ± S.D., $n = 3$)
* PLGA-DC-NP- Docetaxel loaded PLGA nanoparticles
# PLGA-DC-RGD-NP – RGD conjugated Docetaxel loaded PLGA nanoparticles

The release studies of Docetaxel from the optimized nanoparticle batch were conducted in phosphate buffer pH 7.4 + 0.1%w/v polysorbate-80. The release curves of PLGA-DC-NP and PLGA-DC-RGD-NP are shown in Figure: 5.5. For PLGA-DC-NP there was an initial burst release of about 19% in 12hrs and then there was a lag phase and about 80% release resulted in 21 days. The unconjugated nanoparticles showed a high initial burst which can be attributed to the immediate dissociation and dissolution of drug adhered on the surface and located near the surface of the NPs (Magenheim, et al., 1993). While in lag phase, the release is mainly due to the erosion of the polymer matrix and further diffusion of drug molecules through the polymeric matrix of the NPs. The matrix material would require time to erode in the aqueous environment than the release mechanisms of surface release, resulting in the prolonged release. (Esmaeili, F. et al., 2008).The burst effect was absent in PLGA-DC-RGD-NP and the release in 21 days was found to be about 60%. The release studies of Docetaxel from the optimized liposomes batch were conducted in phosphate buffer pH 7.4 + 0.1%w/v polysorbate-80.

Figure: 5.6. In-vitro release of Docetaxel from Liposomes before and after conjugation with RGD

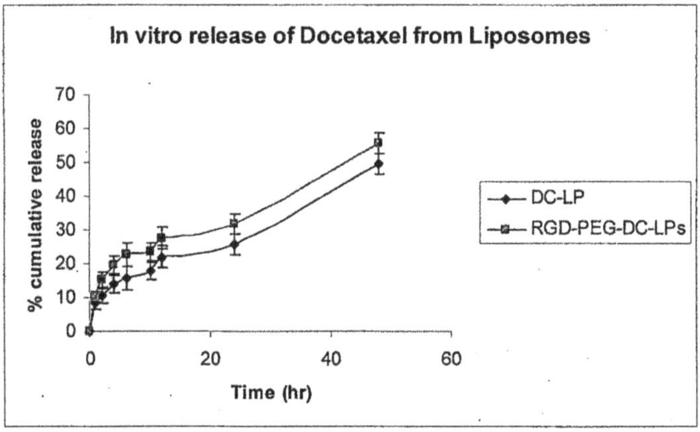

(Mean ± S.D., *n* = 3)
* **LP-DC** Docetaxel loaded Liposomes
# LP-DC-PEG-RGD – RGD conjugated Pegylated Docetaxel loaded Liposomes

In vitro drug release from Docetaxel-loaded, non-pegylated and RGD conjugated pegylated liposomes is summarized in the cumulative percentage release shown in Figure: 5.6. It was found that both formulations produced an initial burst release in which docetaxel release was more than 10 % and 8 % for pegylated and non-pegylated liposomes, respectively, within the initial sampling time (30min). The burst release in both forms of liposomes is related to release of surface adsorbed drug. After the initial burst release, a constant drug release was found and maximum of 75% and 60% drug was released in 48hr of time period with pegylated and non pegylated liposomes respectively. Faster release in pegylated liposomes may be due to the fast hydration process of PEG molecules on the surface of the particles.

Figure: 5.7. In vitro serum drug release for RGD-PEG-DC-NPs and RGD-PEG-DC-LPs

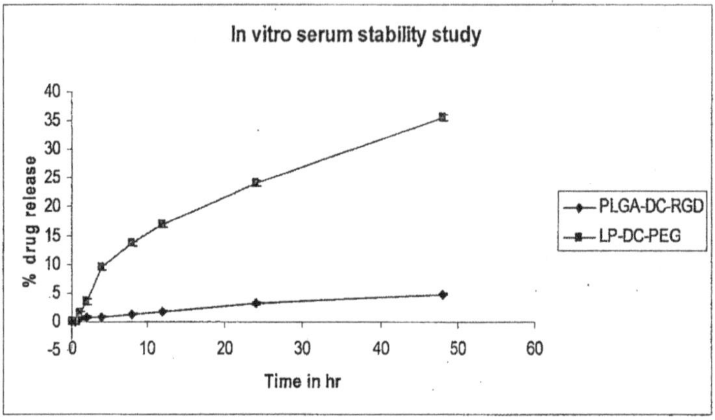

In vitro drug release from DC encapsulated RGD conjugated pegylated liposomes and from DC encapsulated RGD conjugated pegylated nanoparticles was about 35.6% and 4.8% respectively in 48 hrs. The difference of drug release may be attributed to the hydrophobic nature of PLGA.

5.3.3. Transmission Electron Microscopy

The TEM RGD conjugated nanoparticles and liposomes for Docetaxel are shown in Figure: 5.8 and Figure: 5.9, respectively.TEM images NPs & LPs showed spherical NPs & LPs with smooth surfaces.

Figure: 5.8. Morphology of Docetaxel nanoparticles using TEM

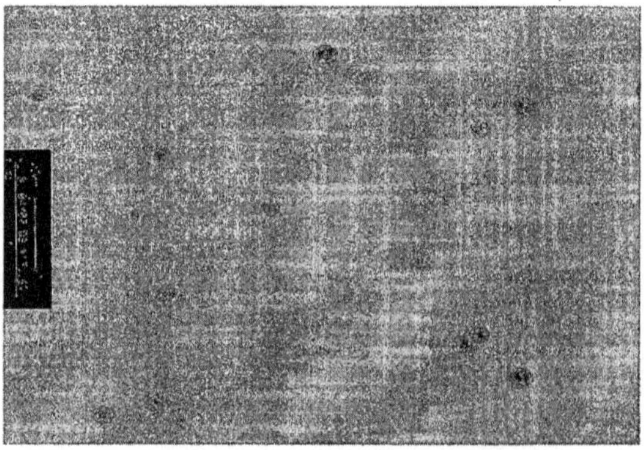

Figure: 5.9. Morphology of Docetaxel liposomes using TEM

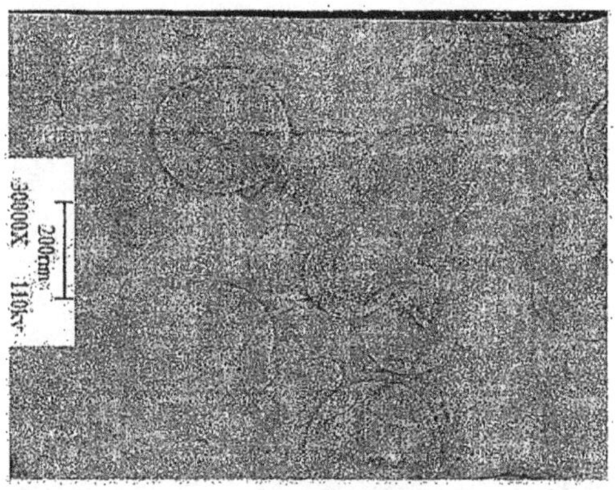

5.3.4. Scanning Electron Microscopy

The SEM images for DC nanoparticles and Liposomes are shown in Figure 5.10 and Figure 5.11, respectively. SEM images of nanoconstructs showed spherical shape with smooth surfaces and the sphericity did not alter significantly after conjugation.

Figure: 5.10. Morphology of Docetaxel nanoparticles using SEM

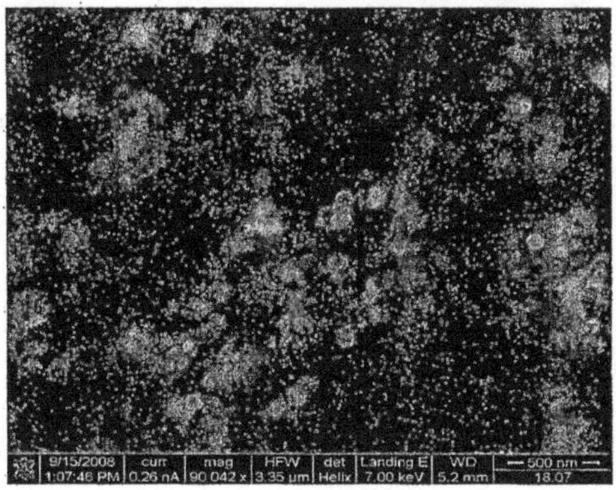

Figure: 5.11. Morphology of Docetaxel liposomes using SEM

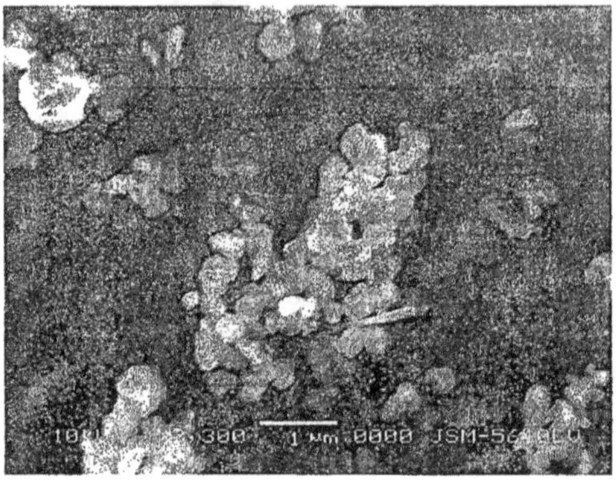

5.2.5. X- ray diffraction studies (XRD)

Crystal diffraction software tools are widely used to simulate XRD patterns as reference standards for individual crystal forms (such as polymorph, solvates, and salts). The XRD pattern of bulk DC showed a total of 12 peaks while the XRD patterns of RGD-DC-PLGA NPs and RGD-DC-LPs did not showed any characteristic peaks. The crystallinity index of DC after conversion into nanoparticles was calculated by considering the intensity of the principle peak obtained with bulk DC as 100%. Results are recorded in Figure: 5.12 and Figure 5.13 for nanoparticles and liposomes, respectively.

Figure: 5.12. XRD photograph of (a) free drug,(b) non PEGylated PLGA NPs, (c) PEG-DC-PLGA NPs and d) RGD-PEG-DC-PLGA NPs

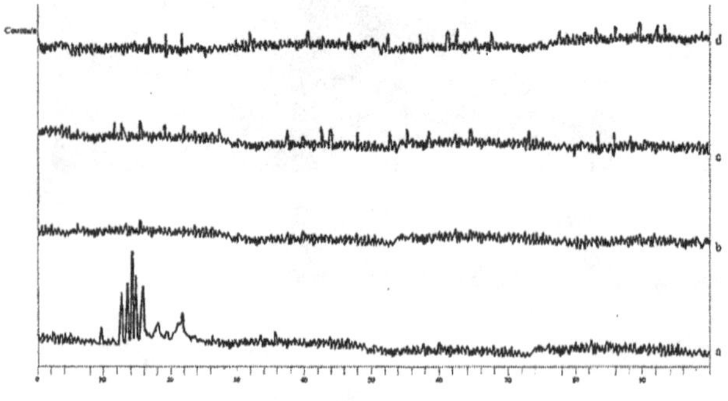

Figure: 5.13. XRD photograph of (a) free drug,(b) non PEGylated liposomes, (c) RGD-PEG-DC liposomes

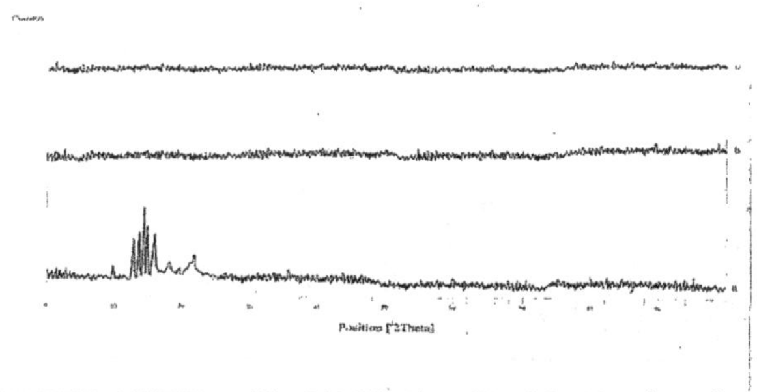

5.3.6. Differential Scanning Calorimetry

The physical state of the drug in nanoparticles can be determined by differential scanning calorimetry (DSC). The drug can exist in different polymorphic forms in the formulations i.e. amorphous or crystalline.

DSC thermogram of plain Docetaxel shown in Figure: 5.15 depicts a sharp melting peak from 169-171°C, indicating the crystalline nature of the drug. The drug in the amorphous form is entrapped in the nanoparticles. For PLGA-DC-NP, as shown in Figure: 5.15, the peak of Docetaxel is absent indicating the conversion of DC into amorphous state during the nanoparticles formulation and thereby entrapped in the PLGA polymer.

Similarly, for LP-DC as in Figure: 5.14, the peak of docetaxel is absent indicating the conversion of DC into amorphous state during the liposome formulation and thereby entrapped in the liposomes.

Figure: 5.14. DSC analysis (b) free drug,(a) PEGylated liposomes, (c) physical mixture of HSPC,SPC,cholesterol,DSPE-PEG2000, (d)HSPC

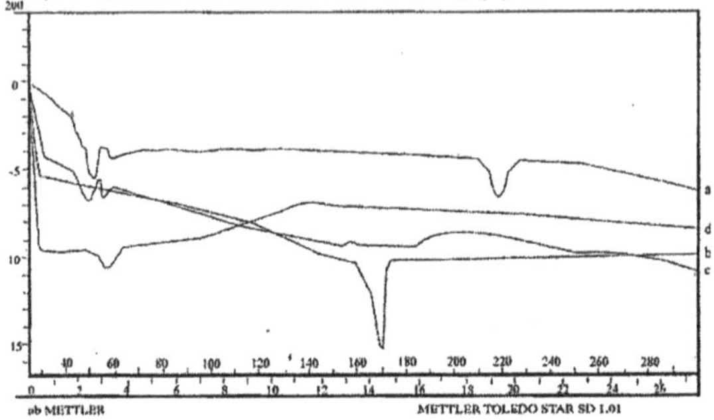

Figure: 5.15 DSC analysis (b) free drug,(a) PEGylated nanoparticles, (c) PLGA (d)RGD-PEG-DC-PLGA NPs

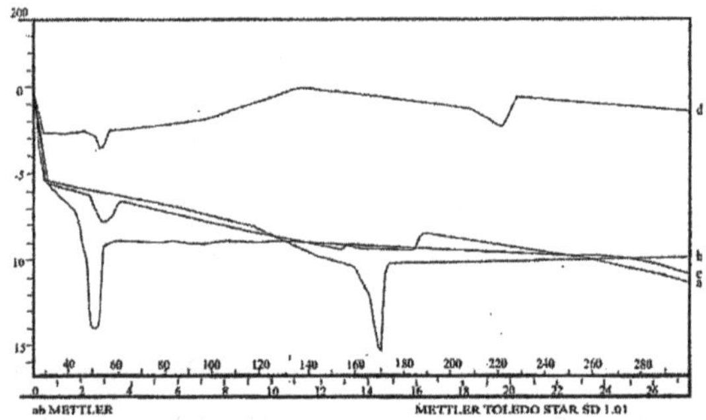

5.3.7. [1H]NMR of the RGD conjugated nanoconstructs

^{1}H-NMR spectroscopy was used to ascertain the conjugation of RGD to the nanoconstructs. The ^{1}H-NMR spectra of PLGA, PLGA-DC-RGD NPs, LPs and RGD-DC-LPs are shown in Figure:5.16 a, b, c and d, respectively.

Figure: 5.16. ^{1}H-NMR spectra of (a) PLGA, (b) PLGA-DC-RGD NPs, (c)RGD and (d) RGD-DC-LPs

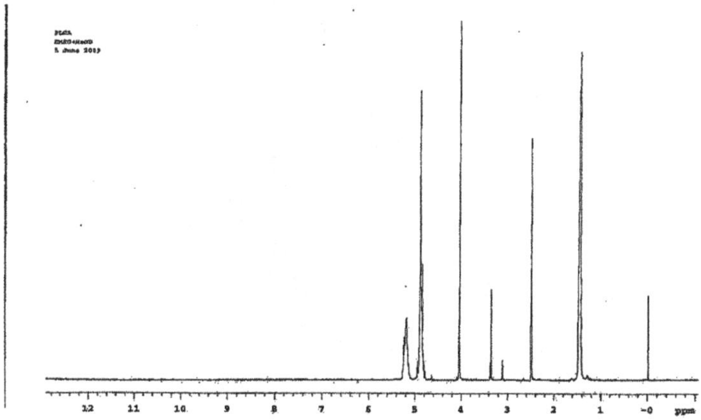

(a)

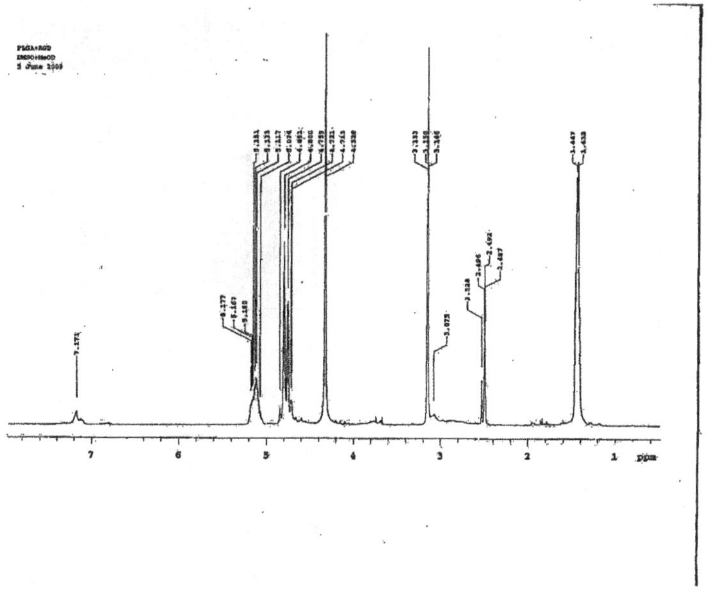

(b)

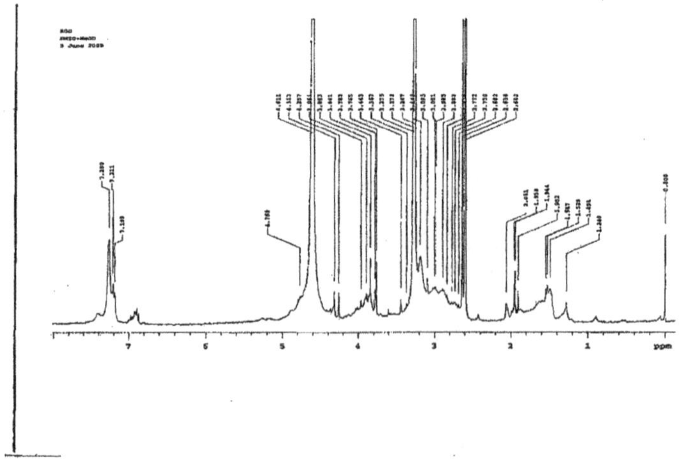

(c)

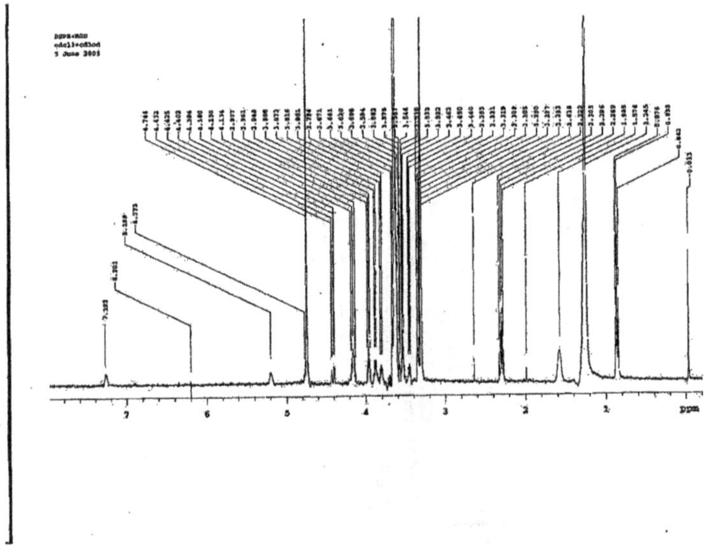

(d)

The presence of characteristic peak at δ value 7.1 reveals the presence of RGD with nanoparticles (Figure 5.16b) and liposomes (Figure 5.16d). The unconjugated PLGA nanoparticles did not show any peak at 7.1, which depicts the absence of RGD.

5.3.8. Infrared spectra of nanoparticles

Infrared spectra of the drug loaded unconjugated and the RGD conjugated nanoparticles and liposomes were obtained (Figure: 5.17 a, b, c and d) and analyzed for confirmation of the RGD conjugation.

Figure: 5.17. FTIR spectra of (a) DC-PLGA NPs,(b) RGD-DC-PLGA NPs, (c) DC-PEG-LPs and (d) RGD-DC-PEG-LPs

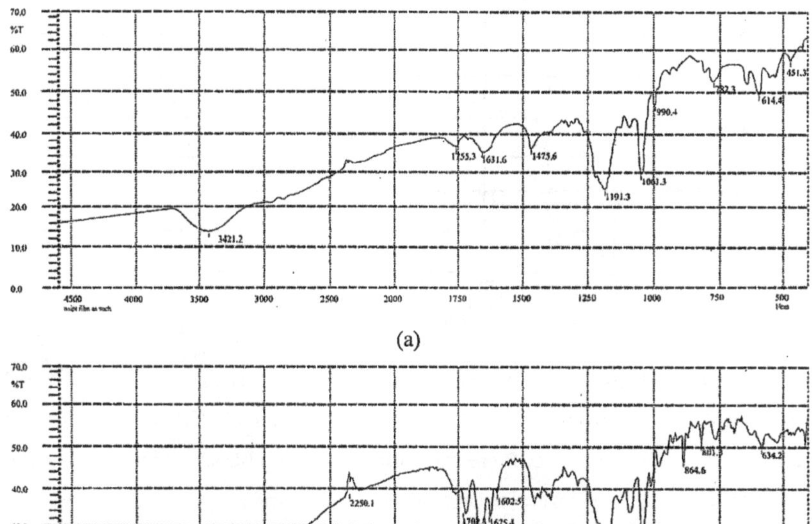

(a)

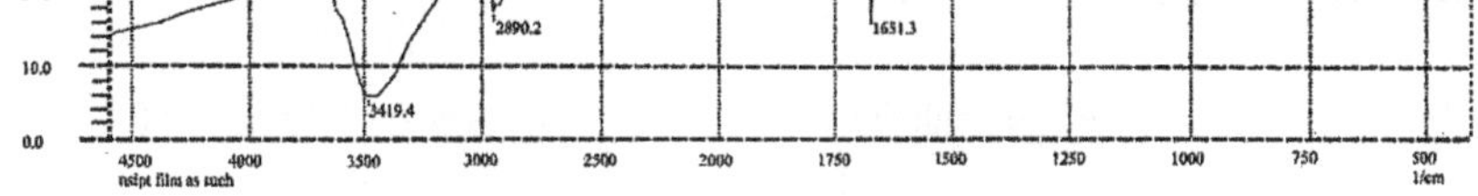

(b)

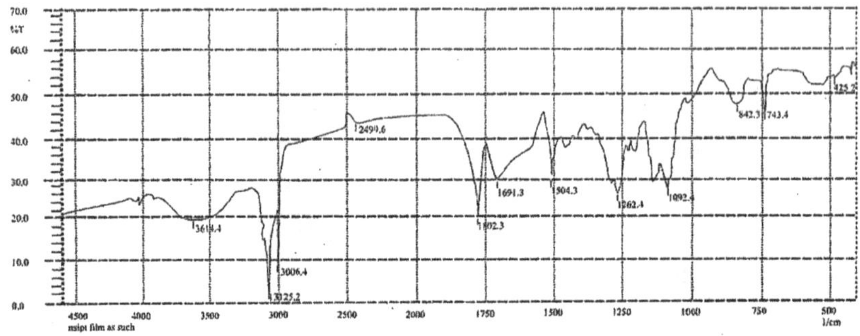

(c)

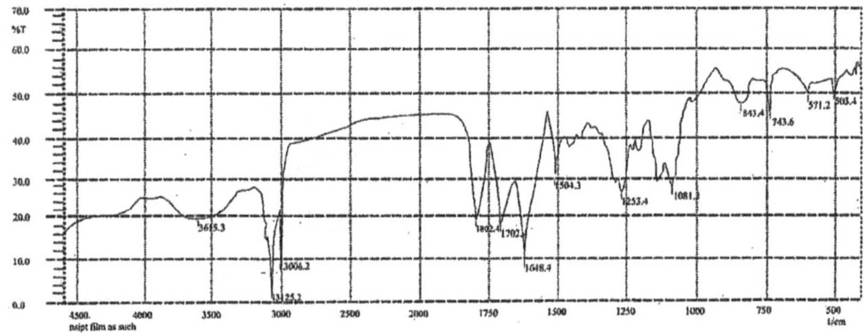

(d)

The peaks at 1625 cm^{-1}, 1651 cm^{-1} and 1648 cm^{-1} in the IR spectra of RGD-DC-NPs and RGD-DC-LPs respectively indicated the presence of amide (CO-NH) group. This confirms the conjugation of RGD onto the surface of nanoconstructs. While the aforesaid peaks are absent in unconjugated nanoconstructs.

5.3.9. Residual PVA

The residual PVA associated with the nanoparticles surface was 7.4 ± 2.1 % and 5.4 ± 1.3 w/w of unconjugated and conjugated docetaxel encapsulated nanoparticles respectively.

5.3.10. Characterization of 6-coumarin nanoparticles

Unconjugated and RGD conjugated fluorescent NPs and liposomes encapsulating 6-coumarin required for studying cellular uptake of NPs by breast cancer cells were prepared and characterized by the same methods used for drug loaded NPs & LPs and the results are recorded in Table:5.4. and Table: 5.5, respectively.

Table: 5.4. Characterization of 6- coumarin nanoparticles

Character	6-coumarin nanoparticles	
	Unconjugated	**RGD conjugated**
Particle size (nm)	247.4 ± 4.5	321.3 ± 8.4
Zeta potential (mV)	-12.6 ± 1.4	-10.3 ± 1.5
Entrapment Efficiency	92.21 ± 3.61	84.47 ± 3.41
Surface RGD (μg /mg)	----	32.3 ± 2.6
Residual PVA (% w/w)	7.4 ± 2.1	5.4 ± 1.3

Table: 5.5. Characterization of 6- coumarin liposomes

Character	6-coumarin nanoparticles	
	Unconjugated	**RGD conjugated**
Particle size (nm)	267.5 ± 5.2	293.6 ±7.3
Zeta potential (mV)	-27.4 ± 2.5	-11.5 ± 3.4
Entrapment Efficiency	90.16 ± 4.22	82.53 ± 4.62
Surface RGD (μg /mg)	----	36.4 ± 3.5

6-coumarin loaded unconjugated NPs and RGD-conjugated NPs had a particle size of 247.4 ± 4.5 nm and 321.3 ± 8.4nm and zeta potential of -12.6 ± 1.4 mV and-10.3 ± 1.5 mV respectively. RGD conjugated NPs had 32.3 ± 2.6 μg RGD /mg of nanoparticles. The entrapment efficiency as evaluated using spectrofluorimetry was found to be 92.21 ± 3.61and 84.47 ± 3.41 for unconjugated and conjugated 6-coumarin nanoparticles. The residual PVA was found to be 7.4 ± 2.1 % and 5.4 ± 1.3 % for unconjugated and transferrin conjugated nanoparticles respectively. The particle size, zeta potential, the surface density of RGD and residual PVA of 6-coumarin NPs were found to be similar to the drug loaded NPs. So it is expected that their cellular uptake would be similar to that of the drug loaded NPs.

5.4. Conclusions

After characterization we can conclude that the unconjugated and RGD conjugated nanoconstructs of docetaxel have small particle size (<300nm) suitable for intravenous administration. A prolonged release was observed for both unconjugated and conjugated nanoconstructs of docetaxel. The smooth and spherical surface of nanoconstructs was confirmed from TEM and SEM. The DSC & XRD studies indicate the presence of the drug in nanoconstructs in the amorphous form.

The unconjugated and RGD conjugated nanoconstructs of Docetaxel were further subjected to stability studies according to ICH guidelines (Chapter 6).

5.5. References:

Anderson, J .M. 1997, Biodegradation and biocom- PLA and PLGA microspheres, Adv. Drug. Deliv. Rev., **28**, 5–24.

Atyabi, F et al., 2009, Preparation of pegylated nano-liposomal formulation containing SN-38: *In vitro* characterization and *in vivo* biodistribution in mice, Acta Pharm.;**59**, 133–144.

Boury, F. et al., 1995, Dynamic properties of poly (D,L-lactide) and polyvinyl alcohol monolayers at the air/water and dichloromethane air/water interfaces. J. Colloid. Interf. Sci., **169**,380–392.

Crotts, G. et al., 1998, Protein delivery from poly(lactic- glycolic acid) biodegradable microspheres: release kinetics and stability issues, J. Microencapsul.. **15**, 699–713.

Esmaeili, F. et al., 2008, PLGA nanoparticles of different surface properties: Preparation and evaluation of their body distribution, International Journal of Pharmaceutics, **349**, 249–255.

Jagdish Singh et al., 2000, Effect of Isopropyl Myristic Acid Ester on the Physical Characteristicsand In Vitro Release of Etoposide from PLGA Microspheres, AAPS. Pharm.Sci.Tech., **1(4)**, article 32.

Joshi, D.P. et al., 1979, Determination of poly (vinyl alcohol) via its complex with boric acid and iodine, Anal. Chim. Acta., **104**, 153–160.

Magenheim, B. et al., 1993, A new in vitro technique for evaluation of drug release profile from colloidal carriers-ultrafiltration technique at low pressure, Int. J. Pharm, **94** , 115–123.

Mu, L. et al., 2002, Vitamin E TPGS used as emulsi.er in the solvent evaporation/extraction technique for fabrication of polymeric nanospheres for controlled release of paclitaxel (Taxols), J. Control. Rel, **80**, 129–144.

Sanjeeb, K. et al., 2002, Residual polyvinyl alcohol associated with poly (lactide-co-glycolide) nanoparticles affects their physical properties and cellular uptake, Journal of Controlled Release, **82(1)**, 105-114.

Shen Gao et al., 2007, Temozolomide/PLGA microparticles and antitumor activity against Glioma C6 cancer cells in vitro, Int. J. of Pharm., **329 (1-2)**, 122-128.

Chapter 6
Stability study

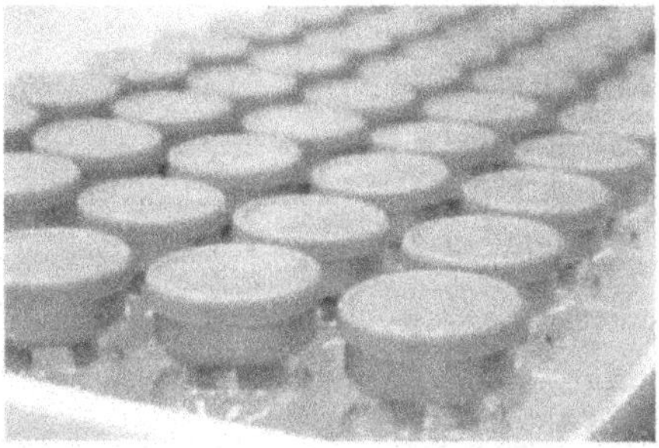

6.1. Introduction

Stability is defined as the capacity of a drug substance or drug product to remain within established specifications to maintain its identity, strength, quality, and purity throughout the retest or expiration dating periods (Draft guidance, Stability Testing of Drug Substances and Drug Products, FDA, 1998). The purpose of stability testing is to provide evidence on how the quality of a drug substance or drug product varies with time under the influence of a variety of environmental factors, such as temperature, humidity, and light, and to establish a retest period for the drug substance or a shelf life for the drug product and recommended storage conditions (Draft guidance, Stability Testing of New Drug Substances and Products, 2003). Physical, chemical, and microbiological data are generated as a function of time and storage conditions (e.g., temperature and relative humidity [RH]). It is a well-known fact that for drug delivery systems, stability of the formulation is one of the most critical parameters from the pharmaceutical aspect. The storage conditions are particularly important to define in order to start biological studies and to make sure that the drug doses used would be preserved. For this purpose, accelerated stability testing at high temperatures and humidity conditions are often employed to predict the shelf life of drugs.

Particulate delivery systems like microparticles and nanoparticles are widely used to deliver a wide range of drugs. The nanoparticles protect the drug from metabolizing enzymes, sustain the release, to be administered orally or injected locally, and target specific tissues by incorporating surface ligand moieties. Poly (lactide), poly(glycolide) and their copolymers approved by the U.S. Food and Drug Administration (FDA) represent a major class of synthetic biodegradable materials essentially useful for the preparation of microparticles and nanospheres. The factors that influence the chemical degradation of PLGA are well known and include polymer molecular weight, ratio of lactic to glycolic acid in the co-polymers, polymer-drug ratio, environmental temperature, pH, and geometry of the delivery system (Burcu Sayin et al., 2004 & Gasper, M.M. et al., 1998). The main mode of degradation for the PLGA polymer is purely through simple hydrolysis of the ester bonds and does not involve any enzymatic activity.(Mauduit, J. et al., 1996) In vivo it degrades into lactic acid and glycolic acid. Lactic acid enters the tricarboxylic acid cycle and is metabolized and subsequently eliminated from the body as carbon dioxide and water. Glycolic acid is either excreted unchanged in the kidney or it enters the tricarboxylic acid cycle and is eventually eliminated as carbon dioxide and water (Burcu Sayin et al., 2004. It has been shown that PLGA nanospheres and microspheres have a shelf-life of more than 3 months (PLGA 50:50, 0.63 dL/g) (Feng, S. et al., 2001).

The liposomes are more susceptible to environmental conditions like temperature/humidity and were affected by oxidation/hydrolysis. Change in environment tends to aggregate and therefore leakage of the drug substance form the lipid vesicles. Liposomal aggregation, bilayer fusion and drug leakage are the main problems of physical stability encountered in any liposomal formulation which could greatly affect the shelf life of liposomes. Unfortunately, liposomal formulations do not meet the required standards for long term stability of pharmaceutical preparations if they are stored as aqueous dispersions (Fransen et al., 1986). The encapsulated drug tends to leak out of the bilayer and the liposomes might aggregate or fuse upon storage.

Here the liposomes were evaluated for the effect of temperature on the particle size and percent entrapment efficiency i.e. aggregation and/or leakage of the DC from the liposomes over the period of 3 months. All the formulations were stable when stored at 2-8°C and there were some aggregation and leakage seen when stored at 25°C.

Although, the instability of the nanoparticles in the dispersion is overcome by lyophilization using cryoprotectants, the influence of the storage conditions like temperature and humidity on the particle size and drug content are important in maintaining the integrity of these delivery systems before use for the biological studies.

6.2. Methodology

The stability studies were carried out in accordance with the ICH guidelines for new drug products. The stability studies were carried out for the nanoparticle formulations at 5°C ± 3°C for 6 months and (25°C ± 2°C/60 ± 5 % RH) up to 6 months. Three batches at optimized process and formulation conditions were prepared and subjected to stability studies. The nanoparticles were filled in glass vials, closed with rubber closures and sealed with aluminum caps.

The samples were withdrawn at predetermined levels and were examined visually for physical appearance. The contents of the vials were evaluated for the particle size, zeta potential and drug content.

Statistical Analysis and Data Interpretation

Three batches of each formulation was evaluated three times, data of nine experiments are expressed as Mean ± SD. The data were compared using ANOVA and student's t-test and difference larger than the value at $p<0.05$ were considered significant.

"Significant change" *was* considered under following conditions

- A 5 percent change in assay from its initial value
- Failure to meet the acceptance criteria for appearance, physical attributes, and functionality test particle size and drug content may be expected under accelerated conditions.

The results of stability studies are recorded in Tables: 6.1 to Table: 6.3 and Figures: 6.1 to Figure: 6.2.

6.3. Results and Discussions

The stability studies of the formulations were performed in order to study the influence of varying environmental conditions on the parameters of the formulation influencing the therapeutic response. The stability studies were carried out in accordance with the ICH guidelines for drug substances intended to be stored in a refrigerator. The stability of the nanoparticles and liposomes were assessed for physical observation, particle size, zeta potential and the drug content (with respect to the initial) at 5°C ± 3°C for 6M and 25°C ± 2°C/60% RH ± 5% RH for 6 months. The drug content in the initial sample was considered as 100 percent. For accelerated condition (i.e. 25°C ± 2°C/60% ± 5 %RH) the sampling was done at 1, 2, 3, 6 months and for 5°C ± 3°C the sampling was done at 1, 3, 6 months.

The results for the stability studies are represented in table 6.1 and 6.2 for PLGA-DC-NP and PLGA-DC-RGD-NP respectively. The graphical representations are given in Figure: 6.1 and Figure: 6.2. The results for LP-DC and LP-DC-RGD are recorded in Table: 6.3.

Table: 6.1. Stability studies data of PLGA-DC-NP

Stability conditions	Description & Redispersibility	Particle size (nm)	Zeta potential (mV)	Drug content %
Initial	Free flowing white powder with easy redispersibility	210.3 ± 2.7	-38.4 ± 2.6	100.0 ± 2.4*
5°C ± 3°C				
1 M	Free flowing white powder with easy redispersibility	209.4 ± 3.6	-38.9 ± 1.5	98.3 ± 2.2
3 M	Free flowing white powder with easy redispersibility	211.7 ± 3.2	-39.2 ± 1.7	97.6 ± 2.2
6 M	Free flowing white powder with easy redispersibility	212.4 ± 2.6	-37.1 ± 2.2	97.4± 1.5
25°C ± 2°C/60% RH ± 5% RH				
1 M	Free flowing white powder with easy redispersibility	210.3 ± 4.5	-38.4 ± 2.8	98.6± 2.2
2 M	Free flowing white powder with easy redispersibility	220.4 ± 6.5	-36.2 ± 3.2	96.8± 2.8
3 M	White powder with poor flow and difficult redispersibility	532.3 ± 9.6	-26.8 ± 2.4	94.5± 2.5
6 M	White powder with poor flow and poor redispersibility	845.6 ± 6.7	-13.6 ± 1.4	93.6 ± 2.2

* Initial drug content was labeled as 100% and the drug content at different time points are with respect to the initial drug content

Table: 6.2. Stability data of PLGA-DC-RGD

Stability conditions	Description	Particle size (nm)	Zeta potential (mV)	Drug content %
Initial	Free flowing white powder with easy redispersibility	230.7 ± 2.3	-10.2 ± 2.8	100.0± 1.6
5°C ± 3°C				
1 M	Free flowing white powder with easy redispersibility	232.5 ± 5.6	-10.5 ± 1.4	99.2 ± 2.6
3 M	Free flowing white powder with easy redispersibility	230.4 ± 4.7	-11.3 ± 1.5	98.8± 2.5
6 M	Free flowing white powder with easy redispersibility	235.6 ± 8.5	-10.5 ± 2.3	98.1± 1.3
25°C ± 2°C/60% RH ± 5% RH				
1 M	Free flowing white powder with easy redispersibility	236.2 ± 6.3	-10.4 ± 1.5	98.2± 2.1
2 M	Free flowing white powder with easy redispersibility	239.4 ± 5.6	-9.2 ± 1.1	96.5± 2.2
3 M	White powder with poor flow and difficult redispersibility	514.8 ± 12.5	-8.4 ± 2.3	96.2± 2.4
6 M	Light pink powder with poor flow and poor redispersibility	861.5 ± 14.5	-4.2 ± 1.4	95.3 ± 2.6

Table: 6.3. Stability data of Docetaxel liposomes

(a) Stability data on % EE

Liposomes	Initial	2-8°C			25± 2 ° C			
		1 month	3 month	6 month	1 month	2 month	3month	6 months
Non-PEGylated	100±2.4	99.1±1.4	98.4±2.6	98.2±2.8	98.8±3.6	97.4±3.4	95.2±3.8	94.3±4.2
PEGylated	100±3.4	99.2±2.1	98.8±2.4	98.4±2.6	98.3±2.3	97.8±2.5	96.4±2.4	94.8±3.5
LP-DC-RGD	100±2.6	99.4±2.2	98.4±2.3	97.9±2.7	99.3±2.5	98.3±2.6	97.4±2.8	94.2±2.2

(b)Stability data on particle size

Liposomes	Initial	2-8°C			25± 2 ° C			
		1 month	3 month	6month	1 month	2 month	3month	6 months
Non-PEGylated	260.6± 2.4	263.2± 1.8	265.4± 4.6	269.2± 4.4	270.8± 5.8	279.4± 5.9	288.2± 7.6	585.6± 12.2
PEGylated	269.6± 3.4	270.2± 3.6	272.8± 4.8	275.4± 5.6	273.3± 6.7	274.8± 5.3	278.4± 3.2	492.2± 11.3
LP-DC-RGD	278.4± 5.2	279.2± 3.4	280.7± 3.4	279.4± 4.5	279.1± 5.3	283.4± 5.2	285.4± 3.4	467.4± 13.8

(c) Stability data on Zeta potential

Liposomes	Initial	2-8°C			25± 2 ° C			
		1 month	3 month	6month	1 month	2 month	3month	6 months
Non-PEGylated	-28.7 ± 1.3	-27.2 ± 2.7	-27.7 ± 1.6	-27.9 ± 1.5	-28.2 ± 2.4	-27.3 ± 1.7	-26.9 ± 2.1	-12.9 ± 2.5
PEGylated	-27.2± 1.8	-27.7 ± 1.8	-27.5 ± 1.4	-28.7 ± 2.2	-28.2 ± 2.3	-27.3 ± 1.5	-26.8 ± 2.9	-16.4 ± 3.1
LP-DC-RGD	-11.6± 1.2	-10.2± 1.4	-11.3± 1.4	-11.7± 1.7	-11.4± 1.5	-10.3 ±1.6	-10.9± 2.1	-18.9 ±2.8

Figure: 6.1. Stability profiles-PLGA-DC-NP (a) particle size (b) zeta potential and (c) drug content Vs time in months

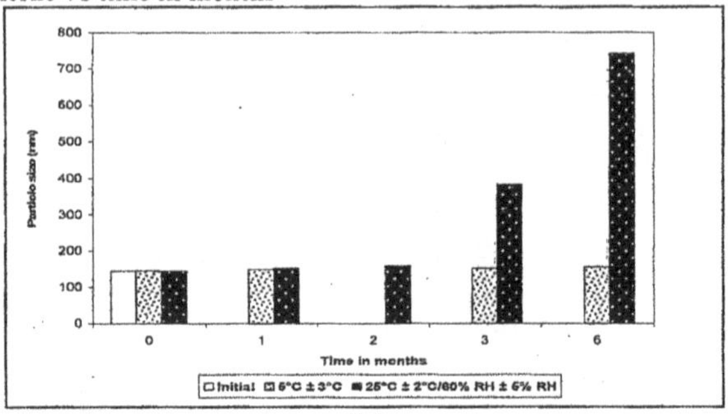

(a)

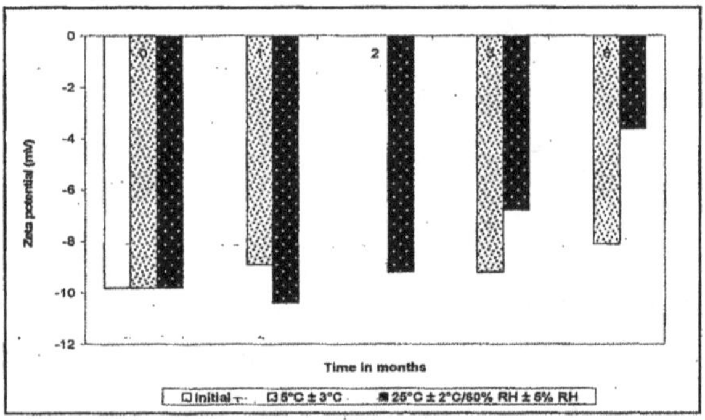

(b)

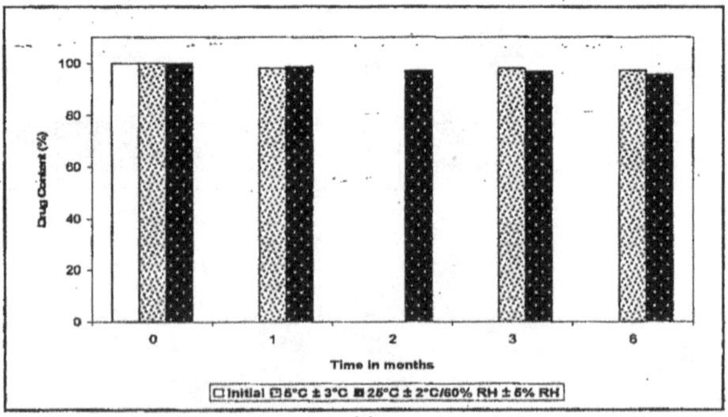

(c)

Figure: 6.2. Stability profiles- PLGA-DC-RGD-NP (a) particle size (b) zeta potential and (c) drug content Vs time in months

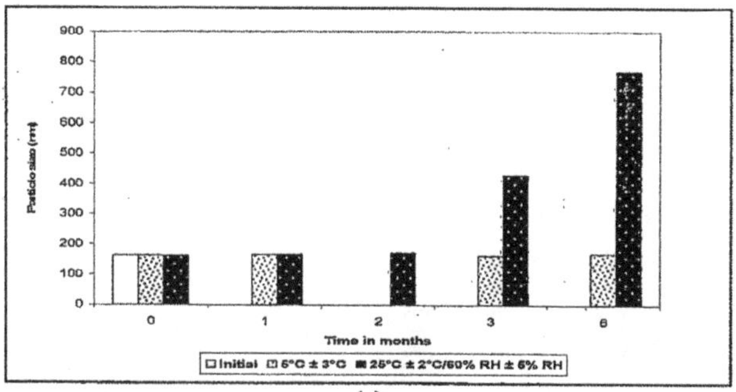

(a)

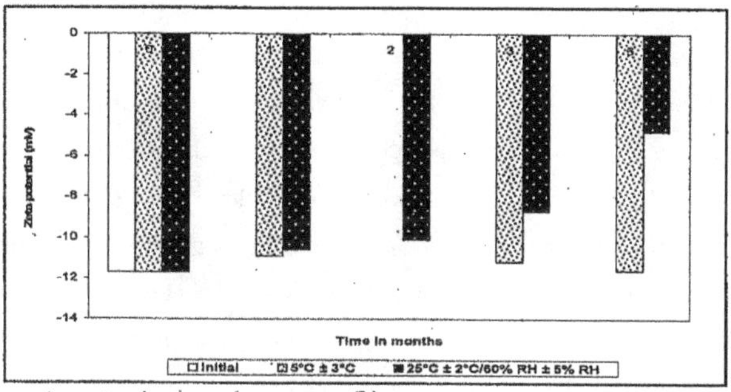

(b)

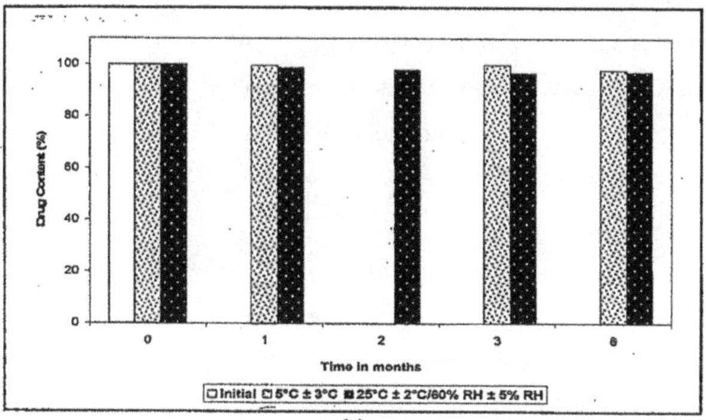

(c)

It was observed that unconjugated and conjugated nanoparticles of docetaxel, there was no significant change (P>0.05) observed in particle size, zeta potential and drug content at 5°C ± 3°C for 6M.

The storage of the unconjugated and conjugated nanoparticles of docetaxel at 25°C ± 2°C/60% ± 5% RH, led to increase in the particle size. The increase in the particle size was not significant during the first month, however became significant and more prominent after 2, 3 and 6 months. During our analysis of samples, the polydispersity index of the nanoparticles stored at 25°C ± 2°C/60% ± 5% RH was found to increase as compared to the initial. The increase in the particle size may be due to the absorption of the moisture by the nanoparticles resulting in the coalescence of the small nanoparticles forming particles larger in size.

The nanoparticles were also observed for physical appearance. After 3 and 6 months the physical appearance was also changed, with loss of the free flowing property followed by the difficulty in redispersibility. Also, the RGD conjugated nanoparticles demonstrated difference in the color than the initial powder. At 6 months the color of the powder was light pink. This could be indicative of the degradation of the surface RGD.

At 25°C ± 2°C/60% ± 5% RH, the zeta potential of the nanoparticles shifted towards the zero for both unconjugated and conjugated nanoparticles. This may be due to the acidic conditions produced due to the degradation of PLGA into lactic and glycolic acid (Sanjeeb, K. et al., 2002). The lowered zeta potential values also might have contributed toward the aggregation of particles.

The drug content of the unconjugated and conjugated nanoparticles was not altered up to 6M at 5°C ± 3°C. However, the drug content was reduced after 6M storage at 25°C ± 2°C/60% RH ± 5% RH. This impact could be due to the moisture absorbed by the nanoparticles upon storage at 25°C ± 2°C/60% RH ± 5% RH, possibly resulting in the degradation of the drug.

The initial drug entrapment was found to be 72.6±2.4% and 69.6±3.4% and initial particle size 260.6±2.4 nm, 260.6±2.4 nm for Non-PEGylated and PEGylated liposomes respectively. Reduction in the entrapment after 3 months, were observed 69.2±2.8% (2-8°C) and 61.2±3.8% (25°C) while particle size was 269.2±4.4 nm (2-8°C) and 288.2±7.6

nm (25°C) for Non-PEGylated. In case of PEGylated liposomes, minor reduction in the drug entrapment was seen (68.2±2.1% and 61.2±3.8%) at 2-8°C and 25°C respectively and increase in the particles size was in the range of 8-12 nm from the initial (Table: 6.3). The release profile of the drug from the nanoparticles was not affected upon storage. The similarity factor calculated for the between the initial and the 6M samples show values greater than 80, indicating high similarity between the initial and 6M.

6.4. Conclusions

From the above study, we can conclude that the unconjugated and RGD-conjugated PLGA nanoparticles and liposomes of docetaxel when stored at 25°C ± 2°C/60% RH ± 5% RH for 6M show instability reflected by change in physical appearance, increase in the particle size, zeta potential and reduction in the drug content. Hence, we can conclusively specify that both unconjugated and conjugated nanoconstructs were stable and can be stored 5°C ± 3°C for 6M retaining its original formulation characteristics. Further, long term stability should be carried our further to assess the influence of the increasing time on the stability of the prepared nanoconstructs at 5°C ± 3°C.

6.5. References

Burcu Sayin et al., 2004, Influence of Accelerated Storage Conditions on The Stability Of Vancomycin-Loaded Poly(D,L-Lactide-Coglycolide) Microspheres, FABAD. J. Pharm. Sci., **29**, 111-116.

Feng, S. et al., 2001, Effects of emulsifiers on the controlled release of paclitaxel (Taxol) from nanospheres of biodegradable polymers, J. Control. Release., **71**, 53-69.

Gasper, M.M. et al., 1998, Formulation of Lasparaginase-loaded poly(lactide-co-glycolide) nanoparticles: influence of polymer properties on enzyme loading, activity and in vitro release, J. Control. Release., **52,** 53-62.

ICH guidelines (www.ich.org)

Mauduit, J. et al., M. Hydrolytic degradation of films prepared from blends of high and low molecular weight poly(DL-lactic acid)s, J. Biomed. Mater. Res., **30**, 201-207.

Sanjeeb K. et al., Residual polyvinyl alcohol associated with poly (lactide-co-glycolide) nanoparticles affects their physical properties and cellular uptake, Journal of Controlled Release, 105-114.

www.fda.gov

Chapter 7
In-vitro Cell Line studies

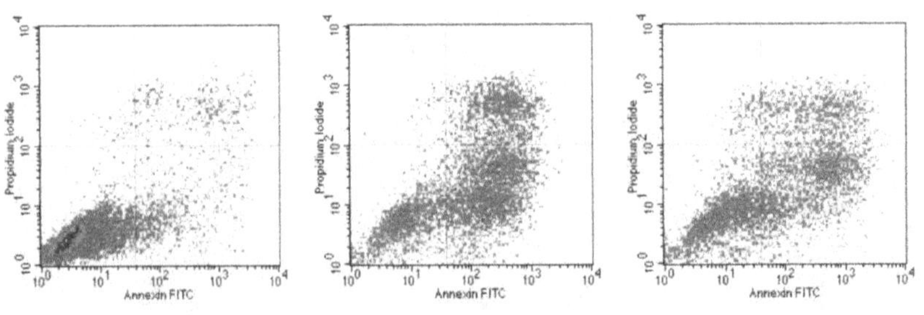

7.1. Introduction

Breast cancer accounts for more deaths of United States women than any other type of malignancy (National cancer Institute 2009). Breast cancer incidence in women in the United States is 1 in 8 (about 13%). There are more than 50 types of different breast cancer cell lines. The criteria considered for the selection of cell lines were Population doubling time (PDT) and expression of receptors for targeting moiety. The MDA-MB-231 and BT-20 cell lines were chosen for the *in vitro* cell culture experiments. The MDA-MB-231 and BT-20 are cell lines of human origin from mammary gland tissue. It was cultured as a monolayer. It is an adherent cell line.

Cell cycle

In order for a living organism to grow their individual cells must increase in size, make exact replicas of all their genetic material, and then go through a process of division. This results in two daughter cells each with one complete copy of the genome. The *eukaryotic cell* of a higher organisms, ranging from yeast to humans, has its genetic material (DNA) is packaged into a membrane bound nucleus. In eukaryotic cells the process of cell growth and division, the cell cycle, is characterized by four distinct phases.

Quiescence: Cells which are not proliferating are said to be quiescent or in "G0" phase.

G1 Phase: During the first phase (G1) cells grow in size in response to mitogenic signals, such as soluble extracellular growth factors and intracellular contact, which may trigger a commitment to entering the next phase of the cell cycle.

The Restriction Point: Late in G1, many cell types become committed to entering the next phase of the cell cycle at a time termed the *restriction point*. The existence of a restriction point can be demonstrated by the simple act by depriving cells from growth factors in their medium. Many types of cells will continue to complete a single cell cycle, if they are in S-phase, G2 or Mitosis, but will then arrest in the next G1 phase.

S-Phase: Soon after the restriction point a cell begins to replicate its genetic material through the activity of a family of enzymes including the DNA polymerases, which are capable of synthesizing an exact replica of the DNA genome. In a mere 6-hours the cell polymerizes exact replicas of all 46 chromosomes, totaling six billion nucleotides, while maintaining the identical sequence of nucleotides as the parental DNA and thus preserving the genetic information. This *"S-phase"* of the cell cycle is thus biochemically distinct from the other phases of the cell cycle and can easily be distinguished from other cells by their ability to stably incorporate fluorescently or radioactively tagged nucleotides, the building blocks of DNA, into their chromosomes.

G2 Phase: At the completion of S-phase, DNA replication ceases and cells enter the G2 phase of the cell cycle.

Mitosis: *Mitosis* is the phase of the cell cycle in which cells physically divide into two separate daughter cells. In order to do so they first dissolve the nuclear membrane which will later reform once cell division is complete. The DNA-containing chromosomes then condense into structures so compact that they can be seen with a light microscope. The chromosomes then precisely segregate to two sides of the cell, such that each half of the cell gets exactly one copy of each chromosome. At the completion of mitosis, cells undergo *cytokinesis* or separation into two halves. This occurs as a band forms around the circumference outer plasma membrane which gradual constricts like a belt until the cell pinches in two and the two daughter cells once again enter G1.

Cell cycle analysis based on measurements of DNA content generates a clear pattern of distribution: G0/G1 phase (one set of paired chromosomes per cell), S phase (DNA synthesis with variable amount of DNA), and G2/M phase (two sets of paired chromosomes per cell, prior to cell division) (Shapiro, H.M. et al., 2003) DNA content can be measured using fluorescent, DNA-selective stains that exhibit emission signals proportional to DNA mass. Flow cytometric analysis of these stained populations is then used to produce a frequency histogram that reveals the various phases of the cell cycle. This analysis is typically performed on permeabilized or fixed cells using a cell-impermeant nucleic acid stain, but is also possible using live cells and a cell-permeant nucleic acid stain. While the choices for fixed-cell staining are varied, there are only a few examples of useful cell-permeant nucleic acid stains.

Nuclear DNA is one of the parameters measured by flow cytometry. This measurement calculates the percentage of a cell population in each phase of the classic cell cycle. The percentage of cells in the S-phase gives an indication of the proliferative activity of that cell population.

The flow cytometer can indicate relative cell size and density or complexity by measuring forward- and side-scattered laser light, respectively. In addition, the flow cytometer can measure relative fluorescence from fluorescent probes which bind to specific cell-associated molecules. These fluorescent probes are often fluorochrome-labeled antibodies specific for cell surface molecules, but may also be nucleic acid probes (e.g. Propidium Iodide), cell function probes (e.g. Indo-1), or fluorescent proteins (e.g. GFP). As the labeled cells flow past a laser beam, the probes fluoresce, and the emitted light is directed to detectors which translate the light signals into information concerning the relative fluorescent intensity associated with each cell.

Flow cytometry measures the percentage of cells in a population with each (or multiple) fluorescent probe(s) attached. The cell sorter is capable of sorting specific cell populations from a mixture of cells based on fluorescence profiles.

The most commonly used dye for DNA content/cell cycle analysis is propidium iodide (PI). It can be used to stain whole cells or isolated nuclei. The PI intercalates into the major groove of double-stranded DNA and produces a highly fluorescent adduct that can be excited at 488 nm with a broad emission centered around 600 nm. Since PI can also bind to double-stranded RNA, it is necessary to treat the cells with RNase for optimal DNA resolution.

Apoptosis

Animal cells can self-destruct via an intrinsic program of cell death (Steller et al., 1995). Apoptosis is a form of programmed cell death that is characterized by specific morphologic and biochemical properties (Wyllie et al., 1980). Morphologically, apoptosis is characterized by a series of structural changes in dying cells: blebbing of the plasma membrane, condensation of the cytoplasm and nucleus, and cellular fragmentation into membrane apoptotic bodies (Steller et al., 1995; Wyllie et al., 1980).

Apoptosis is a complex phenomenon of related morphological and biochemical processes that can vary with tissue and cell type (Zakeri et al., 1995). The protein Bcl-2 appears localized or associated with intracellular membranes of mitochondria, endoplasmic reticulum, and nuclei (Reed et al., 1994). Although the mechanism of Bcl-2 action is unknown, biochemical studies have implicated this protein in the regulation of the redox potential of the cell, as ecotopic expression of bcl-2 suppresses cell death induced by oxidizing agents and appears to affect glutathione levels (Korsmeyer et al., 1993; & Zhong et al., 1993).

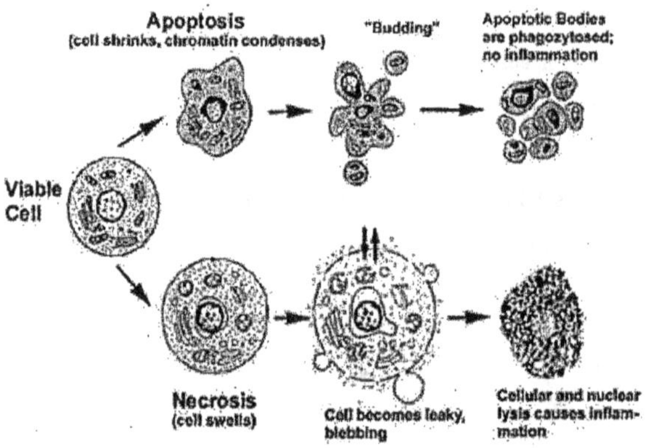

Figure: 7.1. Hallmarks of the apoptotic and necrotic cell death process. Apoptosis includes cellular shrinking, chromatin condensation and margination at the nuclear periphery with the eventual formation of membrane-bound apoptotic bodies that contain organelles, cytosol and nuclear fragments and are phagocytosed without triggering inflammatory processes. The necrotic cell swells, becomes leaky and finally is disrupted and releases its contents into the surrounding tissue resulting in inflammation. Modified from (Cruchten, V. et al., 2002).

Agents like anticancer drugs and ionizing radiation that damage DNA induce apoptosis through a p53-dependent pathway. Binding of p53 and other nuclear proteins to the sites of damage in the DNA appears to trigger the apoptotic process. Another mechanism that can induce apoptosis involves the interaction of proteins such as Fas (CD95) or tumor necrosis factor with their receptors on the surface of cells. Signaling from these so-called death receptors starts the apoptotic process. The characteristic of cells undergoing apoptosis is the capacity to bind the protein Annexin V (AV). AV binds to Phophotydile Serin (PS), which is normally located on the inner leaflet of the plasma membrane, but it is externalized to the outer leaflet during apoptosis. PI staining is widely used to discriminate living cells, which exclude this DNA dye, from dead cells, which are permeable to it. In populations of cells undergoing apoptosis, there are some cells that bind AV but are not stained with PI. This "single-positive" population is thought to represent cells in an early stage of apoptosis because the cells apparently exclude PI and because it appears earlier than DNA ladders can be seen (Eliason, J.F. et al., 2000).

Table: 7.1. Materials and equipments

Material	Source
Water (Double distilled)	Prepared in laboratory by distillation
BT-20 and MDA-MB-231 cells	ATCC
Dulbecco's Modified Eagle Medium (DMEM), HAM's F-10 medium, , fetal bovine serum and streptomycin-penicillin, Phosphate buffer saline	ATCC
6-Coumarin	Gift sample from Neelikon dyes, Mumbai, India
Dimethyl Sulfoxide, Triton X-100	ATCC
Sodium hydroxide	S.D.Fine chemicals, Mumbai, India
CCK-8 reagent	DOJindo Molecular Tech. Inc., Maryland
Nuclepore Polycarbonate membrane0.2, 0.45 and 2 µm 25mm	Milipore, Whatman, USA.
Equipments	**Source/Make**
Calibrated pipettes of 1.0 ml, 5.0 ml and 10.0 ml, volumetric flasks of 10 ml, 25 ml, 50 ml and 100 ml capacity, Funnels (i.d. 5.0 cm), beakers (250 ml) and other requisite glasswares,	Tarsons Ltd., Mumbai
Tissue culture flasks (T 75, T25), 96-well plates, 24-well plates, 35mm PD serological pipettes 1.0 ml, 5.0 ml and 10.0 ml,	Tarsons, Ltd
Micropipette	Brand, Germany
Analytical balance	Precisa 205A SCS, Switzerland
pH meter	Labindia, India
Media Bottles 250ml, 500ml, 1000ml	Durga glasswares Ltd, Baroda
Microtitre plate reader	Synergy HT & Powerwave XS, Biotek, Vermont, USA
Fluoroscent Microscope	Olympus BX61, Japan

7.2. Methods

7.2.1. Intracellular uptake studies

To study the influence of time and concentration on the cellular uptake of Nanoconstructs, following experiments were performed. The cellular uptake studies were carried out using the method reported by *Hu et al 2007*. Briefly, the cells were seeded at a density of 5 X 10^3 cells/well in the 96-well plate (black). At 24hrs, the medium in the plate was changed and plates were kept in the same condition until 80% confluence was reached. The different concentrations (2, 10, 50,100, 200, 500 and 1000μg/ml) of 6-coumarin loaded Nanoconstructs were prepared in culture medium.

To study the influence of the concentration the medium was then replaced with a 100-μl suspension of 6-coumarin loaded nanoparticles of different concentrations. To study the influence of time, the medium was replaced with 100 μl suspensions of 6-coumarin loaded nanoparticles of 100μg/ml & 100 μl of fresh medium and incubated for 0.25, 0.5, 1, 2, 4, 6hrs. For each type of nanoparticles and concentration, a control was kept by adding the corresponding particle concentration in the well. The fluorescence of this well was treated at control i.e. 100%

At the defined time intervals, suspension from the wells was removed and the wells were washed thrice using PBS (pH 7.4). After lysing the cells with 100μl of 0.5% Triton X-100 in NaOH, 100 μl DMSO was added to the wells and the plates were shaken. The plates were read using a microplate reader. The excitation and emission wavelength was 430 and 485 nm, respectively, for 6-coumarin. As 6-coumarin was assumed to be dispersed evenly in the particles, the fluorescence observed was assumed to be linearly proportional to the amount of particles in the cell lysates. The cellular uptake efficiency was given by the ratio between the amount of particles taken up in cells and the amount of those in control and calculated by the following equation

$$\text{Cellular uptake efficiency} = \frac{\text{fluorescence of sample}}{\text{fluorescence of control}} \times 100 \qquad \text{----Equation [7.1]}$$

The results for influence of the incubation time and concentration are shown in Table: 7.3 and Table: 7.2, respectively and in Figure: 7.2 and Figure: 7.1, respectively.

7.2.2. In-vitro Cytotoxicity Studies

The cytotoxicity assay was conducted using CCK-8 assay. The cell viability was determined by a microplate reader. BT-20 and MDA-MB-231 cells were seeded in 96-well plates in Dulbecco's Modified Eagle Medium (DMEM), supplemented with 10% fetal bovine serum, at a density of 5,000 cells/well and allowed to attach overnight. After 24hr, 2X sequential dilutions of each compounds were prepared (DC,PLGA,PLGA-DC,RGD,LP-DC,LP-DC-RGD) in growth medium(GM), blank LP and PLGA in growth medium by using a new 96 well plate at volume of 120 μl/well. The old media from cells was aspirated and fresh 100 μl of GM to cells was added. The diluted compounds prepared from new plate were transferred to old plate in the volume of 100 μl into wells with adhered cells by starting from the lowest concentration. The plate was incubated for one, two and three population doubling time for both types of cells at 37°C in CO_2 incubator. The working dilution of CCK-8 reagent was prepared. For one plate (10x6well), 700 μl CCK-8 was added to 2800 μl GM. The old media from cells was aspirated and washed with PBS 7.4. 100 μl fresh GM was added to the cell and blank wells before adding CCK-8 reagent. Plates were incubated for 1.5~2 hrs at 37°C after adding 50 μl diluted CCK-8 reagent. The plates were observed using microplate reader (Biotek® Powerwave XS, Vermont, USA) at 450nm with blank well correction. All experiments were performed in triplicate. The absorbance of untreated cells was considered as 100% cell viability and with respect to that, the treated cell viability was calculated.

7.2.3. DNA content anlaysis by flow cytometry

The cell suspension of 0.15 x 10^6 cells/ml was prepared for BT-20 cells in growth medium (GM) and was added 2.0 ml/well in 6 well plates. After 24hr, 2X sequential dilutions of each compounds were prepared (DC,PLGA,PLGA-DC,RGD,LP-DC,LP-DC-RGD) in growth medium(GM). The old media from cells was aspirated and fresh 1ml of GM to cells was added. The diluted compounds prepared from new plate were transferred to old plate in the volume of 1ml into wells by starting from the lowest concentration. The plates were incubated for one, two and three population doubling time for both types of cells at 37°C in CO_2 incubator. The non-adherent and adherent cells were harvested in 5ml Falcon (352008) tubes. Cells were detached by using TrypLE solutions. Both types of cells were combined and pellet was made after centrifuging at 1500rpm/min. Cells were washed with ice cold PBS and stored overnight in 0.5ml of cold 70% ethanol (kept at -20°C). Cells were resuspended in 0.2ml of fresh made staining solution and data were acquired on FACScan and analysed by ModFit software. The composition of staining solution for 2000μl was water upto 2000 μl, propadium iodide (0.5mg/ml in water) 100 μl, triton X 100, (10%w/w) 10 μl and RNAse A 2.2 μl.

7.2.4. Apoptosis and Necrosis study

The cell suspension of 0.15 x 10^6 cells/ml was prepared for BT-20 cells in growth medium (GM) and was added 2.0 ml/well in 6 well plates. After 24hr, 2X sequential dilutions of each compounds were prepared (DC,PLGA,PLGA-DC,RGD,LP-DC,LP-DC-RGD) in growth medium(GM). The old media from cells was aspirated and fresh 1ml of GM to cells was added. The diluted compounds prepared from new plate were transferred to old plate in the volume of 1ml into wells by starting from the lowest concentration. The plates were incubated for one, two and three population doubling time for both types of cells at 37°C in CO_2 incubator. The non-adherent and adherent cells were harvested in 5ml Falcon (352008) tubes. Cells were detached by using TrypLE solutions. Both types of cells were combined and pellet was made after centrifuging at 1500rpm/min. Cells were washed with ice cold PBS. The 1X binding buffer solution was made with 10mM HEPES, 140mM NaCl, and 2.5mM $CaCl_2$, pH7.4. The staining solution was prepared in 1X binding buffer with 4µl of Annexin V and 4µl of propadium iodide (100µg/ml) per each 100 µl of cell suspension. The control staining solution with single dye was prepared. 100 µl of staining solution was added to cell pellet. After 15 minutes incubation at room temperature, the 300µl of Annexin V binding buffer was added and samples were analyzed within one hour by flow cytometry. The data were analyzed by cell quest software.

7.2.5. Histological study by TEM

BT-20 Cells were seeded in 96 well plates with wells covered with sterile Acer plastic at the density of $1x10^5$ cells per well. After 24 hrs nanoconstructs dispersion in growth medium was prepared at the 2nM drug equivalent concentration and transferred to well containing cells. After 2 hrs, old medium was aspirated and cells were washed with PBS 7.4pH for three times. After washing cells were fixed in 4% buffered formalin and kept at 4^0C until analyzed by TEM.

7.3. Results and Discussion:

7.3.1. Intracellular uptake of Nanoparticles

Intracellular uptake of nanoparticles is often studied after incorporation of fluorescent dye in to the nanoparticles system. 6-coumarin has been widely used as a fluorescent marker to study the intracellular uptake of nanoparticles. The other advantages of 6-coumarin include the requirement of low dye loading in nanoparticles due to its high fluorescence activity (Panyam, J, et al., 2003). The uptake of these nanoparticles can be easily visualized by fluorescence microscopy. Hence 6-coumarin loaded nanoparticles were used to study the intracellular uptake of the nanoparticles.

The factors affecting the particle cellular uptake primarily include particle size (Panyam, J. et al., 2003, Xie and Wang et al., 2005), different cell lines and cell densities (Jung et al., 2000), different compositions of the particles, surface properties (surface hydrophilicity and surface charge) (Sahoo, S. K. et al., 2002 & Foster et al., 2001). The dye does not leach from the NPs during the experimental time frame and therefore the fluorescence seen in the cells is caused by NPs and not by free dye.

We observed that the entrapment efficiency was 92.21 % (as discussed in chapter 5), suggesting incorporation of most of the dye added in to the nanoparticles. The particle size and zeta potential of 6-coumarin loaded unconjugated nanoconstructs and RGD-conjugated nanoconstructs was similar to that of drug loaded nanoconstructs hence, it is expected that their cellular uptake would be similar to drug loaded nanoconstructs.

Influence of concentration

The results of influence of the concentration on the intracellular uptake are shown in Table: 7.2 and graphically represented in Figure: 7.2.

Table: 7.2. Influence of concentration on the Cellular Uptake Efficiency

Concentration (μg/ml)	Cellular Uptake Efficiency			
	PLGA-DC	**PLGA-DC-RGD**	**LP-DC**	**LP-DC-RGD**
2	63.23± 3.27	84.36± 2.24	68.23± 3.48	85.28± 2.87
50	49.28 ± 3.21	81.18 ± 3.24	52.31 ± 1.82	84.12 ± 1.58
100	33.25 ± 3.73	63.81 ± 3.54	43.68 ± 2.39	78.34 ±3.21
200	26.28 ± 1.62	51.28 ± 1.81	35.26 ± 2.82	72.58 ± 3.75
500	19.83 ± 1.21	41.29 ± 1.42	26.47 ± 2.34	58.61 ±3.52

Figure: 7.2: Influence of Concentration on the Cellular Uptake Efficiency

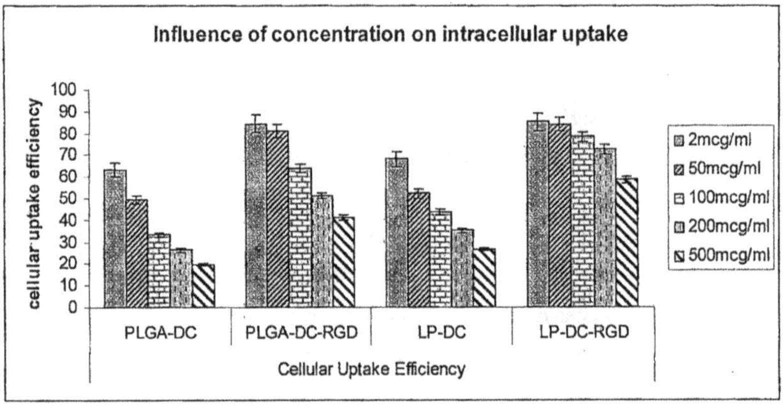

The uptake of the nanoparticles was directly proportional to the concentration of the nanoparticles in the medium. It was observed that the cellular uptake of the nanoparticles increased with increase in the concentration. However, the cellular uptake efficiency was found to be highest at the lowest concentration and found to decrease with increase in concentration. The decrease in the uptake efficiency indicates that the cells might have reached the saturating capacity for uptake. RGD-conjugated nanoconstructs at all concentrations demonstrate 1.6-2.1 folds increased uptake over unconjugated nanoconstructs uptake. The superior uptake of the RGD conjugated nanoparticles could be due to specific active endocytosis process mediated through the RGD adhesion to the integrins.

Influence of Incubation time

The quantitative uptake results of 6-coumarin loaded nanoconstructs are shown in Table: 7.3 representing the influence of the incubation time and graphically shown in Figure: 7.3.

Table: 7.3. Influence of Incubation time on the Cellular Uptake Efficiency

Time (hrs)	Cellular uptake efficiency			
	PLGA-DC	PLGA-DC-	LP-DC	LP-DC-RGD
0	0	0	0	0
0.25	7.31 ± 0.14	15.18 ± 0.12	10.21 ± 0.14	21.56 ± 1.21
0.5	13.54 ± 0.12	27.34 ± 0.38	17.33 ± 0.18	35.67 ± 1.32
1	20.23 ± 0.91	41.27 ± 1.26	25.46 ± 0.72	49.34 ± 2.76
2	29.23 ± 2.12	58.84 ± 1.32	35.67 ± 1.28	68.53 ± 1.48
4	38.45 ± 2.87	71.34 ± 2.18	44.45 ± 2.45	82.45 ± 3.12
5	40.58 ± 2.52	78.62 ± 2.41	48.34 ± 1.78	86.37 ± 2.84

Figure: 7.3. Influence of Incubation time on the Cellular Uptake Efficiency

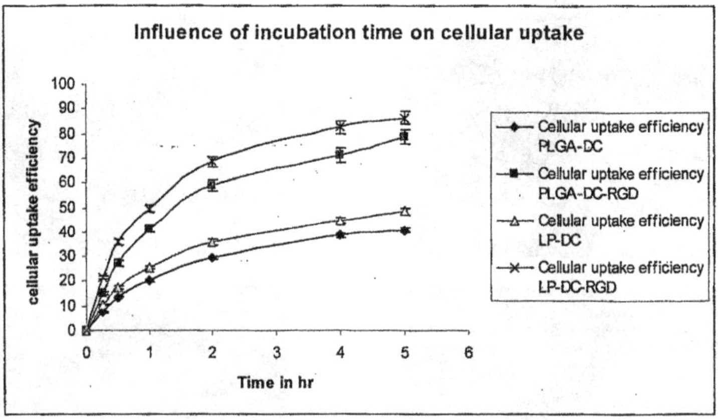

The results of quantitative uptake studies indicate the uptake of the nanoparticles into the cell. The untreated cells did not demonstrate any fluorescence. The nanoconstructs cell uptake efficiency was found to increase with time from 0.25-4hrs for both the unconjugated and RGD conjugated nanoconstructs. At all time points, the uptake efficiency of RGD conjugated systems were approximately 1.6~2.1 folds higher than the unconjugated systems. At 5hrs there was not much increase in the uptake efficiency suggesting the saturation of uptake with time. Hence, the influence of the concentration was performed by keeping the incubation time at 4hrs for all concentrations.

7.3.2. Fluorescent microscopy

The uptake of the nanoparticles in the cells was visualized by fluorescent microscopy (Figure: 7.4).

Figure: 7.4. Intracellular uptake of 6-coumarin loaded PLGA-NP and RGD-PLGA-NP formulations after different time points

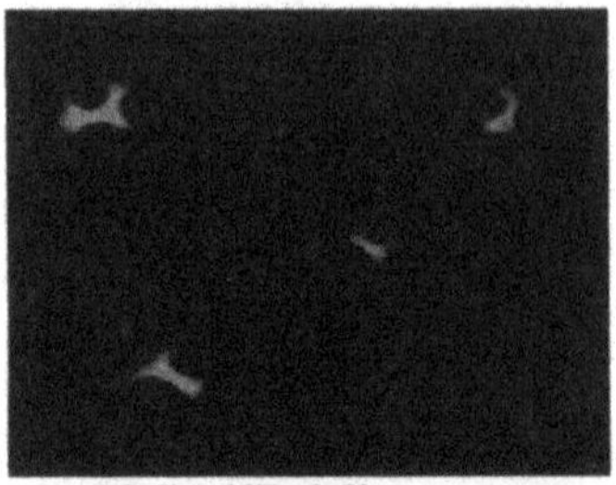

(a) PLGA-NPs-0.5hr

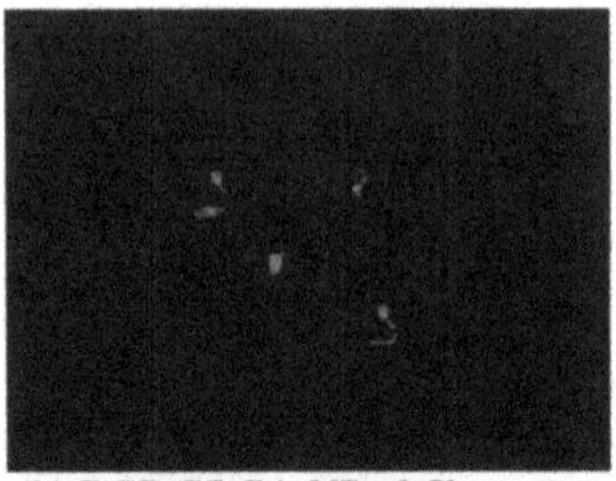

(b) RGD-PLGA-NPs-0.5hr

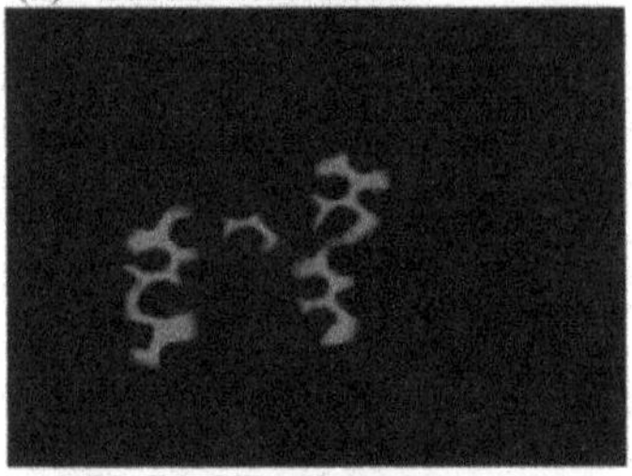

(c) PLGA-NPs-1hr

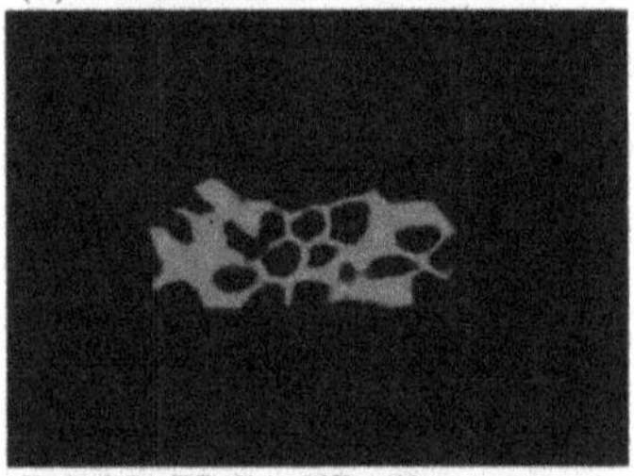

(d) RGD-PLGA-NPs-1hr

(e) PLGA-NPs-1.5hr

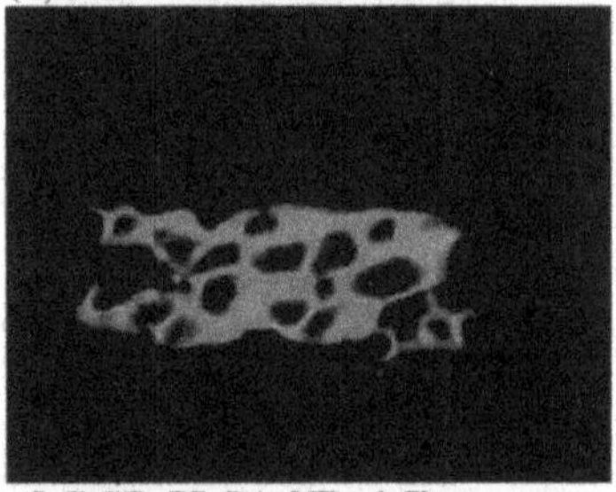

(f) RGD-PLGA-NPs-1.5hr

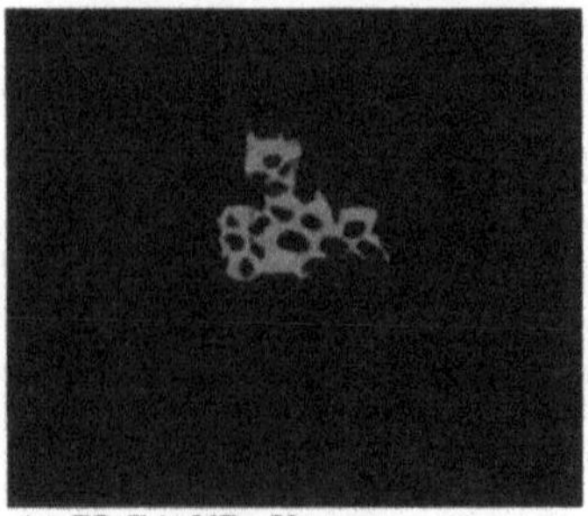

(g) PLGA-NPs-2hr

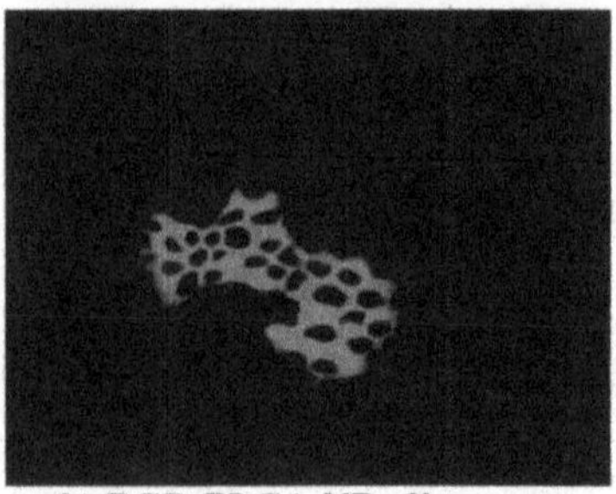

(h) RGD-PLGA-NPs-2hr

The fluorescent microscopic images showed green fluorescence in the cell cytoplasm and around the nucleus which reflects the internalization of the nanoparticles into the cell. Based on this observation, it is reasonable to believe that the nanoparticles may carry the active drug across the cell membrane into the cytoplasm. The RGD conjugated nanoparticles at all the time points demonstrated higher fluorescence intensity than the unconjugated nanoparticles confirming the results of the quantitative uptake studies. Also the RGD conjugated nanoparticles show higher number of the cells showing fluorescence than the unconjugated nanoparticles.

7.3.3. In-vitro Cytotoxicity Studies

The cell cytotoxicity is evaluated by assessment of viable cells after the treatment with drug or the formulation. Measurement of cell viability and proliferation forms the basis for numerous in vitro assays of a cell population's response to external factors. Cell Counting Kit-8 (CCK-8) allows very convenient assays by utilizing Dojindo's highly water-soluble tetrazolium salt. WST-8 [2-(2-methoxy-4-nitrophenyl)-3- (4-nitrophenyl)-5-(2,4-disulfophenyl)-2H-tetrazolium, monosodium salt] produces a water-soluble formazan dye upon reduction in the presence of an electron carrier.

Cell Counting Kit- 8, being nonradioactive, allows sensitive colorimetric assays for the determination of the number of viable cells in cell proliferation and cytotoxicity assays. WST-8 is reduced by dehydrogenases in cells to give a yellow colored product (formazan), which is soluble in the tissue culture medium. The amount of the formazan dye generated by the activity of dehydrogenases in cells is directly proportional to the number of living cells. The detection sensitivity of CCK-8 is higher than other tetrazolium salts such as MTT, XTT, MTS or WST-1.

To facilitate the basis of comparison the drug solutions, drug loaded nanoparticles & liposomes and drug loaded RGD conjugated nanoparticles & liposomes were added at same concentrations.

From the initial experiments, it was found that as compared to control (untreated cells), there was no significant cytoxicity observed for blank PLGA nanoparticles and blank liposomes and RGD itself at the highest concentration used in the study.

The cell viability results of Docetaxel and its nanoparticles formulations on BT-20 and MDA-MB-231 cells are given in Table: 7.4 & Table: 7.5 and graphically represented in

Figure: 7.5, and Figure: 7.6, respectively. The IC_{50} values observed for docetaxel and docetaxel nanoparticles are recorded in Table: 7.8 and Table: 7.9.

Similarly the cell viabilities for docetaxel and its liposomal formulations on BT-20 and MDA-MB-231 cells are given in Table: 7.6 & Table: 7.7 and graphically represented in Figure: 7.7 and Figure: 7.8. The IC_{50} values observed for docetaxel and docetaxel liposomes are recorded in Table: 7.10 and Table: 7.11.

Table: 7.4. Cell viability of Docetaxel and Docetaxel Nanoparticles on BT-20 cells

Conc. nM	Cell Viability (%) ± SD (n=3)								
	24hr			48hr			72hr		
	DC	PLGA-DC	PLGA-DC-RGD	DC	PLGA-DC	PLGA-DC-RGD	DC	PLGA-DC	PLGA-DC-RGD
50	45.6±2.3	44.4±1.8	41.4±1.05	24.9±1.2	15.8±1.3	10.8±0.82	5.2±0.56	2.8±0.14	1.8±0.22
25	51.7±4.1	52.8±2.9	49.3±2.1	35.8±2.5	29.4±1.7	12.4±0.56	7.4±0.63	6.4±0.34	3.6±0.45
12.5	71.6±3.5	70.4±1.6	68.4±2.7	52.5±2.6	42.8±2.1	18.5±1.4	13.7±0.92	11.4±0.91	5.4±0.43
6.25	81.4±4.5	79.2±2.3	76.4±3.2	62.4±3.1	59.4±2.6	29.6±1.3	21.6±1.6	15.4±0.98	11.5±0.93
3.125	91.3±4.8	85.4±3.8	83.2±4.2	72.6±3.7	69.8±3.2	41.8±2.1	44.1±2.6	29.8±1.6	19.7±1.2
1.5625	95.2±3.6	92.8±3.6	89.2±3.9	81.6±4.3	79.4±2.4	54.3±2.5	71.3±2.5	39.6±2.1	26.8±1.6
0.78125	96.3±2.9	94.3±2.8	92.5±4.1	89.4±4.7	85.4±4.1	65.6±3.1	83.4±4.1	48.4±2.1	39.4±2.1
0.390625	98.4±5.1	96.5±4.6	94.4±4.9	95.2±3.9	91.2±4.2	79.4±3.6	90.2±3.8	85.4±4.1	51.8±3.9
0.195313	99.4±4.7	98.4±4.2	96.2±5.2	98.2±5.3	94.2±3.8	89.4±4.3	94.6±5.3	90.2±4.2	88.7±4.1
0	104.2±3.8	103.4±5.2	104.8±5.5	106.4±5.2	105.4±5.4	102.8±4.2	106.8±5.1	102.7±3.8	103.2±4.5

(Mean±S.D., n=3)

Table: 7.5. Cell viability of Docetaxel and Docetaxel Nanoparticles on MDA-MB-231 cells

Conc. nM	Cell Viability (%) ± SD (n=3)								
	24hr			48hr			72hr		
	DC	PLGA-DC	PLGA-DC-RGD	DC	PLGA-DC	PLGA-DC-RGD	DC	PLGA-DC	PLGA-DC-RGD
50	41.3±0.98	39.5±2.7	21.4±1.7	19.5±0.78	11.6±0.32	10.5±0.21	1.2±0.05	1.5±0.03	1.4±0.05
25	49.6±1.4	45.4±1.1	41.4±1.8	25.4±0.45	19.4±1.2	15.4±0.43	2.4±0.11	2.1±0.02	1.8±0.04
12.5	59.2±1.5	56.8±1.2	52.8±1.5	39.8±0.79	33.8±2.1	23.8±0.35	4.8±0.31	3.5±0.05	2.5±0.03
6.25	64.2±1.9	61.7±3.2	58.7±2.1	52.7±1.6	42.4±1.7	32.7±1.1	9.4±0.25	5.7±0.12	4.9±0.45
3.125	75.4±2.3	72.3±2.4	69.3±1.3	69.6±1.7	51.2±1.5	41.4±2.1	19.8±0.98	11.8±0.23	10.4±0.67
1.5625	84.6±3.2	81.8±2.9	79.4±1.5	75.4±2.6	73.2±2.6	49.4±2.4	29.5±0.76	22.4±0.63	19.3±0.98
0.78125	91.5±2.9	87.4±3.2	85.6±2.3	83.4±2.8	80.1±3.8	71.6±3.1	52.2±2.1	41.4±1.3	35.5±2.1
0.39063	95.4±2.7	91.4±4.2	89.4±2.6	91.8±3.2	89.4±3.6	88.4±4.1	71.6±3.4	53.8±2.5	41.4±1.5
0.19531	97.2±3.8	95.2±3.4	94.9±4.3	95.4±4.2	93.3±6.1	91.6±5.2	89.7±5.6	89.2±5.1	52.8±3.4
0.09766	99.3±3,6	99.4±4.3	98.2±3.4	98.5±4.7	97.8±4.5	96.4±7.1	96.4±6.1	95.2±6.1	95.8±4.6
0	104.2±5.3	103.6±5.2	104.8±5.3	102.8±5.1	106.9±6.2	102.8±4.8	104.7±6.3	103.6±5.6.1	103.2±7.2

(Mean±S.D., n=3)

Table: 7.6. Cell viability of Docetaxel and Docetaxel Liposomes on BT-20 cells

Conc. nM	Cell Viability (%) ± SD (n=3)								
	24hr			48hr			72hr		
	DC	LP-DC	LP-DC-RGD	DC	LP-DC	LP-DC-RGD	DC	LP-DC	LP-DC-RGD
50	41.3±1.2	36.7±1.6	29.2±1.8	19.5±0.95	5.8±0.56	2.4±0.12	1.2±0.04	1.2±0.05	1.2±0.07
25	49.6±2.1	41.4±1.3	39.8±0.83	25.4±0.98	12.8±0.87	10.8±0.45	2.4±0.07	1.8±0.04	1.4±0.08
12.5	59.2±2.3	51.4±2.5	48.9±1.4	39.8±2.1	23.6±1.1	19.7±1.4	4.8±0.13	2.9±0.24	2.5±0.23
6.25	64.2±1.7	59.6±3.4	51.8±3.2	52.7±1.6	32.8±2.1	29.8±1.1	9.4±0.45	4.2±0.54	3.4±0.89
3.125	75.4±3.2	65.8±1.4	61.7±3.1	69.6±4.2	45.2±1.4	36.6±1.3	19.8±0.97	10.4±0.97	9.4±0.43
1.5625	84.6±2.8	72.6±2.8	68.6±4.9	75.4±5.6	65.2±3.2	46.8±1.2	29.5±1.1	19.8±1.1	15.8±0.85
0.78125	91.5±3.6	81.4±2.4	78.9±2.6	83.4±5.2	76.7±3.9	71.4±3.4	52.2±3.1	35.8±2.1	29.7±1.4
0.39063	95.4±2.3	85.4±4.9	81.4±4.1	91.8±4.3	85.8±4.7	84.6±2.7	71.6±4.2	45.8±3.1	39.4±3.2
0.19531	97.2±5.1	91.6±4.6	87.6±6.1	95.4±3.9	91.6±3.4	89.7±3.6	89.7±3.4	57.8±2.1	48.9±2.4
0.09766	99.3±5.3	97.4±3.7	95.7±4.9	98.5±5.8	95.4±5.1	94.9±4.6	96.4±5.1	75.7±4.5	74.6±3.3
0.04883	99.5±6.7	99.1±4.8	99.4±5.6	99.6±6.2	98.9±5.6	98.2±6.3	98.4±4.7	99.7±6.3	95.6±4.1
0	104.2±4.9	103.6±5.4	104.8±6.2	102.8±5.4	106.9±3.8	102.8±5.9	104.7±4.9	103.6±7.1	103.2±5.6

(Mean ± S.D., n=3)

Table: 7.7. Cell viability of Docetaxel and Docetaxel Liposomes on MDA-MB-231 cells

Conc. nM	Cell Viability (%) ± SD (n=3)								
	24hr			48hr			72hr		
	DC	LP-DC	LP-DC-RGD	DC	LP-DC	LP-DC-RGD	DC	LP-DC	LP-DC-RGD
25	51.7±2.3	41.4±1.2	35.4±2.3	35.8±1.3	13.7±0.76	5.8±0.45	7.4±0.56	1.5±0.04	1.5±0.04
12.5	71.6±3.6	49.2±3.2	48.1±2.5	52.5±1.4	25.9±1.4	11.2±0.75	13.7±0.87	2.9±0.06	3.1±0.06
6.25	81.4±2.8	68.5±3.4	66.5±1.3	62.4±3.2	39.4±1.2	17.6±0.56	21.6±0.99	9.4±0.32	5.9±0.11
3.125	91.3±3.1	75.4±4.1	73.8±4.2	72.6±2.5	52.8±2.3	27.2±2.3	36.4±1.4	13.8±0.15	10.5±0.24
1.5625	95.2±3.8	83.2±4.2	81.4±4.8	81.6±4.1	61.9±3.1	40.4±3.5	49.2±2.8	28.4±1.3	15.8±0.56
0.78125	96.3±5.3	89.4±4.8	88.6±3.5	89.4±3.4	71.8±2.3	53.9±2.8	83.4±3.9	37.8±3.2	24.7±1.3
0.39063	98.4±3.5	91.2±5.1	91.4±3.2	95.2±5.1	81.6±5.6	64.2±4.3	90.2±4.1	49.5±3.4	38.4±2.1
0.19531	99.4±4.2	95.4±4.3	93.2±5.1	98.2±3.2	89.4±4.3	78.6±3.5	94.6±4.9	84.6±5.1	49.6±2.5
0.09766	99.8±3.6	97.4±5.5	95.6±4.2	99.2±2.5	93.8±5.3	90.8±4.2	96.8±5.6	90.5±5.4	87.5±3.4
0	104.2±6.2	103.4±7.2	104.8±5.3	106.4±5.6	105.4±6.1	102.8±3.2	106.8±7.1	102.7±6.1	103.2±6.5

(Mean±S.D., n=3)

Figure: 7.5. **Cell viability of Docetaxel and Docetaxel Nanoparticles on BT-20 cells at a) 24hrs, b) 48hrs and c) 72hrs**

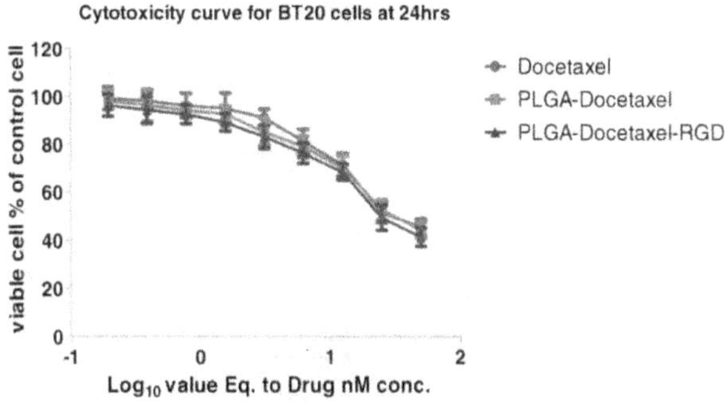

(a)

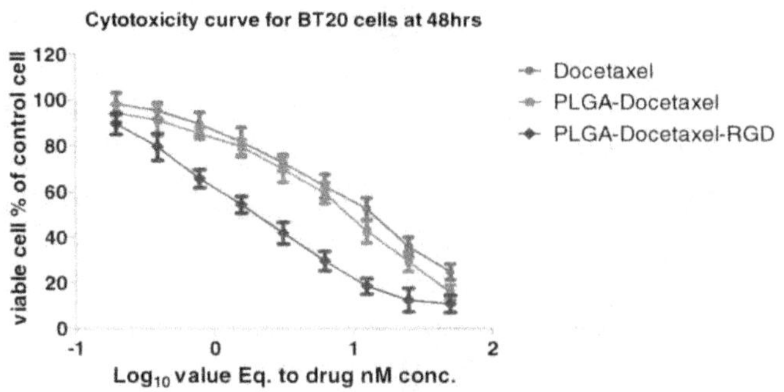

(b)

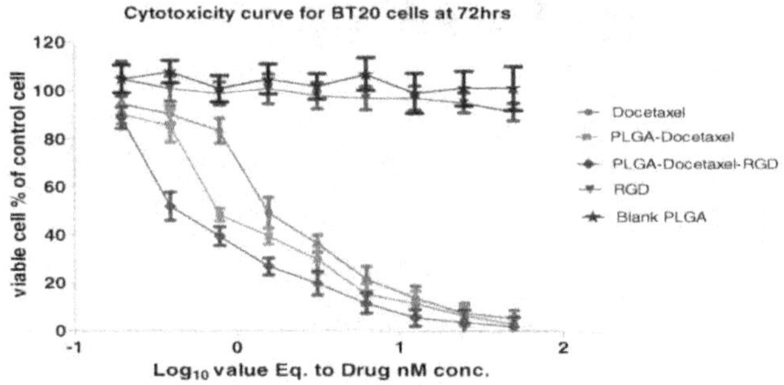

(c)

Figure: 7.6. Cell viability of Docetaxel and Docetaxel Nanoparticles on MDA-MB-232 cells at a) 24hrs, b) 48hrs and c) 72hrs

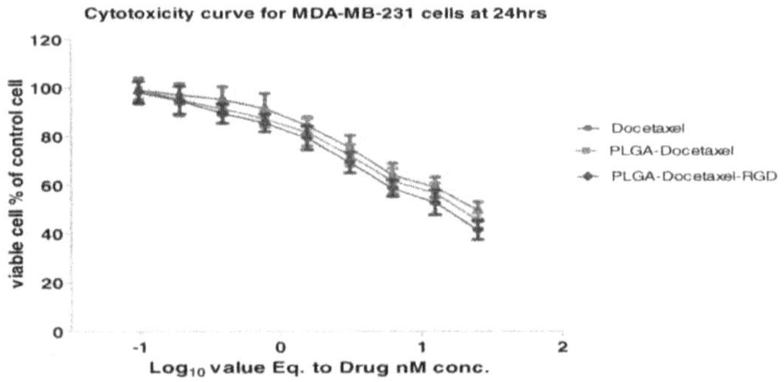

(a)

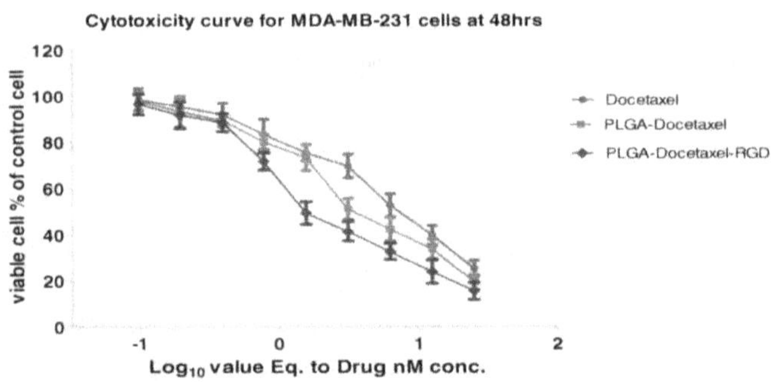

(b)

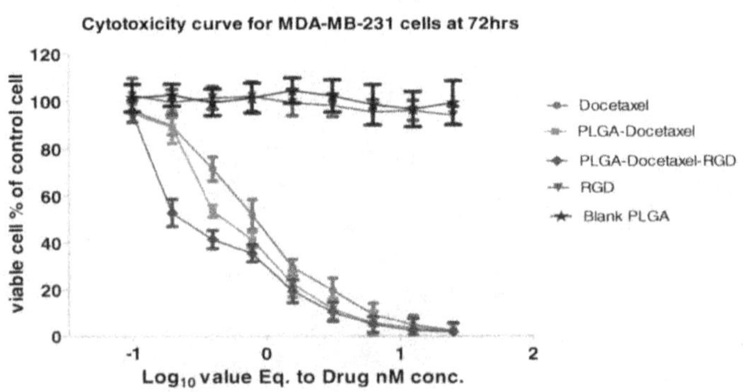

(c)

Figure: 7.7. **Cell viability of Docetaxel and Docetaxel Liposomes on BT-20 cells at a) 24hrs, b) 48hrs and c) 72hrs**

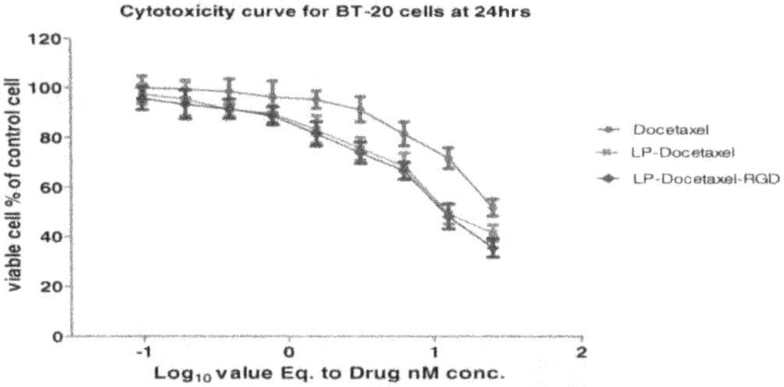

(a)

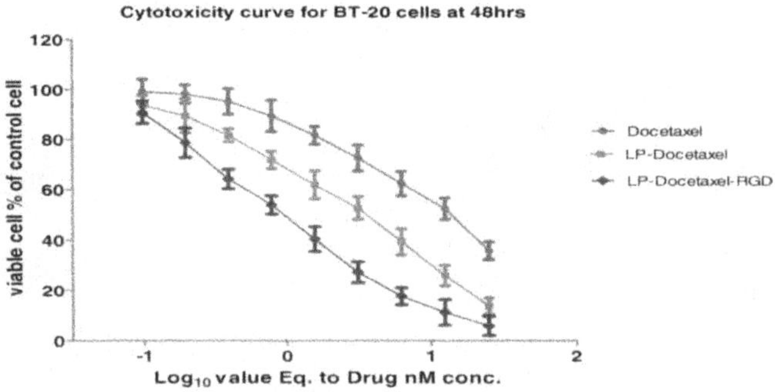

(b)

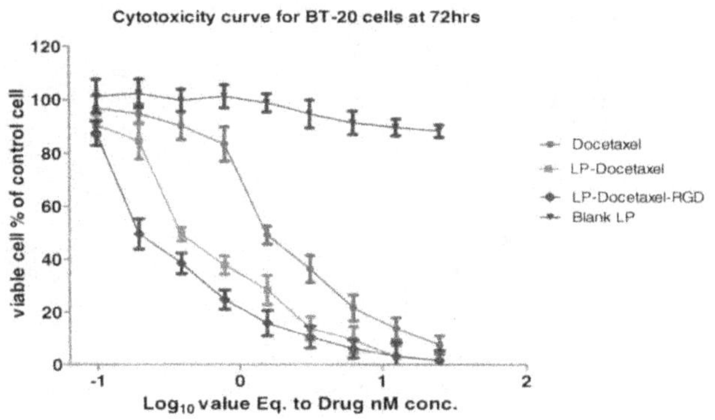

(c)

Figure: 7.8. Cell viability of Docetaxel and Docetaxel Liposomes on MDA-MB-231 cells at a) 24hrs , b) 48hrs and c) 72hrs

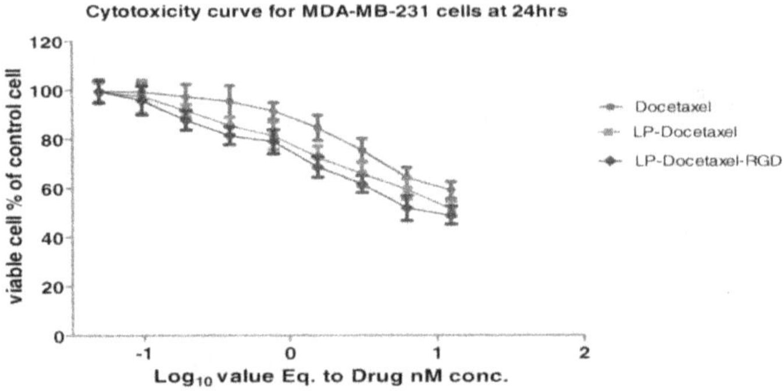

(a)

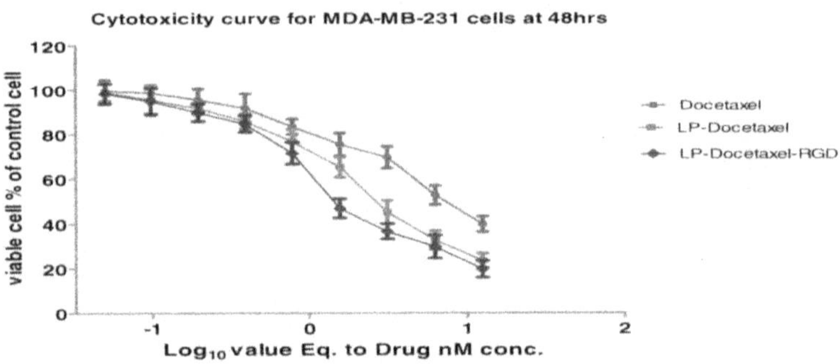

(b)

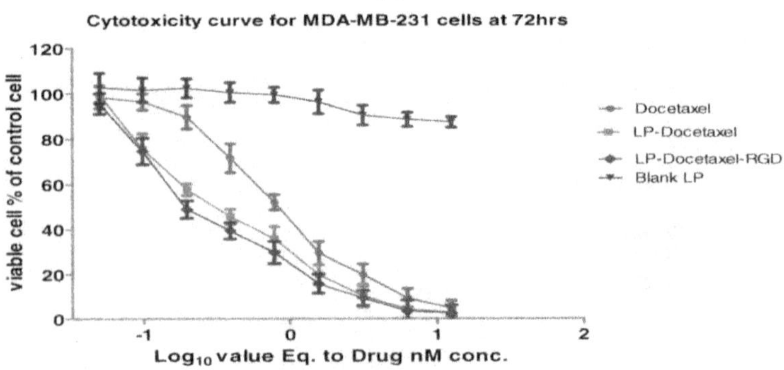

(c)

Table: 7.8. IC50 values for Docetaxel and Docetaxel Nanoparticles for BT-20 cell

Time (hr)	IC_{50} (nM)		
	DC	PLGA-DC	PLGA-DC-RGD
24	24.8±1.1	19.5±0.67	14.6±0.23
48	7.3±0.73	3.2±0.21	1.4±0.03
72	2.62±0.02	0.41±0.01	0.21±0.01

Table: 7.9. IC50 values for Docetaxel and Docetaxel Nanoparticles for MDA-MB-231 cells

Time (hr)	IC_{50} (nM)		
	DC	PLGA-DC	PLGA-DC-RGD
24	26.2±1.2	27.5±0.98	23.4±0.99
48	11.6±1.1	9.35±0.32	2.2±0.07
72	1.5±0.12	0.72±0.01	0.4±0.01

Table: 7.10. IC50 values for Docetaxel and Docetaxel Liposomes for MDA-MB 231 cells

Time (hr)	IC_{50} (nM)		
	DC	LP-DC	LP-DC-RGD
24	24.8±1.1	14.6±0.56	8.3±0,23
48	5.8±0.12	2.7±0.12	1.3±0.02
72	0.81±0.03	0.31±0.01	0.17±0.01

Table: 7.11. IC50 values for Docetaxel and Docetaxel Liposomes for BT-20 cells

Time (hr)	IC_{50} (nM)		
	DC	LP-DC	LP-DC-RGD
24	24.8±1.1	12.3±0.78	12.2±0.98
48	5.8±0.23	3.6±0.06	0.81±0.02
72	1.5±0.03	0.38±0.01	0.18±0.01

The cytoxicity of the drug loaded PLGA nanoparticles, RGD conjugated PLGA nanoparticles, liposomes and RGD conjugated liposomes formulations were significantly higher ($p<0.05$) than the docetaxel solution itself for both cell lines. The cytotoxicity was found to be dose dependent. The results demonstrate that the cell viability decreases with increase in drug concentration, indicating increase in the cytotoxicity of the drug and the Nanoconstructs. It was also observed that the cytotoxicity increased with incubation time. The cytotoxicity at all the time points i.e 24, 48 and 72 hrs was found to be in descending order as RGD conjugated drug loaded nanoconstructs > drug loaded nanoconstructs > drug solution.

For PLGA nanoparticles as shown in Table: 7.4 & Table: 7.5, at 24 hrs though the conjugated nanoparticles (PLGA-DC-RGD) showed higher toxicities than drug solution and unconjugated nanoparticles (PLGA-DC), the difference was insignificant ($p>0.05$). The drug solution was found to be more cytotoxic than the unconjugated nanoparticles (PLGA-DC) but the difference was insignificant ($p>0.05$). Any significant difference was not observed in cytotoxicity after 24hrs between any forms of drugs on BT-20 cell lines. However in case of MDA-MB-231 cells, the PLGA-DC-RGD showed significantly ($p<0.05$) higher toxicity than the unconjugated nanoparticles and drug solution. With increase in the incubation time, the toxicities of the drug and the nanoparticles were found to increase.

At 48 hrs, docetaxel solution produced significantly low toxicity than both unconjugated and RGD conjugated nanoparticles. Among the nanoparticles, the RGD conjugated nanoparticles showed significantly higher toxicity than unconjugated nanoparticles for both types of cell line.

At 72hrs, i.e. after three population doubling time, the RGD conjugated nanoparticles at dose of 1.5nM showed greater toxicities with about ~74% & ~80% cytotoxicity (26% & 20% viability) compared to ~60% & 78% and ~50% & ~73% cytotoxicity for unconjugated nanoparticles and drug solution for BT20 and MDA-MB-231 cell lines respectively. At higher concentrations there was not much difference between the cytotoxicites of drug solution and the nanoparticles formulations (at 72hrs).

The IC_{50} values of the solution and nanoparticles formulations as shown in Table: 7.8 & Table: 7.9, indicating decrease in IC_{50} values with increase in incubation time. The cytotoxicity indicated by IC_{50} values suggests that RGD conjugated nanoparticles at 72hrs are 2.1 and 4 time more cytotoxic than unconjugated nanoparticles and drug solution for BT-20 cell lines. Similarly, for MDA-MB-231 cells, the RGD conjugated nanoparticles are 2 and 10 time more cytotoxic than unconjugated nanoparticles and drug solution.

For liposomes, as shown in Table: 7.6 & Table: 7.7 at 24hrs the unconjugated liposomes (LP-DC) and RGD conjugated liposomes (LP-DC-RGD) showed a significant ($p<0.05$) high toxicity with compared to drug solution for both types of cells. While the RGD conjugated liposomes (LP-DC-RGD) showed a significant high toxicity with compared to untargeted liposomes for MDA-MB-231 cells but in case of BT-20, this difference is insignificant. The DC loaded liposomes and RGD conjugated DC liposomes expressed significant cytotoxic effect ($p<0.05$) at all other time points compared to the drug solution and unconjugated nanoparticles for both types of cell lines. As observed for PLGA nanoparticles, the cytotoxicity for drug loaded unconjugated and RGD conjugated liposomes also increased with increase in the dose and the incubation time. The RGD conjugated and unconjugated liposomes of DC depicted high cytoxicity than the free drug solution at high dose of 25nM for both types of cell lines.

The IC_{50} values are shown in Table: 7.10 & Table: 7.11 for docetaxel encapsulated liposomes. The cytotoxicity indicated by IC_{50} values suggests that RGD conjugated liposomes at 72hrs are 1.875 and 8.3 time more cytotoxic than unconjugated liposomes and drug solution for BT-20 cell lines. Similarly, for MDA-MB-231 cells, the RGD conjugated liposomes are 1.82 and 4.7 time more cytotoxic than unconjugated liposomes and drug solution.

Docetaxel being a substrate to P-gp could have been exocytosed and thereby reduced intracellular levels and hence lower cytotoxicities. The higher cytotoxicity with the nanoconstructs formulation for docetaxel may be attributed to the enhanced intracellular levels of drug available after internalization of the nanoparticles. The nanoparticles after intracellular uptake act as drug reservoir and release the drug with sustained action.

The superior antiproliferative/cytotoxic effect action with RGD conjugated nanoparticles could be because of greater intracellular uptake of RGD conjugated nanoparticles via $\alpha_v\beta_3$ integrins compared with unconjugated nanoparticles and drug solution. The BT-20 and MDA-MB-231 cells are reported to show over expression of the $\alpha_v\beta_3$ integrins. (MD. Anderson cancer unit). The over expression of the $\alpha_v\beta_3$ integrins leads to selective receptor mediated endocytosis of the RGD conjugated nanoparticles and thereby resulting greater intracellular delivery than the unconjugated nanoparticles and drug solution. Additionally, *in vitro* release study (as discussed in chapter 5) indicates that about 36.8% and about 19.4% docetaxel is released from unconjugated and RGD conjugated nanoparticles respectively in 3 days. For liposomes, the release was found to be 49.7% and 55.6% for unconjugated and RGD conjugated liposomes respectively, in 2 days. This indicates the release of drug is rapid with liposomal system with compared to PLGA nanoparticles. This might contribute to high toxicity of the drug encapsulated liposomes compared to drug containing nanoparticles.

It was found that nanoparticles and liposomes were more toxic for MDA-MB-231 cells compared to BT-20 cells. The one of the difference between both the cell lines is population doubling time (PDT). The BT-20 has 48 hrs of PDT while MDA-MB-231 has 24hrs of PDT. The cell repair mechanism are believed to be more active with cells having long PDT as each phase of cell cycle is longer than the usual. This might be one of the reasons that the toxicity of drug is also high with MDA-MB-231 as compared to BT-20 cells.

The greater availability of the RGD conjugated nanoparticles combined with the sustained release has led to the superior cytotoxicity. In one of the reports suggested by *Kim et al. 2006*, that the cytotoxicity of the anticancer drugs is more at repeated low metronomic doses than a high conventional dose. The sustained release from the nanoparticles could have acted as low metronomic doses and demonstrated higher cytotoxicity than the drug solution acting as conventional high dose.

7.3.4. Cell cycle study:

Cell cycle analysis was done to determine the growth phase in which the cells were accumulating due to inhibition of cell cycle progression. Docetaxel inhibits cell growth and proliferation primarily through its effect on the cell cycle and induction of apoptosis and necrosis (Khuri, F.R. et al., 2003). In our studies, the mechanism of inhibition of cell proliferation was found to be mediated through inhibition of cell-cycle progression with a relatively higher percentage of cells in the G_2 phase and lower percentage of cells in the S phase in the group that was treated with drug-loaded nanoconstructs and with the drug in solution (Table: 7.12 to Table: 7.16).

Table: 7.12. Cell cycle arrest study with Docetaxel

	24hrs			48hrs		
Component	**G1**	**S**	**G2**	**G1**	**S**	**G2**
Control A	62.7±2.5	21.5±1.5	15.8±0.76	57.2±1.4	25.5±1.2	17.2±0.87
DC 10nM	40.2±1.2	24.6±1.8	35.2±1.3	7.3±0.11	3.9±0.23	88.6±3.9
DC 30 nM	31.6±1.1	19.7±1.2	48.7±1.4	3.80±0.12	3.5±0.12	92.6±4.8
DC 50 nM	19.5±3.1	15.8±0.99	64.7±3.5	3.4±0.54	4.6±0.11	91.8±5.3

Table: 7.13. Cell cycle arrest study with Docetaxel Nanoparticles (PLGA-DC)

Components	24hr			48hrs		
	G1	**S**	**G2**	**G1**	**S**	**G2**
Control	57.2±2.3	20.5±0.78	13.2±0.77	57.2±2.3	20.5±0.23	13.2±0.56
5nM	44.4±1.3	25.3±2.1	30.3±0.99	25.6±1.1	8.9±0.11	65.5±2.8
10nM	33.8±1.1	21.6±0.76	44.6±2.3	2.6±0.07	1.2±0.02	96.2±5.4
20nM	21.6±1.3	16.8±0.87	61.6±3.1	2.4±0.03	1.3±0.03	96.3±6.4
Blank PLGA	-	-	-	56.3±3.8	21.325±1.1	22.31±1.1

Table: 7.14. Cell cycle arrest study with RGD conjugated Docetaxel nanoparticles (PLGA-DC-RGD)

Components	G1	S	G2
5nM 24hrs	31.5±1.2	16.8±0.98	51.7±2.4
10nM 24hrs	17.6±0.45	14.2±0.89	68.2±2.9
5nM 48hrs	10.4±0.12	15.5±0.88	74.1±3.6
10nM 48hrs	2.3±0.05	1.4±0.01	96.3±5.5
RGD	58.8±3.2	21.9±1.1	19.3±0.56

Table: 7.15 Cell cycle arrest study with Docetaxel Liposomes (LP-DC)

	24hrs			48hrs		
Components	**G1**	**S**	**G2**	**G1**	**S**	**G2**
Control	57.2±2.3	20.5±1.4	13.2±0.95	59.2±2.3	24.5±0.53	16.2±0.73
5nM	38.6±1.2	15.7±1.5	45.7±1.5	23.4±0.62	9.7±0.13	66.9±3.2
10nM	25.6±1.4	12.8±1.1	61.6±3.1	3.1±0.04	1.4±0.03	95.6±4.2
20nM	15.6±0.25	11.7±0.22	72.7±3.3	2.1±0.05	1.5±0.04	96.4±4.5
Blank LP	-	-	-	59.7±3.2	23.6±0.72	16.7±0.94

Table: 7.16. Cell cycle arrest study with RGD conjugated Docetaxel Liposomes (LP-DC-RGD)

Component	G1	S	G2
5nM 48hrs	8.6±0.56	15.8±0.34	75.6±4.3
10nM 48hrs	2.5±0.06	1.2±0.02	96.3±4.8
5nM 24hrs	30.4±1.3	14.2±0.04	55.4±1.3
10nM 24hrs	13.5±0.98	5.6±0.78	80.9±5.6

Figure: 7.9. Cell cycle arrest study after 24hrs with DC (a) and after 48hrs with DC (b)

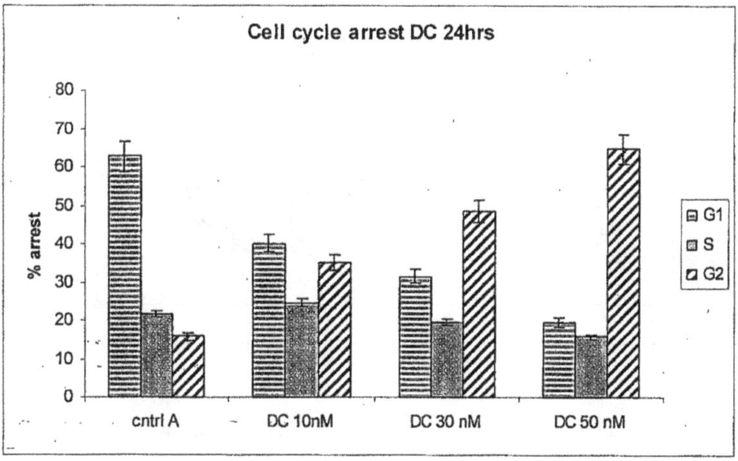

(a)

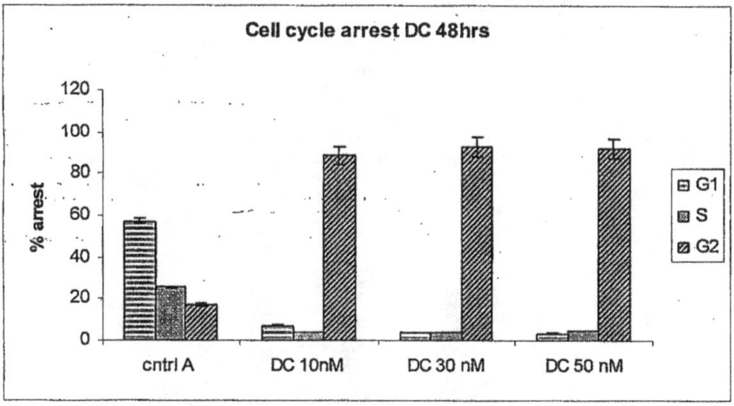

(b)

Figure: 7.10. Cell cycle arrest study after 24hrs with PLGA-DC (a), after 48hrs with PLGA-DC (b) and with PLGA-DC-RGD(c)

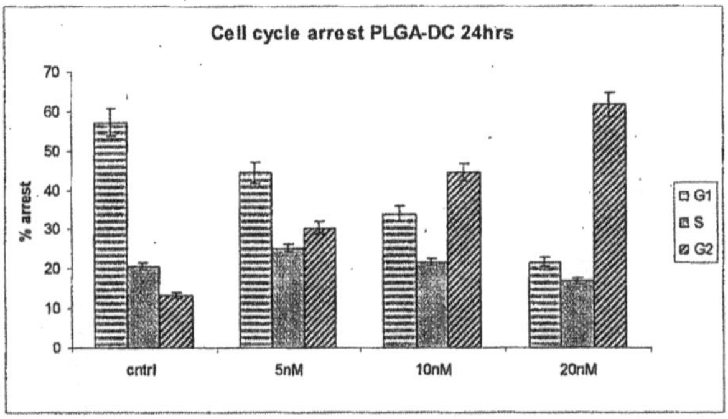

(a)

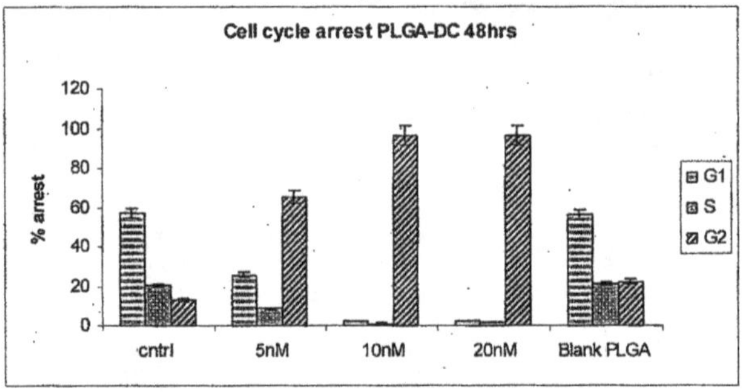

(b)

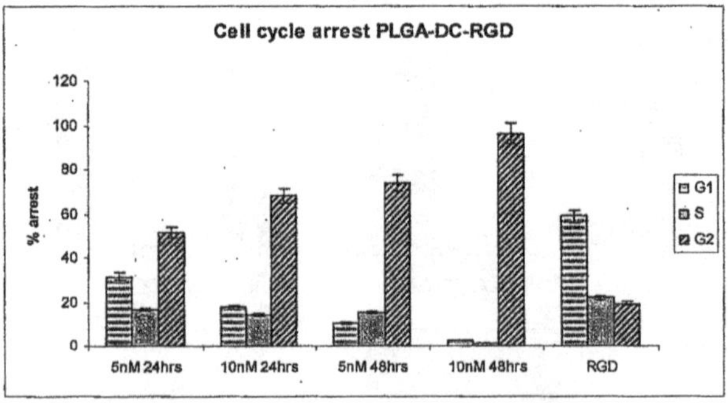

(c)

Figure: 7.11. Cell cycle arrest study after 24hrs with LP-DC (a), after 48hrs with LP-DC (b) and with LP-DC-RGD(c)

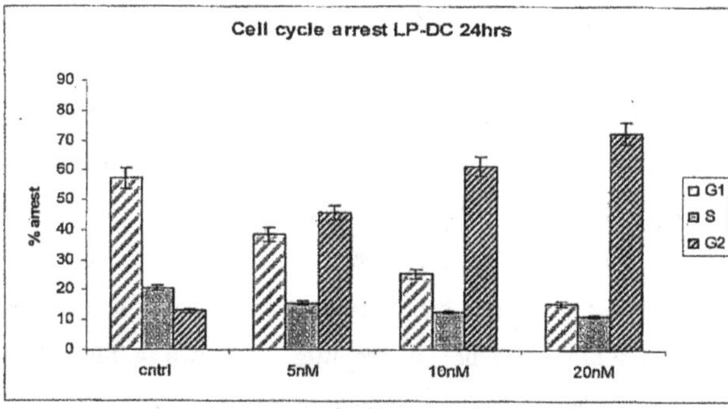

(a)

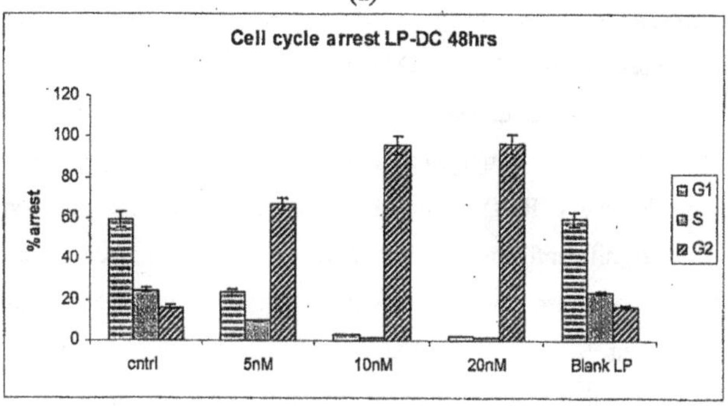

(b)

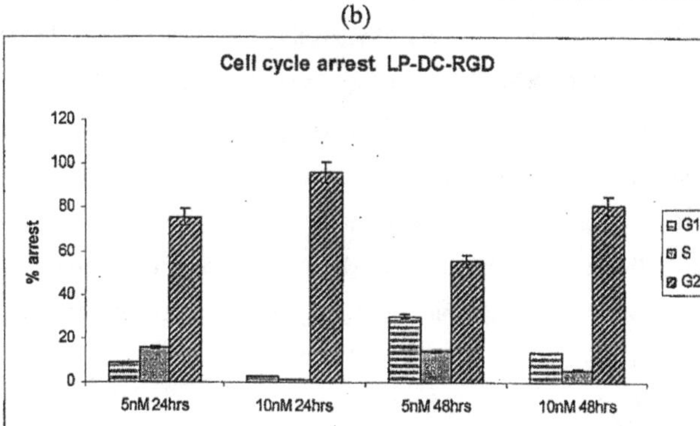

(c)

The study was done to find the effect of concentration and time. In case of free drug, the arrest in G2 phase was observed at lower concentration of 1nM and 2 nM but due to the high amount of debris, the exact percentage of each phase was difficult to calculate by Modfit software. At 24hrs, the cell cycle arrest in G2 phase was increasing significantly ($p<0.05$) as increase in concentration from 10nM to 30nM (Table: 7.12) for free drug. However, the difference was insignificant ($p>0.05$) at 48hrs between intra concentrations of free drug at 48hrs (Table: 7.12). It was observed at 48hrs, that with 10nM of free drug solution, the percentage G2 phase arrest was increased significantly compared to 24hrs effect. But the difference was insignificant with 30nM and 50nM of free drug. As shown in Table 7.14 the RGD conjugated nanoparticles at the drug equivalent concentration of 5nM showed 51% G2 phase arrest as compared to 30% G2 phase arrest with unconjugated nanoparticles at the same concentration at 24hrs (Table: 7.13). The block in G2 phase was found to be time and concentration dependent. At 48hrs, there is no significant difference between the effects of conjugated and unconjugated nanoparticles at 10nM concentration. Similarly, RGD conjugated drug encapsulated liposomal system was found to have significantly high arrest of cell cycle as compared to unconjugated system at same concentrations. The cell cycle arrest was found to be concentration and time dependent.

Cell cycle analysis demonstrated that all free DC, PLGA-DC and PLGA-DC-RGD arrested BT-20 cells in the G-2 phase of the cell cycle. However, in cells treated with PLGA-DC and PLGA-DC-RGD, the appearance of populations shown to be in G-2 was found to be more by at least 2 fold as compared to those treated with free DC. Further, the accumulation of cells in G-2 was accompanied by a 7–8 fold decrease in the number of cells in S phase compared to control cells, an indication of DNA replication inhibition. Blank PLGA and RGD peptide alone had no effect on cell cycle progression when applied using the same range of concentrations as PLGA-DC and PLGA-DC-RGD.

Figure: 7.12. **DNA content analysis for BT-20 cells (a) control cell (b) Treated with IC50 eq. concentration of drug nanoparticles (c) Treated with 10nM drug eq. concentration of nanoparticles.**

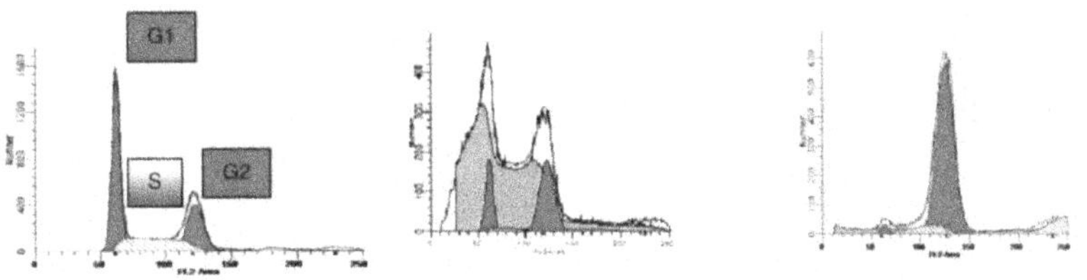

(a) (b) (c)

7.3.5. Apoptosis and Necrosis study:

The Apoptosis and Necrosis study was carried out to study the mode of cell death after the cell treatment with free drug solutions and drug containing nanoconstructs.

Figure: 7.13. **Apoptosis and necrosis study with BT-20 cells (a) control cell (b) Treated with 0.5nM eq. concentration of drug nanoparticles (c) Treated with 0.25nM drug eq. concentration of nanoparticles.**

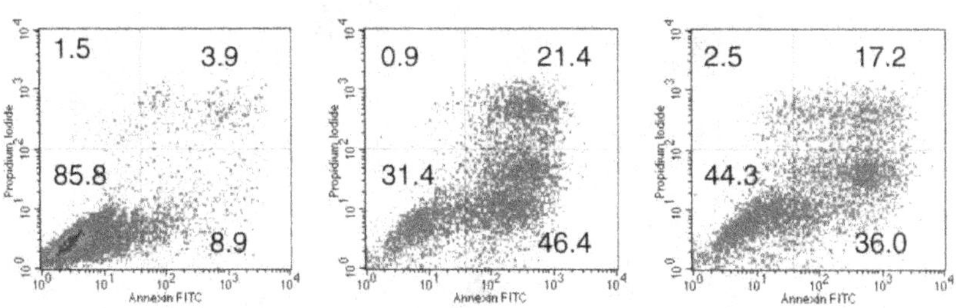

(a) (b) (c)

Table: 7.17. Apoptosis Necrosis study with Docetaxel, Docetaxel Nanoparticles and RGD conjugated Docetaxel Nanoparticles

Concentration	Components	24hr			48hr			72hr		
		Alive	Necrotic	Apoptotic	Alive	Necrotic	Apoptotic	Alive	Necrotic	Apoptotic
5nM	DC	85.3±3.2	13.6±0.45	1.1±0.01	65.4±3.2	22.4±1.1	2.2±0.06	30.4±2.1	66.2±4.1	3.4±0.04
	PLGA-DC	69.3±3.1	5.1±0.22	25.6±0.89	52.3±2.1	6.4±0.44	43.3±1.8	21.5±1.4	7.3±0.05	69.2±2.1
	PLGA-DC-RGD	65.3±1.2	6.4±0.11	28.3±1.1	35.2±0.69	5.6±0.35	59.2±1.1	15.4±1.1	3.3±p.06	81.3±3.4
10nM	DC	55.5±2.1	10.2±0.88	34.3±2.1	25.4±0.99	10.3±0.55	64.3±2.2	14.4±0.99	10.3±0.34	75.3±3.9
	PLGA-DC	44.2±1.1	8.4±0.56	47.4±2.3	15.3±0.57	10.3±0.23	74.4±3.4	10.3±0.33	11.3±0.25	78.4±5.1
	PLGA-DC-RGD	42.1±2.5	10.7±0.77	48.3±1.1	9.6±1.4	10.2±0.33	81.2±5.6	6.4±0.22	8.2±0.31	85.4±4.2

Table: 7.18. Apoptosis Necrosis study with Docetaxel, Docetaxel Liposomes and RGD conjugated Docetaxel Liposomes

Concentration		24hr			48hr			72hr		
	Components	Alive	Necrotic	Apoptotic	Alive	Necrotic	Apoptotic	Alive	Necrotic	Apoptotic
5nM	DC	85.3±4.5	13.6±0.05	1.1±0.02	65.4±3.2	22.4±1.2	2.2±0.02	30.4±1.2	66.2±3.2	3.4±0.03
	LP-DC	68.2±1.2	5.2±0.08	24.3±0.87	45.6±1.4	3.2±0.01	41.2±1.4	15.2±0.99	2.4±0.01	82.4±4.1
	LP-DC-RGD	64.3±1.6	6.5±0.23	29.7±0.98	20.8±1.1	2.1±0.03	77.1±2.2	7.3±0.55	3.3±0.03	89.4±3.4
10nM	DC	55.5±1.9	10.2±0.33	34.3±0.89	25.4±0.99	10.3±0.22	64.3±3.1	14.4±0.67	10.3±0.13	75.3±4.1
	LP-DC	38.4±2.1	11.4±0.55	50.2±1.6	15.5±0.79	9.3±0.31	75.2±3.7	7.2±0.15	7.4±0.23	85.4±3.8
	LP-DC-RGD	35.3±1.2	12.5±0.56	52.2±3.8	7.2±0.23	8.4±0.21	84.4±4.3	5.4±0.11	4.2±0.08	91.4±5.3

Figure: 7.14. Apoptosis Necrosis study with (a) Docetaxel, (b) Docetaxel Nanoparticles and (c) RGD conjugated Docetaxel Nanoparticles

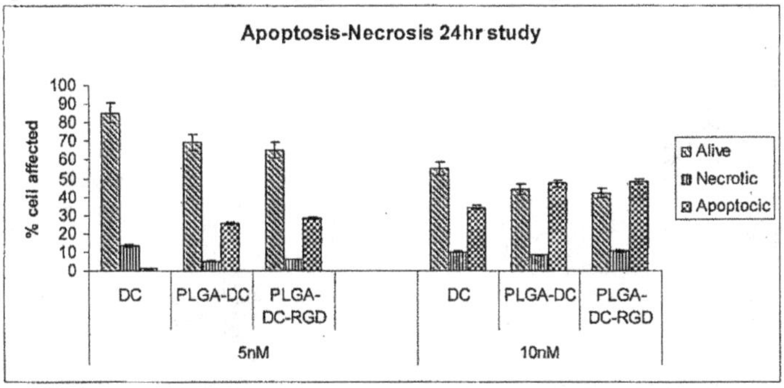

(a)

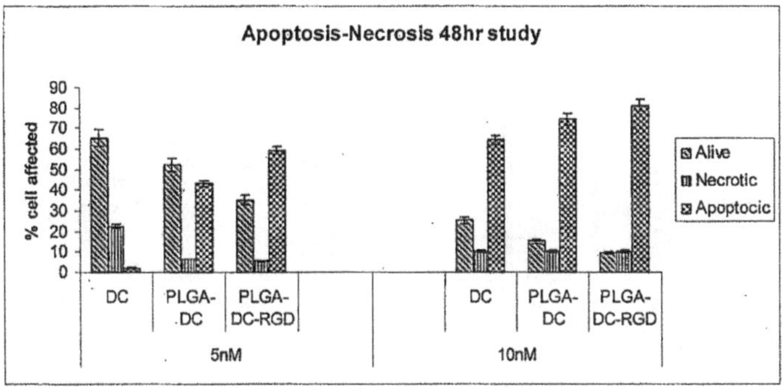

(b)

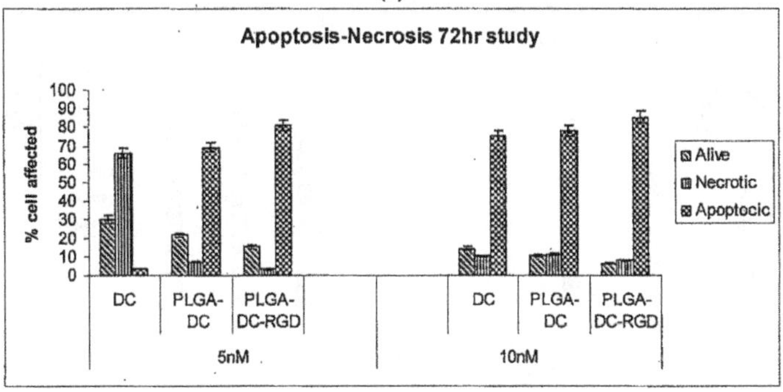

(c)

Figure: 7.15. Apoptosis Necrosis study with (a) Docetaxel, (b) Docetaxel Liposomes and (c) RGD conjugated Docetaxel Liposomes

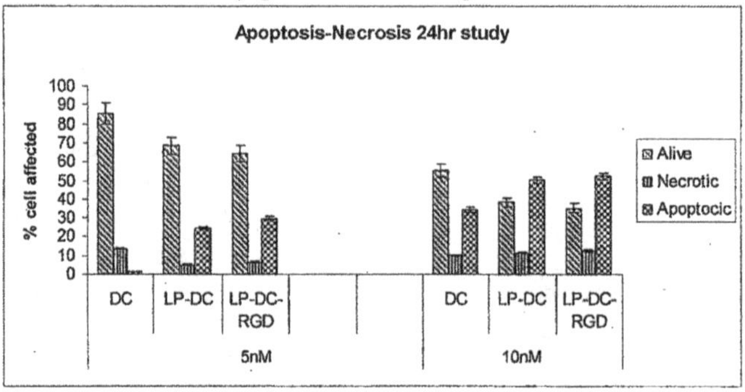

(a)

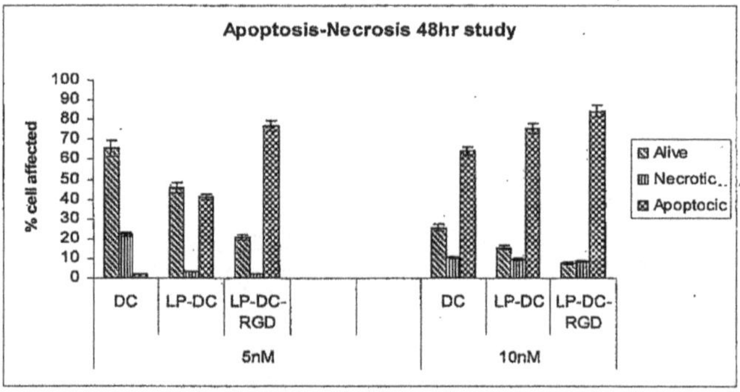

(b)

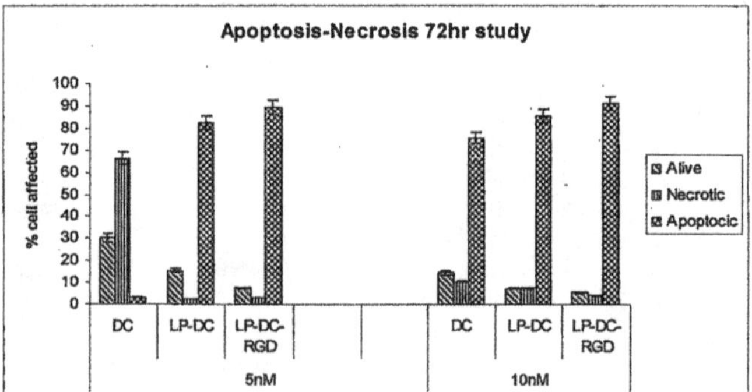

(c)

The apoptosis and necrosis effect was found to be concentration and time dependent for both types of drug delivery systems. In case of nanoparticles, the RGD conjugated nanoparticles have more apoptotic cell fragments than the unconjugated nanoparticles and drug solution at the same drug equivalent concentrations. At 24 hrs, the treatment of 5nM of drug solution with cells resulted in 13.6% & 3.4 % necrotic & apoptotic cell fragments, respectively. While at similar drug equivalent concentration, the PLGA-DC-RGD and PLGA-DC nanoparticles showed 6.4% & 28.3% and 5.1% & 25.6% necrotic & apoptotic cell fragments respectively. At 72hrs, the percent apoptotic cell fragments were significantly high for targeted nanoparticles as compared to untargeted nanoparticles and drug solution at 5nM concentration (Table: 7.17). While at 72hrs, the 5nM drug solution had significant high necrotic cell fragments as compared to targeted and untargeted Nanoparticulate systems. The free drug has found to have two mode of action at two different concentrations. At 5nM concentration it produces significantly high necrosis and low apoptosis. While at 10nM concentration the observed effect was reversed i.e. high apoptosis and low necrosis. The necrosis effect was significantly low in case of targeted and untargeted nanoparticles at both concentrations. At 10nM drug eq. concentration, the PLGA-DC-RGD nanoparticles have shown to be significantly high percentage of apoptosis with compared to same concentration of drug solution at all time points i.e. 24hrs, 48hrs and 72hrs. However the difference is insignificant with compared to PLGA-DC nanoparticles. Similar kinds of effects were observed with liposomal systems also (Table: 7.18).

We have shown that differences in the concentration of docetaxel will influence its mechanism of action at the molecular level, including cell cycle and cell death. In contrast, lower concentrations of free drug (2–4 nM) induce a high amount of cell debris. According to *Vargas H.H et a, 2007*, who has studied the dependency of this effect on cell cycle phase and concluded that docetaxel at lower concentrations is able to induce aberrant mitosis and aneuploidy. Currently, there are no experimental data to explain these findings, although several lines of evidence can shed light onto this issue. Docetaxel is easily accumulated in cells and produces impairment of microtubules. This impairment produces a moderate stabilization of p53 protein, followed by an induction of p53 transactivation activity once mitotic arrest is overcome. In contrast, docetaxel accumulation after higher doses of the drug induces a sustained arrest in mitosis with the consequent inhibition of transcription and higher p53 accumulation. Owing to an unknown mechanism, this difference in mitotic arrest duration also affects the postmitotic consequences, that is, aberrant mitosis with production of hypodiploid cells (at 2–4 nM docetaxel) vs mitosis slippage without cytokinesis producing large multinucleated cells (at 10-100 nM docetaxel). Moreover, as a consequence of this, the type of cell death will also be different, that is, mainly non-apoptotic after asymmetrical division, and mainly apoptotic after multinucleation. According to *Blagosklonny, et al 2006* model, mitotic arrest will induce p53 accumulation owing to the lack of transcriptional regulation of p53 during mitosis. After slippage, cells recover transcriptional ability and p53 protein will induce transcriptional targets, including p21. In agreement with Blagosklonny hypothesis, our data point to a mechanism regulating the different consequences of Docetaxel exposure according to the duration of mitotic arrest, depending on the accumulation of proteins (including p53 family of transcription factors) in a moment of the cell cycle when there is no transcriptional activity. Timing of arrest would determine the amount, and probably also the quality or type, of protein/s that will accumulate.

The consequences of a better understanding of the mechanisms of action of docetaxel are important. Mitotic perturbations will determine the main mechanism of cell death after docetaxel exposure. Similar to our results, *Fabbri et al 2006* found that lower concentrations of docetaxel were not able to induce early apoptosis (Annexin V, PI cells) in a bladder cancer cell line, and instead it induced a necrotic type of cell death. In a similar way, the ability of paclitaxel to induce cell death by independent mechanisms has been studied in more detail than docetaxel. It has been described that paclitaxel-dependent cytotoxicity requires cells to be first arrested at mitosis and upon mitotic slippage to enter apoptotic cell death (Blajeski et al., 2001). Moreover, differences in mechanism of action according to drug concentration have also been described with paclitaxel. In the early work of *Torres K, et al 1998*, aberrant mitosis was induced by low concentrations of paclitaxel followed by nonapoptotic cell death, and high concentrations induced mitotic arrest with apoptosis. In addition, according to *Giannakakou et al 2001*, low concentrations of paclitaxel (between 6 and 12 nM) induce p53, p21 and G1/G2 arrest in MCF7 cells, instead of mitotic arrest.

7.3.6. Histology study by TEM:

The results are shown in Figure: 7.16a, Figure: 7.16b and Figure: 7.16c for Control cell, LPs-DC-RGD and PLGA-DC-RGD-NPs, respectively. Photomicrograph by TEM depicted that the RGD conjugated drug encapsulated liposomes were able to enter the nucleus of the BT-20 cells. While nanoparticles were found to be present in cell cytoplasm of breast cancer cells.

Figure: 7.16. Histology studies by TEM (a) Control cell (b) LPs-DC-RGD (c) PLGA-DC-RGD-NPs

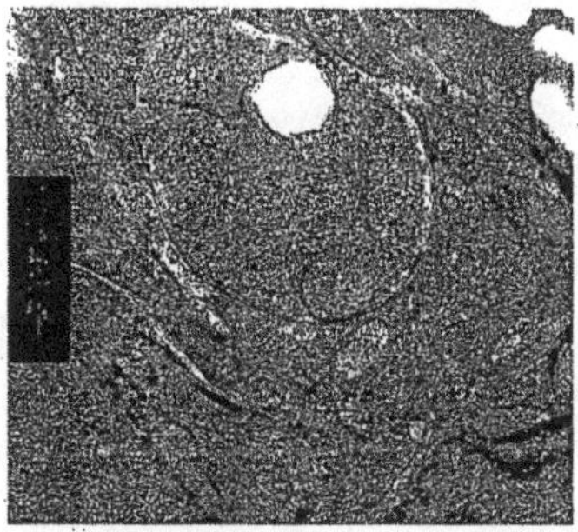

(a)

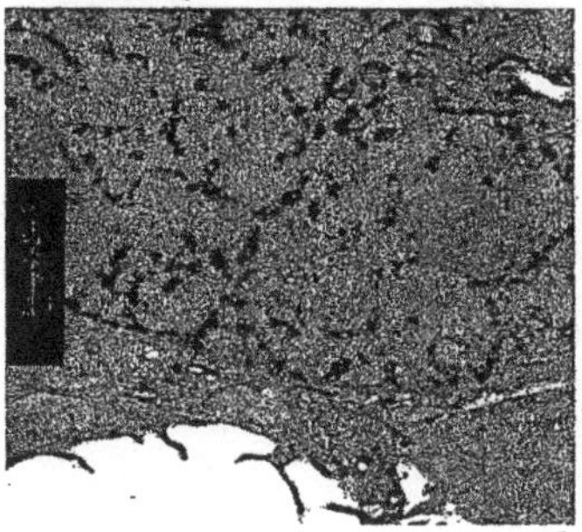

(b)

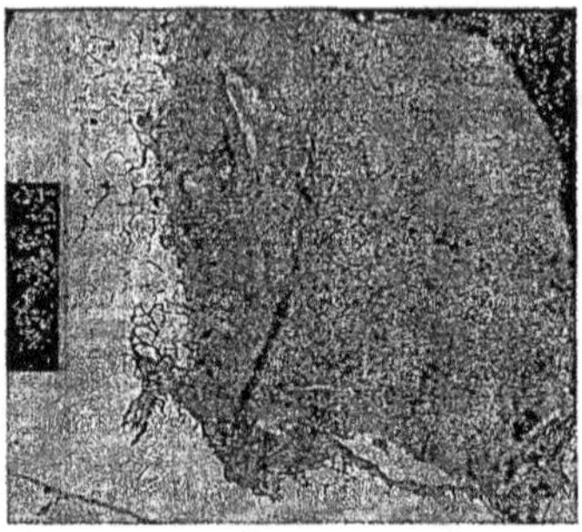

(c)

7.4. Conclusions

The blank PLGA nanoparticles and liposomes demonstrated no cytotoxicity on breast cancer cells suggesting the use of these nanoconstructs for safe delivery of anticancer agents. These nanoconstructs demonstrated higher cytotoxicity than drug solution due to high intracellular uptake of nanoconstructs and the prolonged release of drug from the nanoconstructs. RGD conjugated nanoconstructs due to receptor mediated uptake demonstrated significantly higher intracellular uptake and cytoxicity than unconjugated nanoconstructs and drug solution. The higher intracellular uptake of the RGD conjugated nanoparticles was confirmed by fluorescence microscopy. At the same drug equivalent concentrations, targeted docetaxel encapsulated nanoparticles and liposomes have shown high DNA content in G2 phase of cell cycle and more apoptotic cell fragments than untargeted systems and free drug solutions. Hence, it can be concluded that these nanoparticles and liposomes are suitable carriers to deliver docetaxel intracellularly for higher and prolonged cytotoxic effect.

7.5. References

Blagosklonny, M.V. et al., 1996, Taxol-induced apoptosis and phosphorylation of Bcl-2 protein involve c-Raf-1 and represent a novel c-Raf-1 signal transduction pathway, Cancer. Res., **56**, 1851–1854.

Blajeski, A.L. et al., 2001, A Multistep Model for Paclitaxel-Induced Apoptosis in Human Breast Cancer Cell Lines, Exp. Cell. Res., **270**, 277–288.

Foster K. A. et al., 2001, Microparticulate uptake mechanism of in-vitro cell culture models of the respiratory epithelium, J. Pharm. Pharmacol., **53**, 57-66.

Giannakakou, P. et al.,2001, Low concentrations of paclitaxel induce cell type-dependent p53, p21 and G1/G2 arrest instead of mitotic arrest: molecular determinants of paclitaxel-induced cytotoxicity, Oncogene, **20**, 3806–3813.

Jung T. et al., 2000, Biodegradable nanoparticles for oral delivery of peptides: is there a role for polymers to affect mucosal uptake, Eur. J. Pharm. Biopharm., **50**,147-160.

Khuri, F.R. et al., 2003, Mode of action of docetaxel – a basis for combination with novel anticancer agents, Cancer Treatment Reviews, **29**, 407–415.

Kim, et al., 2006, Metronomic treatment of temozolomide inhibits tumor cell growth through reduction of angiogenesis and augmentation of apoptosis in orthotopic models of gliomas, Oncology reports, **16**, 33-39.

Korsmeyer, S.J., et al., 1993, Sem. Cancer Biol., **4**, 327-332.

Panyam, J. et al., 2003, Fluorescence and electron microscopy probes for cellular and tissue uptake of poly(D,L-lactide-co-glycolide) nanoparticles, Int. J. Pharm., **262**, 1-11.

Reed, J.C. et al., 1994, J. Cell Biol., **124**, 1-6.

Sahoo, S. K. et al., 2002, Residual polyvinyl alcohol associated with poly (D,L-lactide-co-glycolide) nanoparticles affects their physical properties and cellular uptake, J. Control. Rel., **82**, 105-114.

Sahoo, S. K. et al., 2004, Efficacy of transferrin-conjugated paclitaxel-loaded nanoparticles in a murine model of prostate cancer, Int. J. Cancer, **112**, 335–340.

Sahoo, S. K. et al., 2005, Enhanced Antiproliferative Activity of Transferrin-Conjugated Paclitaxel-Loaded Nanoparticles Is Mediated via Sustained Intracellular Drug Retention, Molecular Pharmaceutics, **2 (5)**, 373-383.

Steller, H. et al., 1995, Science, **267**, 1445-1449.

Torres, K. et al., 1998, Mechanisms of Taxol-induced cell death are concentration dependent, Cancer Res., **58**, 3620–3626.

Vargas, H. H. et al., 2007, Molecular profiling of docetaxel cytotoxicity in breast cancer cells: uncoupling of aberrant mitosis and apoptosis, Oncogene, **26**, 2902–2913.

Wyllie, A.H. et al., 1980, Int. Rev. Cytol., **68**, 251-306.

Xie J. et al., 2005, Self-Assembled Biodegradable Nanoparticles Developed by Direct Dialysis for the Delivery of Paclitaxel, Pharmaceutical Research, **22(12)**, 2079-2090.

Zakeri, Z. et al., 1995, Death and Differentiation, **2**, 87-96.

Zhong, L.T. et al., 1993, Proc. Natl. Acad. Sci. USA, **90**, 4533-4537.

Zsolt Bacso et al., 2000, Cancer Research, **60**, 4623–4628.

Chapter 8
HPMA -Docetaxel copolymer peptide conjugated system

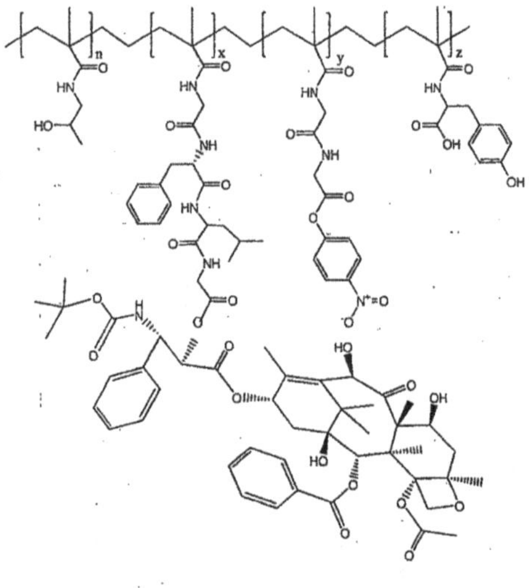

8.1. Introduction

Polymer conjugates, especially those prepared using N- (2-hydroxypropyl) methacrylate (HPMA) have been extensively studied for intracellular and cytoplasmic drug delivery .HPMA conjugated to oligonucleotides via lysosomally degradable spacers were shown to enter the cytoplasm and nucleus of the cells (Jensen, K.D. et al., 2003). The polymer conjugates offer the flexibility of attaching specific targeting molecules that enable their accumulation in specific intracellular compartments. For example, efficient cytoplasmic and nuclear accumulation of the HPMA conjugates can be obtained by attaching either a NLS (Nuclear localization sequences) or a TAT peptide to the conjugate (Jensen, K.D. et al., 2003).

Polymeric conjugates have been used for targeted delivery of drugs to tumor sites because the attachment of drugs to water soluble polymer increases their solubility, reduces the side effect, and overcomes multi-drug resistance; the large size of conjugates increases blood half life and significantly alters the drug properties and pharmacokinetics; the conjugates can be tailor-made (i.e., side-chain content, molecular weight, charge etc.) for specific targeting and delivery needs; they can be designed to passively (EPR) or actively target tumor sites; and site specific drug release can be achieved by designing biodegradable spacers that can be enzymatically cleaved or that are pH sensitive. The advantages have led to the development of a wide range of polymer-anticancer drug conjugates, some of which are currently in clinical trials.

HPMA copolymer has been employed to modify the in vivo biodistribution of chemotherapeutics agents and enzymes. The advantage of HPMA copolymer over other water soluble polymers is that they can be tailor-made with simple chemical modification to regulate drug and targeting moiety content for biorecognization, internalization, or subcellular trafficking depending on specific therapeutics needs. The over all molecular weight of HPMA copolymers is determined by the polymerization conditions, particularly the concentration of initiator and chain transfer agents. Various side chain moieties (isotope chelator, targeting moieties and drug) may be directly linked to the polymer chain via a biodegradable or non-biodegradable spacer.

Polymeric based delivery systems have been used as carriers for passive and active targeting of drugs in the treatment of various diseases and as novel imagine agents. Without a specific targeting ligand moderate-size (> 30 kD) polymer can passively (via

EPR) accumulate in tumor tissues. The EPR effect has been used to deliver macromolecular bioactive agents to solid tumors including anti-angiogenic drugs. Peptide-targeted delivery has a basis in nature as many peptides are used as attachment ligands by bacteria and viruses. The use of peptides as ligands for receptor targeting has been investigated by several groups (Shadidi et al., 2003). Peptide ligands have a number of advantages. These include their lower antigenic potential, making them less likely to cause an immune reaction. They are also easier to synthesize and characterize. Their smaller size means multiple peptides could be attached to a single nanoparticle conferring multivalent attachment. The most widely investigated receptor family for targeting with peptide ligands is the integrin family. These receptors are expressed on the neo-vasculature of various tumours and are involved in adhesion and cell signaling (Vander et al., 1994). Their peptide ligands are defined as arginine-glycine-aspartic acid (RGD) peptides, and comprise a range of linear and cyclic peptides containing the RGD motif (Arap et al., 1998). *Arap et al 1998* found that mice treated with RGD-targeted doxorubicin had greater survival than mice treated with doxorubicin alone in a murine tumour model. Many other targets are being investigated with peptide ligands targeting the tumour vasculature, cancer cell surface and surface immunoglobulins (Shadidi et al., 2003).

8.2. Preparation of copolymer

8.2.1. Preparation of HPMA monomer

To a solution of 1-amino-2-propanol (23.98ml, 0.3 mol) in 90 ml of acetonitrile, freshly distilled methacryloyl chloride (MA-Cl) (14.8ml, 0.15 mol) was added dropwise under vigorous stirring and cooling to -5^{0}C. A small amount of inhibitor, tertiary octyl pyrocatechine was added. The reaction mixture was stirred for an additional 30 min at room temperature. 1-amino-2-propanol hydrochloride formed as a byproduct was precipitated and filtered off. The filtrate was cooled to -70^{0}C and the HPMA precipitated. After equilibrating to room temperature the product was filtered off and washed with pre-cooled acetonitrile. Recrystallization was from acetone and the pure product was isolated.

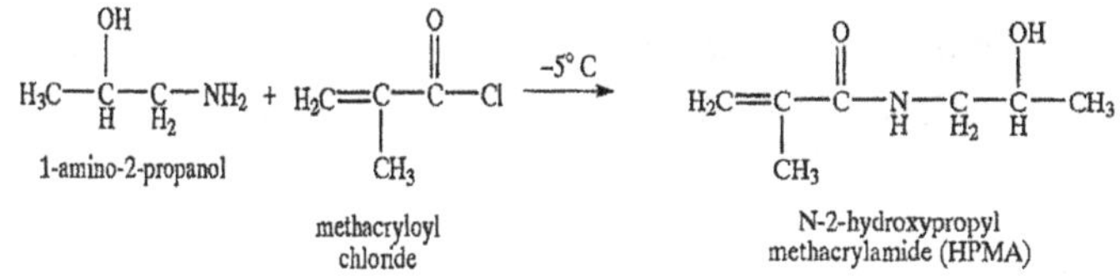

---- Reaction (1)

8.2.2. Preparation of MA-GF-OH

Glycylphenylalanine (Gly-Phe, 11.85gm, 0.0532mol) was dissolved in 4N NaOH (0.05mol) and cooled to 0^0C. Freshly distilled MACl (7gm, 0.612mol) in 10ml of dichloromethane was added dropwise. A small amount of inhibitor, tertiary octyl pyrocatechine was added to prevent polymerization of monomers. Simultaneously but with slight delay, 0.6 mol of 4N NaOH was added dropwise to the reaction mixture. After addition of MACl and NaOH the reaction mixture was warmed upto room temperature and allowed to react for one hour. The pH was maintained at around 6-7. The dichloromethane layer was separated from water layer, washed with 10ml of water and discarded. The collected water layer was acidified with citric acid to pH 3 and this white emulsion was extracted with ethyl acetate (3x150ml) in presence of inhibitor. The collected organic layer was washed with aq. NaCl and dried over anhydrous sodium sulfate. The organic layer was removed by Rota evaporator to obtain product as a white powder and recrystallized from EtOAc.

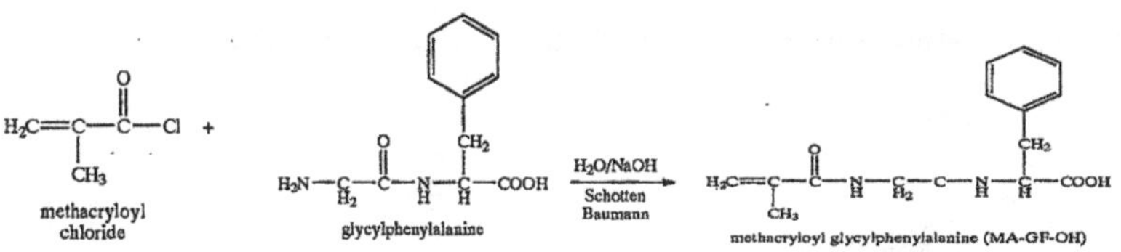

-----Reaction (2)

8.2.3. Synthesis LG-OMe.HCl

Leucylglycine (Leu-Gly, 10gm 53.31mmole) was dissolved in 80ml of methanol and cooled to -5^0C. 4.2ml (55mmole) of $SOCl_2$ was added dropwise under stirring. After equilibrating to room temperature the mixture was refluxed for three hours. The solvent was evaporated to dryness and the residue was dissolved in methanol and evaporated to remove HCl and $SOCl_2$. The residue was redissolved in toluene and evaporated to obtain white amorphous solid. This was used in subsequent steps without purification.

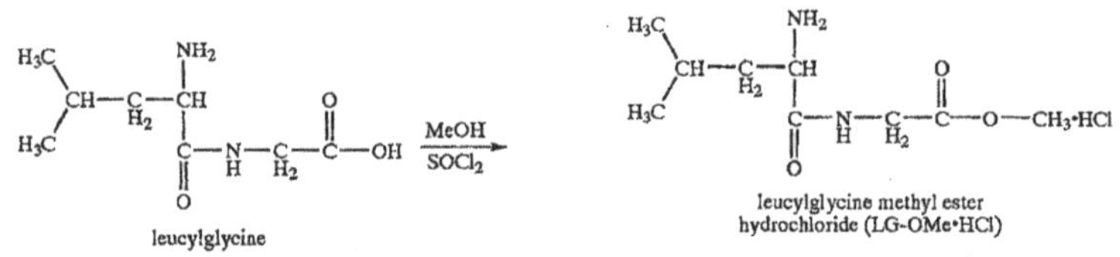

-----Reaction (3)

8.2.4. Synthesis of MA-GFLG-OMe

To a solution of Leu-Gly-OMe.HCl (9.8gm, 0.0410mole) in 80ml of DMF, was added 6gm(45mmole) of HOBT, 7.83ml of DIEA (45mmole) and the MA-GF-OH (10.74gm, 0.037mol). The reaction mixture was stirred and cooled to -10^{0}C. 9.28gm of DCC in 50ml of DMF was added dropwise within five minutes. The solution was stirred for two hours at 0^{0}C and then for 24hrs at room temperature. After overnight stirring the precipitated byproduct dicyclohexyl urea (DCU) was filtered off. The filtrate was rota-evaporated to remove the DMF completely. The residue was mixed with 100ml of 5% $NaHCO_3$ solution and extracted with EtOAC three times (3x150ml). The extract was washed with (3x100ml) of citric acid 5% solution, 5% $NaHCO_3$ solution and 3x50ml of saturated brine and dried over anhydrous sodium sulfate for two hours. After filtering off the drying agent and addition of a small amount of inhibitor, the filtrated was concentrated under vacuum to obtain the product. Recrystallization was done from EtOAC.

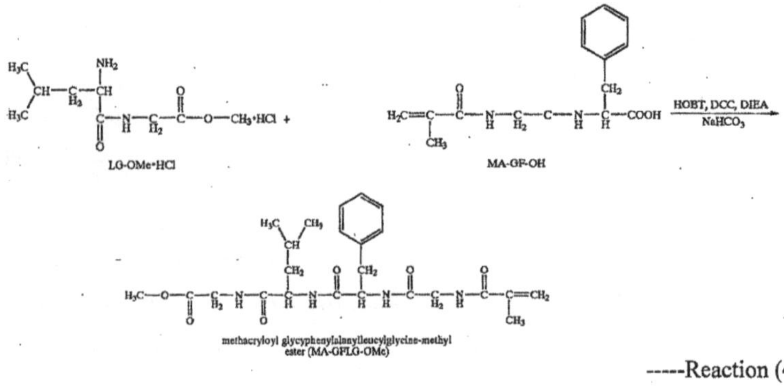

-----Reaction (4)

8.2.5. Synthesis of MAGFLG-OH

To a solution of MA-GFLG-OMe (16.71gm) in 80ml of methanol and cooled to 0^0C., excess of 2N NaOH was added dropwise under stirring. After addition of a small amount of inhibitor the reaction mixture was stirred for one and half hours at 0^0C and then for two hours at room temperature. The reaction mixture was concentrated under vacuum to remove methanol. 160ml of distilled water was added and the mixture was acidified with concentrated citric acid to pH 2. The free acid was extracted with 4x250ml of EtOAC, washed with saturated brine and dried over anhydrous sodium sulfate overnight. After evaporation of the solvent under vacuum the tetrapeptide product was re-crystallized from EtOAc.

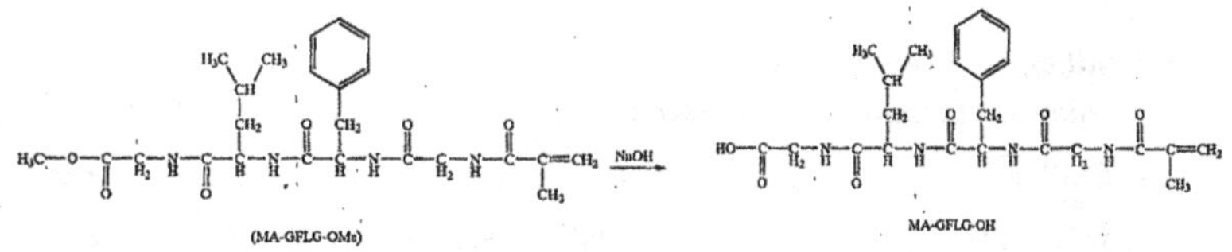

-----Reaction (5)

8.2.6. Synthesis of MA-GG-OH

Glycyleglyceine (Gly-Gly, 26.2gm, 0.2mol) was dissolved in 4N NaOH (0.2mol) and cooled to 0^0C. Freshly distilled MACl (0.2mol) was added dropwise. A small amount of inhibitor was added to prevent polymerization of monomers. Simultaneously but with slight delay, 0.2 mol of 4N NaOH was added dropwise to the reaction mixture. After addition of MACl and NaOH the reaction mixture was warmed up to room temperature and allowed to react for one hour. The pH was maintained at around 6-7. The product was precipitated by acidification with HCl (1:1) at pH 2 in presence of inhibitor. The final product was recrystallized from ethanol: H_2O (50:50) as MA-GG-OH.

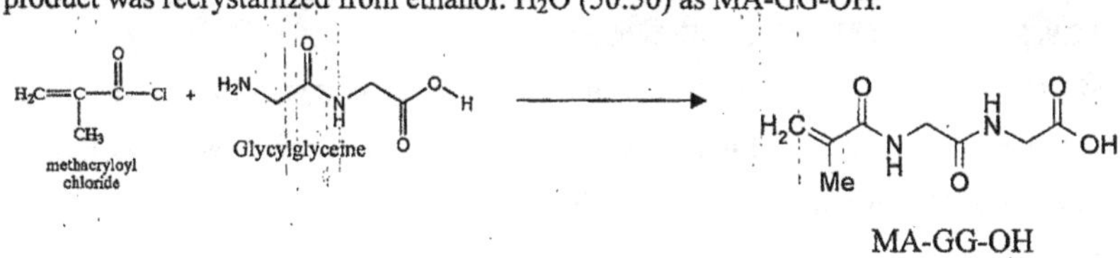

MA-GG-OH

-----Reaction (6)

8.2.7. Synthesis of MA-GG-ONp

To a solution of MA-GG-OH (9gm, 0.45mol) in 150 ml of DMF a solution of 6.15g of p-nitrophenol in 30ml of DMF was added under stirring and cooling to -10^{0}C followed by a solution of 10.31gm of DCC in 10ml of DMF. The reaction mixture was stirred for six hours at -10^{0}C and then overnight at 4^{0}C. The precipitated byproduct DCU was filtered off and the DMF was removed by rotary evaporation. The residue was dissolved in EtOAc and the remaining byproduct was filtered off. EtOAc was evaporated to dryness. The product was soaked in ether to remove excess p-nitrophenol. This procedure was repeated several times and the purity of the final product was determined by calculating extinction coefficient in DMSO.

8.2.8. Synthesis of MA-Tyr-OMe

To a solution of Tyrosine methyl ester (1 gm, 5.16mmol) in 100ml of Acetonitrile a freshly distilled MA-Cl (0.55gm, 5.16mmol) was added dropwise at -5^{0}C. The reaction mixture was brought to room temperature and allowed to react for 2 hours. The solution was concentrated on rota-evaporator to about half of the total volume. The precipitates were extracted with dichloromethane. The organic layer was washed with 5% citric acid solution.

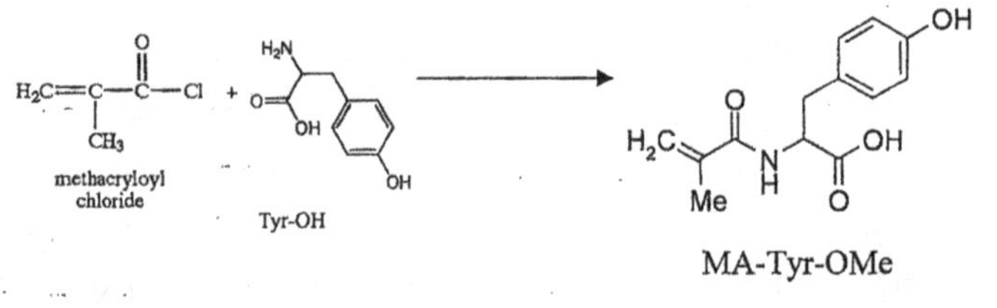

-----Reaction (7)

8.2.9. Synthesis of MA-GFLG-Docetaxel:

MA-GFLG-OH, Docetaxel and DMAP were weighed and kept in dessicator for 1 hr. This solid mixture was dissolved in anhydrous DMF and to this solution at 0°C DIPC (1.2x) was added. The resulting solution was allowed to warm to room temperature and left for 16 hrs. The completion of reaction was checked by TLC & Mass analysis.

Table: 8.1. Feed ratio of compounds for Docetaxel comonomer reaction

Compound	Mwt	Density	Wt taken(gm)	# of Moles	Molar ratio
MA-GFLG-OH	460.52	-	0.1	6.51438E-05	1
Docetaxel	805.91	-	0.210	7.81725E-05	1.2
DMAP	122.17	-	0.01591722	.000130288	2
DIPC	126.2	0.815	0.00986537	7.81725-05	1.2

MA-GFLG-OH + Docetaxel —DMF→ MA-GFLG-Docetaxel

-----Reaction (8)

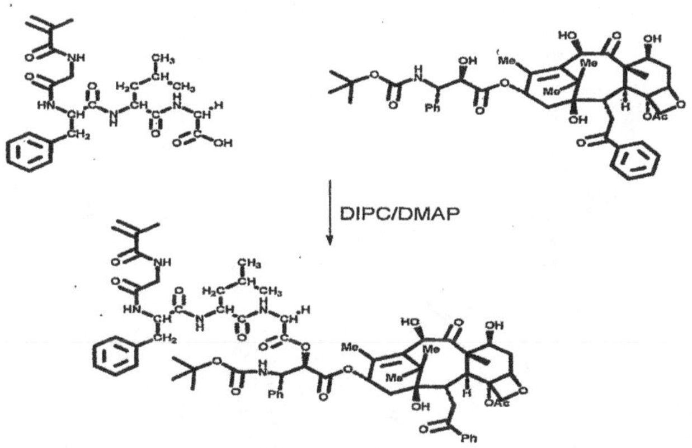

N-methcryloyl-glycyl-phenylanalyl-leucyl-glycyl-docetaxel

8.2.10. Polymerization of co-monomers

The polymerization was carried out using mixtures of n-HPMA, MA-GG-ONp,MA-GFLG-DC and MA-Tyr.OMe at various molar ratio as shown in Table: 2 using the initiator (2,2-azobisisobutyronitrile, AIBN). The solution containing the monomers in desired molar ratios dissolved in acetone with 1%DMSO and mixed with the initiator was transferred to an ampoule and bubbled with nitrogen for 5 min. The ampoule was sealed and put in an oil bath at 50^{0}C for 24 hrs under stirring. After 24hrs the copolymer was precipitated out of solution and the ampoule was cooled to room temperature to increase the yield of the precipitated polymer further. The reaction mixture with precipitated copolymer was added dropwise to ether to improve the yield. It was vacuum dried and further characterized by size exclusion chromatography.

Table: 8.2. Composition of comonomer feed ratio

Compound	Mole percentage	Weight in mg
HPMA	80.5	275
MA-GG-ONp	15	125
MA-GFLG-DC	2.5	57
MA-Tyr-OH	2	11.9
AIBN	-	23
Acetone	-	2.6ml

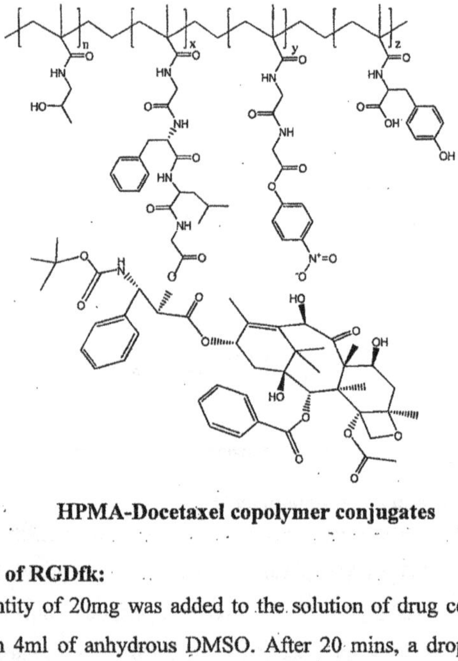

HPMA-Docetaxel copolymer conjugates

8.2.11. Attachment of RGDfk:

The RGDfk in quantity of 20mg was added to the solution of drug containing polymer (20mg) dissolved in 4ml of anhydrous DMSO. After 20 mins, a drop of Pyridine was added to the reaction mixture. After 48hrs, 100μl of 0.1N NaOH was added dropwise through syringe pump and allowed to stir for 2 hrs to quench the reaction. The peptide conjugated drug containing polymer was obtained after complete removal of solvent via vacuum drying.

8.3. In vitro characterization and biological evaluation of HPMA-docetaxel- RGDfk copolymer conjugates:

8.3.1. Characterization of comonomers by Mass spectrometry

The n-HPMA, MA-GG-OH, MA-GF-OH, LG-OMe, MA-GLFG-OMe, MA-GFLG-OH, MA-GFLG-DC and MA-Tyr-OH were dissolved in methanol to a final concentration of 1mg/ml and analyzed for their respective mass by mass spectrometer.

8.3.2. Characterization of comonomers by NMR

1H NMR spectra were obtained on a Mercury 400 spectrometer (300 MHz for 1H) in CD_3OD solvent for Docetaxel, MA-GFLG-DC, HPMA-DC and blank HPMA. Chemical shifts were reported in ppm with CH_3OH as the internal standard.

8.3.3. Determination of drug content

5 mg of untargeted copolymer conjugates were hydrolyzed by 1 ml of 1 N NaOH. The copolymer was separated from hydrolyzed p-nitrophenyl by Sephadex G-10 (PD 10) column. The collected fractions of copolymer were lyophilized and Docetaxel content was measured by UV spectrophotometer at λmax260nm in DMSO solvent.

8.3.4. Determination of ONp content

2 mg of untargeted copolymer conjugates were hydrolyzed by 1 ml of 1 N NaOH. Serial dilutions were prepared in 1 N NaOH and analyzed by UV spectrophotometer at λmax 400nm for free p-nitrophenol. The ONp content was calculated from the standard plot of pure p-nitrophenol in 1 N NaOH.

8.3.5. Determination of Molecular weight of the copolymer

10 mg of untargeted copolymer conjugates were hydrolyzed by 1 ml of 1 N NaOH. The copolymer was separated from hydrolyzed p-nitrophenyl by Sephadex G-10 (PD 10) column. The collected fractions of copolymer were lyophilized. 5 mg of the dry copolymer was solubilized in 0.5 ml PBS 7.4 pH and injected the Sepharose 12 column for size exclusion chromatography with multi-angle light scattering detector from Wyatt technology. The targeted polymer was directly injected without hydrolysis in 0.5ml of PBS pH 7.4.

8.3.6. Determination of peptide content

1 mg of targeted polymer was dissolved in 1 ml of PBS pH 7.4. The attached peptide was hydrolysed to its individual amino acids and evaluated by amino acid analysis.

8.3.7. Drug release studies

The in vitro release of Docetaxel from HPMA copolymers was evaluated using the model lysosomal enzyme cathepsin B (CPB) according to previously described procedures with minor modifications (Kasuya, Y. et al., 2002, Wang, D. et al., 2000 & Pan, H. et al.,2006) Enzyme incubation mixture consisted of CPB stock solution (0.98 ml, 0.572 mg/ml in 0.1 M ammonium acetate buffer pH=5.5, 1 mM EDTA) and cysteine solution (0.02 ml, 250 mM in acetate buffer pH=5.5, 1 mM EDTA). 5 mg of HPMA copolymer-Docetaxel conjugates P1 and P2 (Table: 8.3) were dissolved in the incubation mixture (1ml, 5 min preincubation at 37°C). At 15, 60 and 180 min, 100 µl samples were removed, drug extracted twice with 1 ml ethyl acetate, organic layer separated and dried under nitrogen. Resulting residue was dissolved in 0.5ml of mobile phase and evaluated for drug content using reverse-phase high performance liquid chromatography (HPLC). Docetaxel was analyzed by HPLC method as previously described method B. *Mallikarjuna Rao et al* with slight modification. The mobile phase consisted of deionized water and HPLC grade acetonitrile, with 34% acetonitrile in deionized water held for 5 min, then linear gradients to 58% acetonitrile in 16 min, then linear gradients to 70% acetonitrile in 2 min, then linear gradients to 34% acetonitrile in 4 min and 34% acetonitrile held for 5 min and was delivered at a flow rate of 1.0 ml/min. UV detection was performed at 227 nm.

8.3.8. In vitro cytotoxicity assay

In vitro cytotoxicity and IC_{50} dose of free drug and copolymers was evaluated on BT-20 and HCT116 cells using a CCK-8 procedure. 6,000 cells per well were seeded in 96-well micro titer plates and plated for a total of 96hrs. On 24hrs cells were treated with drug and copolymer solutions in complete media lasting for 72h. Following treatments, CCk-8 solution was added for 1.5h, media gently aspirated, and absorption measured at 450 nm with blank well correction. Cell growth inhibition was determined by the cell viability at after 72h treatment and expressed as % cell viability compared to untreated cells.

Experiments were routinely conducted in the exponential growth phase. IC_{50} values were determined by nonlinear regression analysis using GraphPad Prism software.

8.3.9. DNA Content Analysis study by Flowcytometer

Cells were plated at the initial density of 0.15 X 10^6 six well plates. After 24hrs cells were exposed to DC and HPMA-DC with the concentration of 10, 30, 60 and 100nM for 24hrs. Cells pellets were collected and washed with PBS pH 7.4 after detaching with Tripsin Like enzyme. Cells were kept in 70% ethanol for overnight. Cells pellet were resuspended in 200µl of staining solution made of Propadium Iodide after washing with PBS and acquired for DNA content by Flow cytometer (FAScan, Becton Dickinson). The data were analyzed by Modfit Software.

8.3.10. Confocal Microscopy

Cells were seeded at the density of 2x 10^4 and 1x10^4 in 35mm glass bottom microwell dishes. After 24hrs both forms of drugs were added in the concentration of 1xIC_{50} and 2x IC_{50}. Control and treated cell were examined under the laser scanning confocal microscope.

8.3.11. Stability studies in mice serum and PBS pH 7.4

HPMA-DC conjugates were dissolved in 1 ml of 100% mice serum, 10%serum and PBS pH 7.4 respectively in the concentration equivalent to 1 mg of free Docetaxel. The solutions of conjugates were incubated at 37^0C with continuous stirring. At predetermined time intervals, 100µl of sample was withdrawn and free drug was extracted with 300 µl of chloroform. The extraction was repeated three times and the collected choloroform layer was evaporated to dryness under nitrogen. The residue obtained was dissolved in 100 µl of mobile phase and the amount of Docetaxel was analyzed by HPLC.

8.4. Results and Discussion:

8.4.1. Characterization of monomers by Mass spectrometer

Results for analysis of mass are shown in Figure: 8.1 to Figure: 8.7 for respective monomers. In each figure, (a) and (b) denotes mass spectra of mixture and of individual monomer, respectively.

Figure: 8.1. Mass spectra of matrix (a) and MA-GF-OH (b)

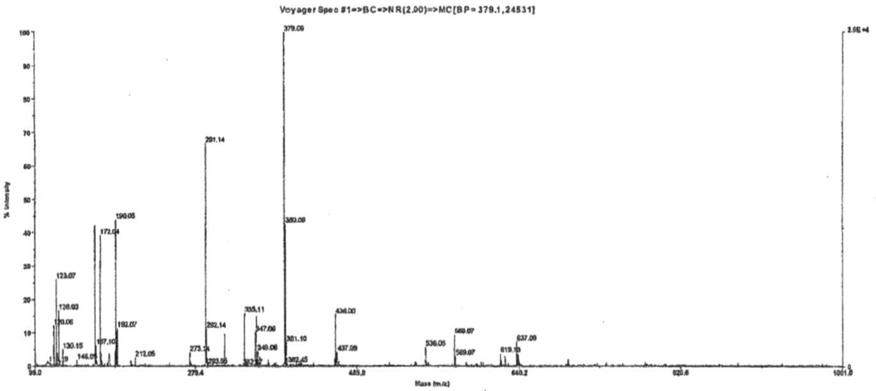

(a)

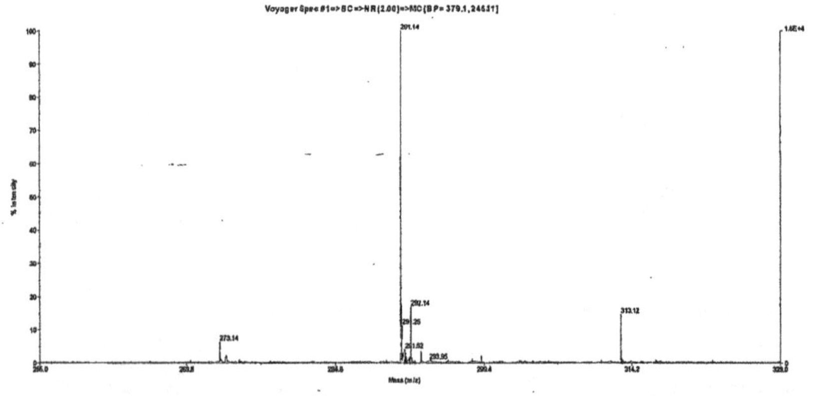

(b)

Figure: 8.2. Mass spectra of matrix (a) and LG-OMe (b)

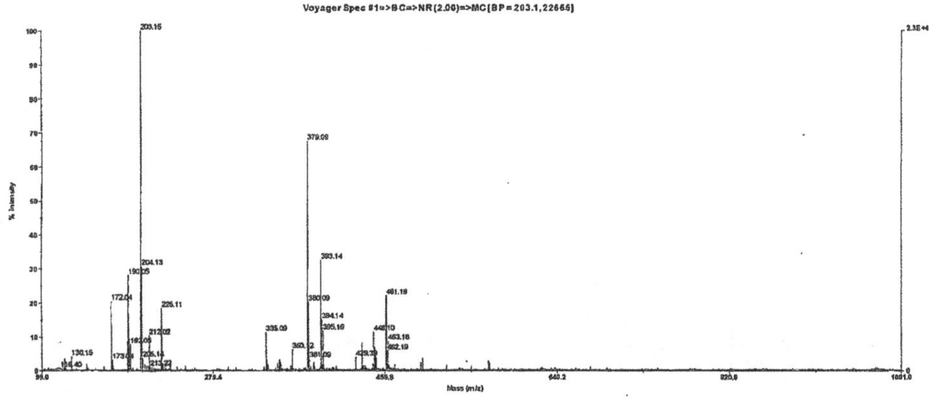

(a)

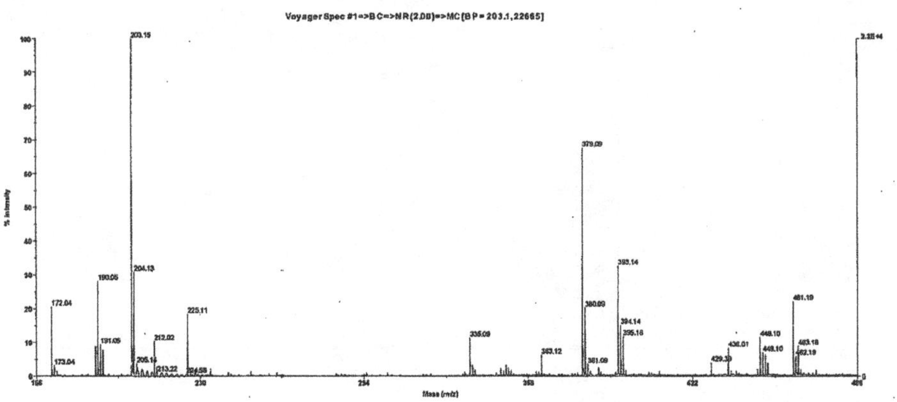

(b)

Figure: 8.3. Mass spectra of matrix (a) and MA-GG-OH (b)

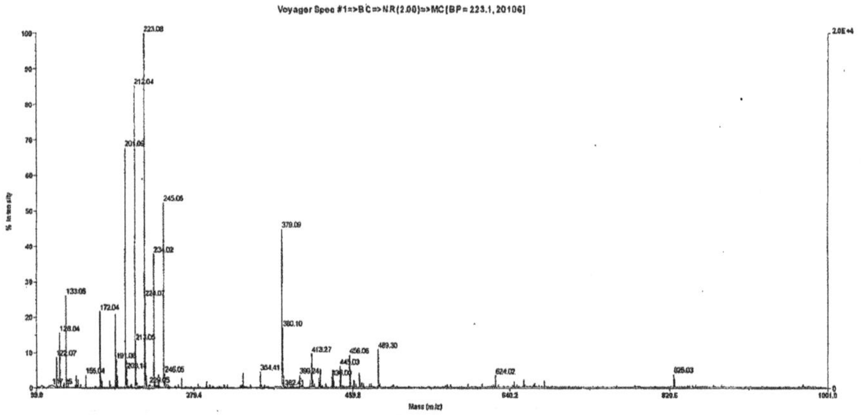

(a)

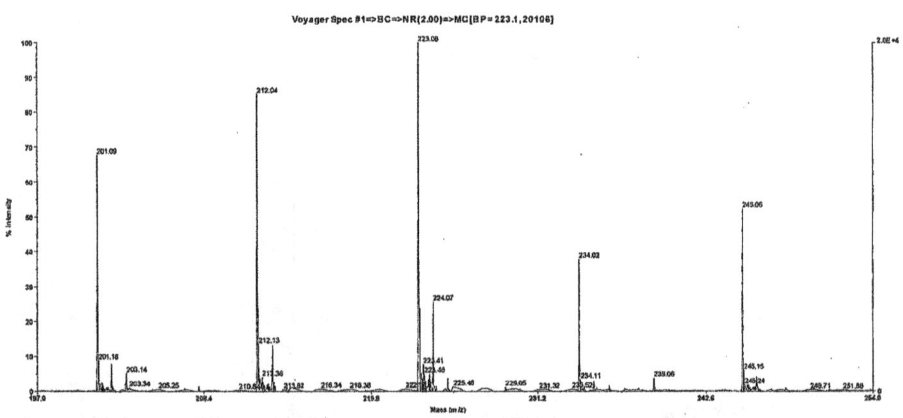

(b)

Figure: 8.4. Mass spectra of matrix (a) and MA-GFLG-OH (b)

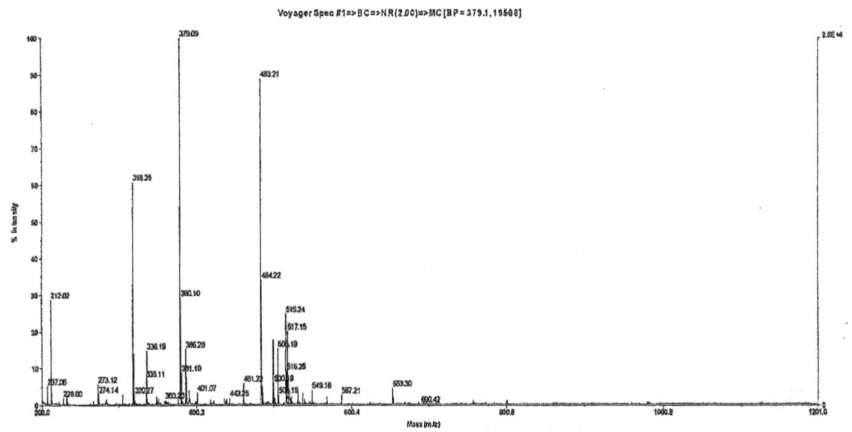

(a)

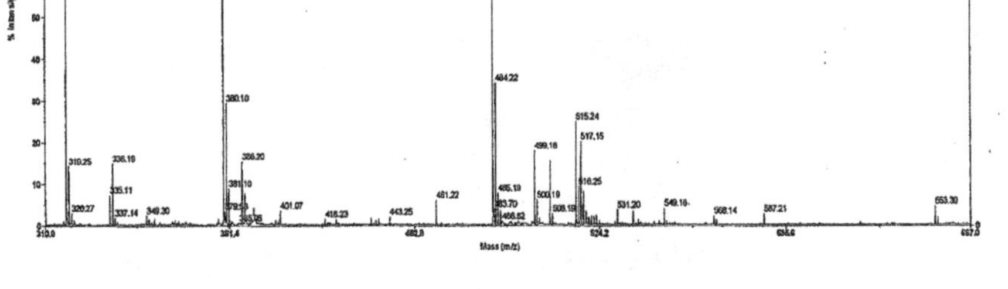

(b)

Figure: 8.5. Mass spectra of matrix (a) and MA-GFLG-DC (b)

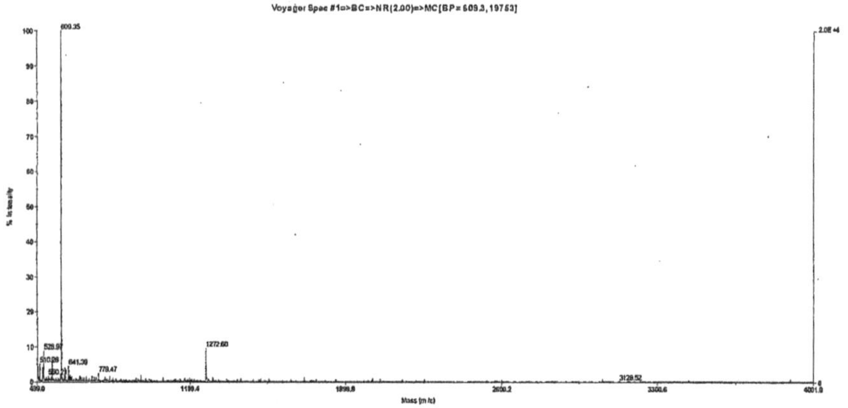

(a)

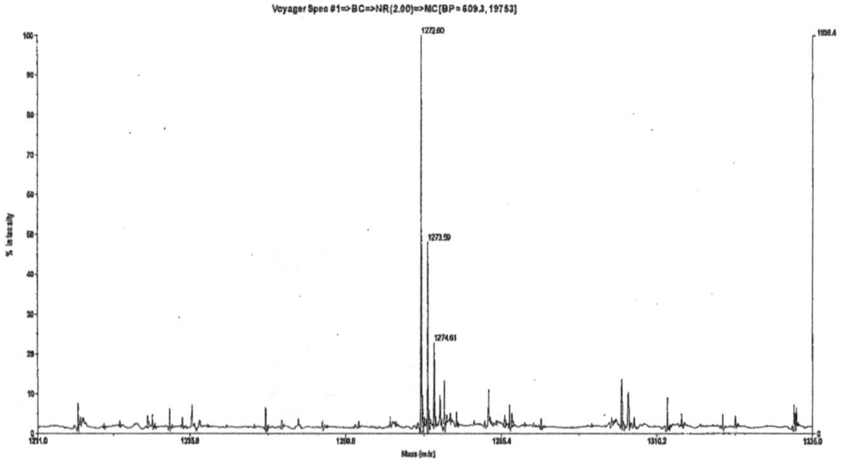

(b)

8.4.2. Characterization of drug attachment by NMR

The ^{1}H NMR analyses as shown in Figure: 8.6 depicts that the presence of drug in monomer as well as in polymer drug conjugates. The characteristic peak of drug at δ 8.1 is present in all drug containing moieties. However, the peak is absent in blank copolymer.

Figure: 8.6. ^{1}H NMR spectra of a) free Docetaxel b) MA-GFLG-Docetaxel and c) HPMA-Docetaxel d) Blank HPMA

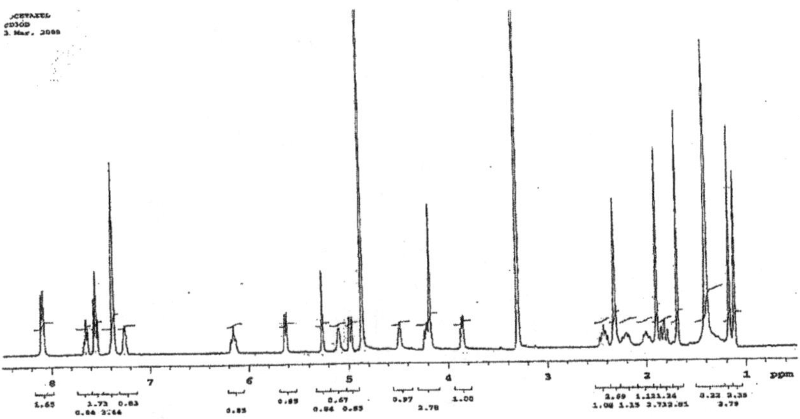

(a)

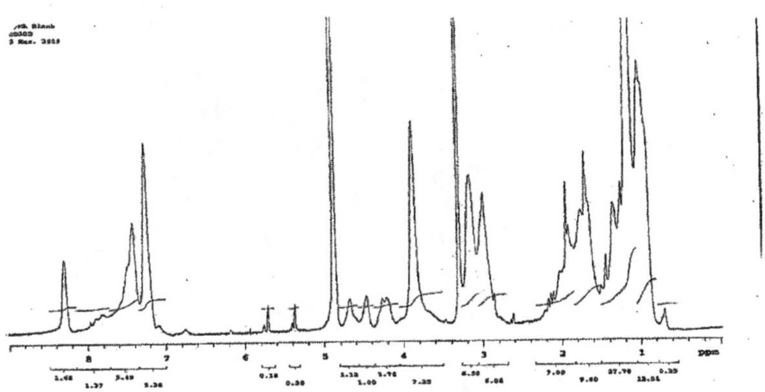

(b)

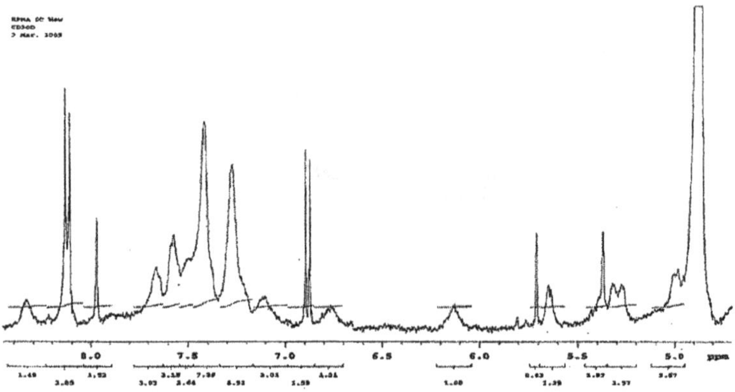

(c)

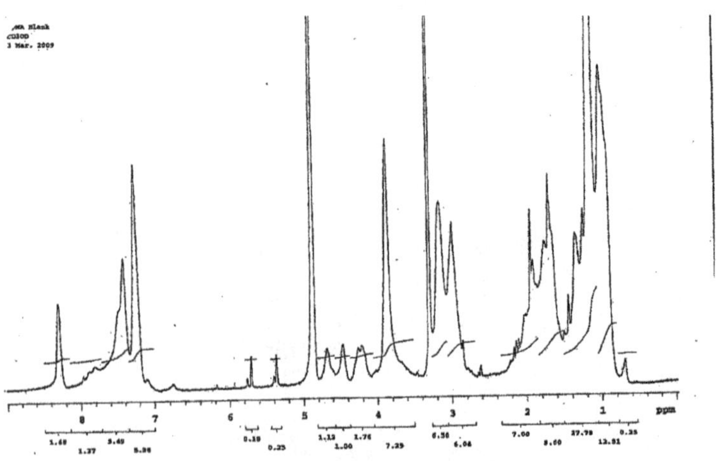

(d)

8.4.3. Determination of drug, peptide content and molecular weight of copolymer

The amount of drug and peptide attached, composition of comonomer feed ratio and molecular weight of copolymer synthesized is enumerated in Table: 8.3. Drug containing copolymers without (P1) and with (P2) RGDfK peptide targeting moiety were synthesized with an estimated molecular weight of *57.0* kDa (for precursor) with 10.3% (wt/wt) drug content. The ^{1}H NMR analyses as shown in Figure: 8.6 depicts that the presence of drug in monomer as well as in polymer drug conjugates.

Table: 8.3. Characterization of copolymer

Polymer no.	Structure	Comonomer Feed Composition (mol %)				Estimated M_w (kD)[a]	M_w/M_n[a,b]	DC content[c]		RGDfK content[d]	
		HPMA	MA-GG-ONp	MA-GFLG-DC	MA-Tyr			mmol /g	% wt/wt	mmol/g	peptides/ backbone
1	P-(GFLG-DC-GGOH) (p1)	80.5	15	2.5	2	28.0	1.4	0.128	10.3	-	-
2	P-(GFLG-DC-GG-RGDfk) (p2)	80.5	15	2.5	2	57.0	0.99	-	-	0.123	7.04

a. Molecular weight, molecular weight distribution (polydispersity) by FPLC
b. Polydispersity
c. Drug content analysis by HPLC method
d. Peptide content determination by amino acid analysis and SEC

8.4.4. Cathepsin B catalyzed drug release from HPMA copolymer-DC conjugates

Extent of drug release from HPMA copolymer products was evaluated at 15, 60,180,720 and 1440 minutes (Table: 8.4 & Figure: 8.7). The Docetaxel released by CPB catalyzed hydrolysis was quantified by RP-HPLC. Extraction efficiency was calculated to be 97%. The total drug release after 1 and 24hr was found to be 34.5±3.2% and 59.2±0.4% respectively.

Table: 8.4. Cathepsin B release study

Time (hrs)	% release (avg.)	SD
0	0	0
0.25	18.96	1.429452
0.5	25.26	1.817507
1	34.5	3.214032
2	39.03	1.41892
3	45.3	1.873499
12	51.1	0.707107
24	59.2	0.458258

Figure: 8.7. Cathepsin B Release Study

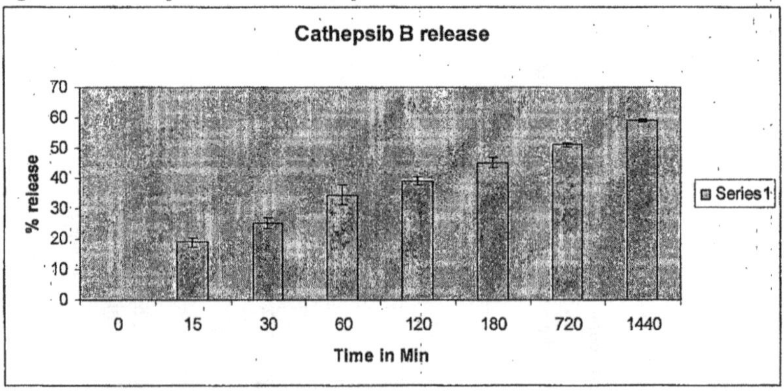

8.4.5. In vitro growth inhibition

Antiproliferative activity of drug and copolymer-drug conjugates in BT-20 and HCT 116 cells are shown in Figure: 8.8a & Figure: 8.8b. IC_{50} values for all treatments were determined by non-linear regression and are given in Table: 8.5 & Table: 8.6 and Figure: 8.8a & Figure: 8.8b. Results for DC drug treatments show that the attachment of DC to HPMA copolymer- conjugates improves its efficacy as compared to blank polymer.

Figure: 8.8. **Cytotoxicity curves**

a) Cell toxicity study (Free Docetaxel (DC), HPMA-GFLG-DC, HPMA-GG-DC, HPMA-GFLG-DC-RGD,HPMA) for BT-20 cells

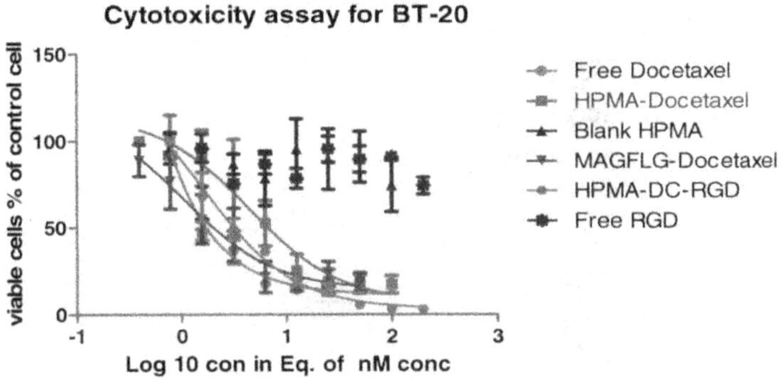

Table: 8.5. **IC_{50} for BT-20 cell line**

(Mean ± S.D., *n* = 3)

Components	IC 50 values in nM
Free Docetaxel	2.65±0.3
HPMA-Docetaxel conjugates	7±1.2
MAGFLG-Docetaxel monomer	3.6±0.5
HPMA-DC-RGD conjugate	3.8±0.1

b) For HCT 116 cells (Free Docetaxel (DC), HPMA-GFLG-DC, MAGFLG-DC, blank HPMA without drug)

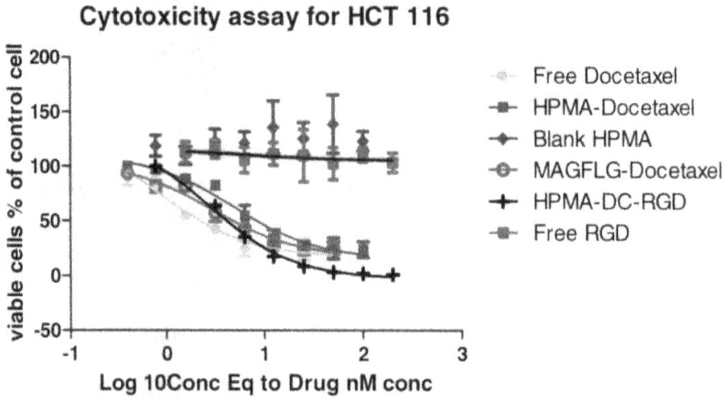

Table: 8.6. **IC_{50} values for HCT 116 cell line (Mean ± S.D., n = 3)**

Components	**IC 50 values in nM**
Free Docetaxel	1.74±0.12
HPMA-Docetaxel conjugates	4.45±0.21
MAGFLG-Docetaxel monomer	4±1.97
HPMA-DC-RGD conjugate	3.7±0.1

8.4.6. DNA Content Analysis study by Flowcytometery

The amounts of DNA content in cells are shown in Figure: 8.9a, Figure: 8.9b & Figure: 8.9c. The data shown hereby are for the higher concentration of both Free DC and HPMA-DC. Results show the both forms for drug arrest cell cycle in G2 phase. However, the percent cell cycle block in G2 phase was insignificant between the 10nM to 100nM concentration for both free and polymer bound drug. The influence of blank HPMA without drug was found to be similar as that of the untreated cells. It was also found that the data at lower concentration was inconclusive because of the difficulties in analysis due to high amount of debris.

Figure: 8.9. **DNA content analysis**

(a) BT- 20 cells with free DC

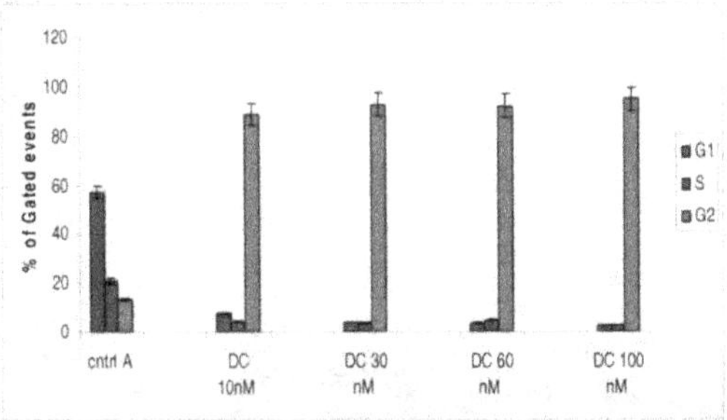

(b) BT- 20 cells with HPMA-DC and Blank HPMA

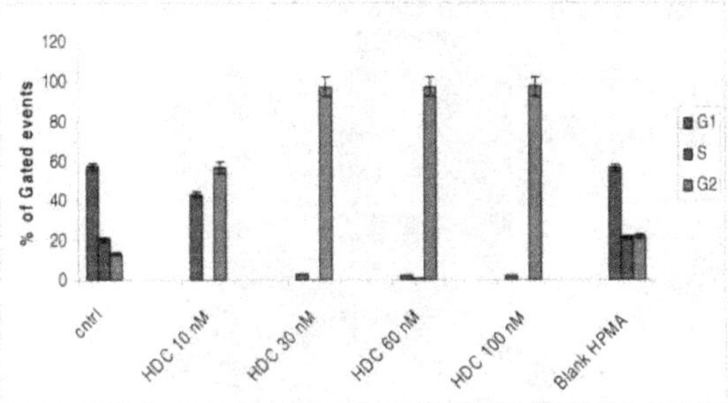

(c) HCT 116 cells with free DC and HPMA-DC:

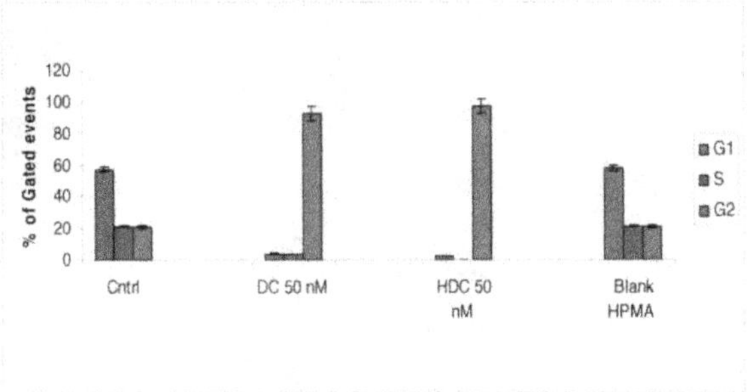

8.4.7. Confocal Microscopy

The results are shown in Figure: 8.10a and Figure: 8.10b. The multinuclear cells were observed for both types of cancer cells with free drug and polymer bound drug.

Figure: 8.10a

HPMA-GFLG-Docetaxel Induce Mitosis Aberration in Human Breast Cancer BT-20 Cells

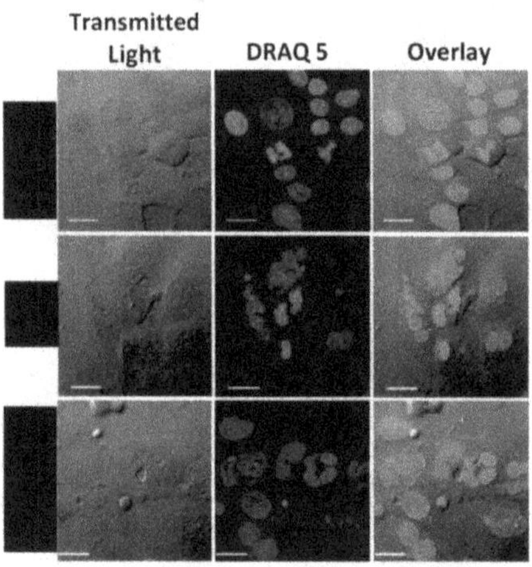

Treatment with both forms of docetaxel produces a large multinucleated cells.

Cells are shown after 48 h incubation. Similar cell morphology was observed after 24 h incubation.

Figure: 8.10b. **HCT 116 cell line**

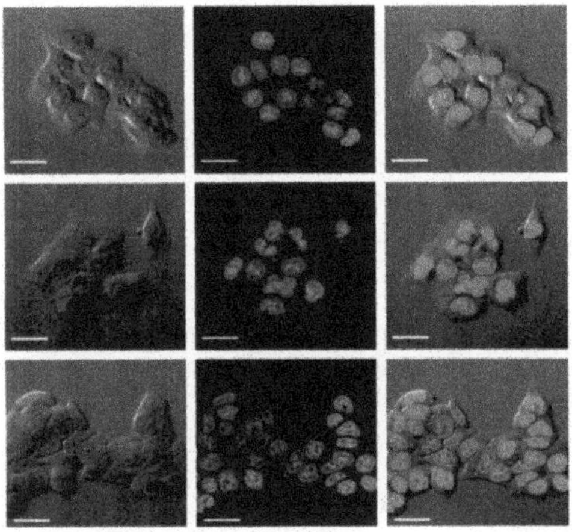

Cells are shown after 24 h incubation. Similar cell morphology was observed after 48 h incubation.

Nucleus stained with DRAQ 5 (magenta).

Scale bar is 20 μm

8.4.8. Stability study

As shown in Table: 8.7 and Figure: 8.11, the Docetaxel conjugated via ester bond with HPMA backbone was found to be stable in PBS pH 7.4 for 24 hrs. While the liberated amount of free drug from the conjugate was 62.6% and 7.29% in serum and 10% serum respectively. The results suggest that the ester bond was instable in the presence of esterase enzymes in serum and the amount of drug cleaved was less in 10% serum than the 100% serum. The rate of drug release was found to be decrease with increase in time with 100% serum.

Table: 8.7. Stability studies in 100% serum, 10% serum and PBS pH 7.4

Time in hr	Serum	PBS 7.4pH	10%serum
0	0	0	0
0.5	18.83±3.06	0	0
1	30±5.54	0	4.39±0.62
2	37.56±5.06	0	5.16±0.58
3	43.46±4.46	0	6.33±0.56
24	62.6±8.88	0	7.29±0.75

(Mean ± S.D., *n* = 3)

Figure: 8.11. Stability studies in 100% serum, 10% serum and PBS pH 7.4

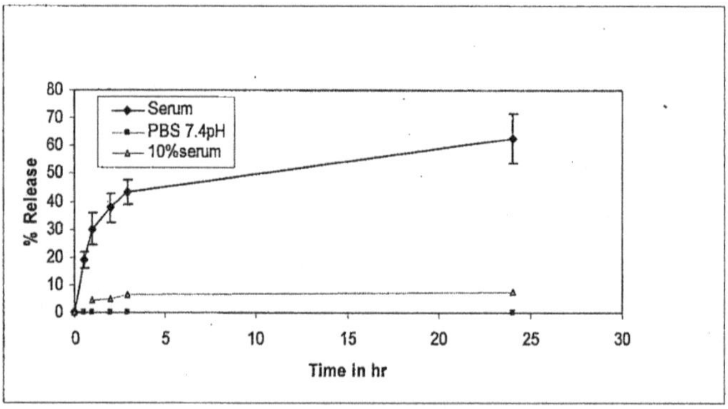

8.4. Discussion:

The synthesis, characterization, in vitro growth inhibition, and cell cycle arrest study of a new HPMA copolymer-RGDfK-Docetaxel conjugate was evaluated in this study. This is the first report of using HPMA copolymer-RGD conjugates for delivery of docetaxel. These copolymer conjugates can be used to actively deliver therapeutic agents to a broad spectrum of cancers with tumor angiogenesis. This work has focused on the synthesis and in vitro cytotoxicity and stability evaluation of HPMA copolymer docetaxel to breast & colon cancer cells.

HPMA copolymers were successfully synthesized and characterized containing RGDfK and docetaxel. The Docetaxel was conjugated via an ester bond with HPMA copolymer backbone. The monocyclic RGDfK was chosen for targeting to $\alpha_v\beta_3$ integrins. This peptide has a higher affinity than linear RGD sequences and greater solution stability than other doubly cyclized or linear peptide versions (Assa-Munt, N. et al., 2001). The RGDfK peptide ligand actively targets the $\alpha_v\beta_3$ integrin and can enhance the cellular entry of HPMA copolymer conjugates through receptor-mediated internalization of conjugates bound to the $\alpha_v\beta_3$ integrin (Schraa. A. J. et al., 2002). This should result in drug release from the copolymers that occurs via enzymatic degradation of GFLG peptide sequences in the lysosomal compartment.

Drug release from the conjugates was evaluated in vitro with the model lysosomal enzyme CPB to understand the release profiles of copolymer. RP-HPLC was employed to accurately quantify the released drug.

Growth inhibition results showed that the IC50 values for free drug is low for both cell lines as compared with the targeted and non targeted polymer drug conjugates. However the HPMA copolymer-DC-RGDfK conjugates affected cell proliferation more that the nontargeted one. This difference may be due to the presence of the RGDfK on the copolymer side chains causing an increased amount of intracellular accumulation of the conjugates due to receptor mediated uptake. The difference in cytotoxicity of free drug and polymer bound drug may be attributed to the lysosomally degradable linker which delays the liberation of free drug from the conjugates. The BT-20 cells were found to be more sensitive towards all forms of drugs than the HCT-116 cells. The difference in population doubling time might be the responsible for aforesaid difference.

Cell cycle analysis demonstrated that both free DC and HPMA-DC arrested BT-20 and HCT 116 cell in G2 phase of cell cycle. There was no obvious difference in the population appeared the G2 phase in the cells treated with different concentration of both forms of drugs. Hence, cell cycle arrest was not concentration dependent. However, due to the high amount of debris we were unable to determine the cell cycle arrest in the cells treated with 1 to 5nM concentration of free and polymer bound drug.

The stability studies of the conjugates showed that the ester bond between drug and polymer backbone was not stable in serum. The percent drug release was more in 100% serum than the 10% serum. However, this bond was found to be stable in PBS pH 7.4. The study suggests that the amount of drug release was dependent on the available concentration of the esterase enzymes. Hence, the drug release was more with 100% serum. However, hydrolytic cleavage was not found for polymer drug conjugate which reveals the stability of bond in plain buffer.

The mitosis aberration was observed in both types of cells with both forms of conjugates. Docetaxel being a microtubule stablilizing agent, produces mitosis aberration which subsequently leads to formation of multinucei as nuclear envelop forms around chromosomes or group of chromosomes.

8.5. Conclusions:

HPMA copolymer-DC-RGDfK conjugates showed growth inhibition activity in vitro against Breast and Colon cell lines. Our study also demonstrated the cell cycle arrest of cancer cells. The cell cycle analysis study and in vitro stability study reveals the fact that polymer conjugated drug shows toxicity as a result of combined effect of hydrolyzed drug in the medium and enzymatically cleaved drug inside the cancer cells.

8.6. References

Arap, W. et al., 1998, Science, **279**, 377–380.

Assa-Munt, N. et al, 2001, Solution structures and integrin binding activities of an RGD peptide with two isomers, Biochemistry, **40**, 2373-8.

Bogdanowich-Knipp, S. J. et al., 1999, Solution stability of linear vs. cyclic RGD peptides, J. Pept. Res., **53**, 530-41.

Jensen, K.D. et al, 2003, J.Control. Release, **87**, 89-105.

Kasuya, Y. et al., 2002, Influence of the structure of drug moieties on the in vitro efficacy of HPMA copolymer-geldanamycin derivative conjugates, Pharm. Res., **19**: 115-23.

Koivunen, E. et al., 1995, Phage libraries displaying cyclic peptides with different ring sizes: ligand specificities of the RGD-directed integrins, Biotechnology (N Y), **13**, 265-70.

Mallikarjuna Rao, B. et al., 2006, A stability-indicating HPLC assay method for docetaxel, J. Pharma. Bio. Anal., **41(2)**, 676-681.

Pan, H. et al., 2006, Water-soluble HPMA copolymer--prostaglandin E1 conjugates containing a cathepsin K sensitive spacer, J. Drug. Target, **14**, 425-35.

Shadidi, M. et al., 2003, Selective targeting of cancer cells using synthetic peptides. Drug Resist Updat, **6(6)**, 363-371.

Schraa, A. J. et al., 2002, Endothelial cells internalize and degrade RGD-modified proteins developed for tumor vasculature targeting, J. Control. Release., **83**, 241-5.

Wang, D. et al., 2000, Synthesis of starlike N-(2-hydroxypropyl)methacrylamide copolymers: potential drug carriers, Biomacromolecules, **1**, 313-319.

Chapter 9
Summary and Conclusion

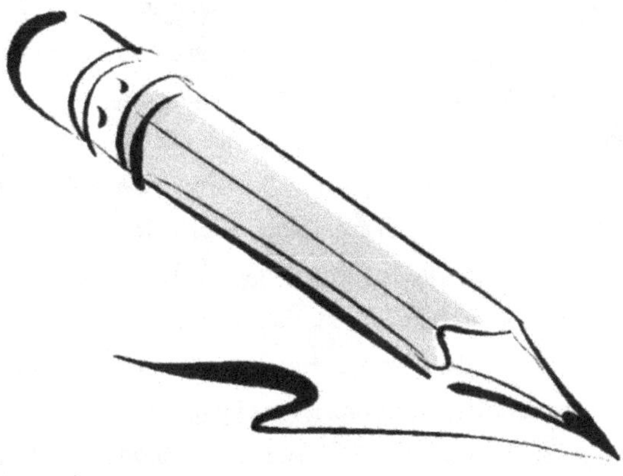

9.1. Summary

In the past few decades, rapid advances in cell and molecular biology have allowed us to develop a better understanding of the pathophysiology of Cancer. Despite tremendous efforts made to conquer cancer in recent decades, it still remains the second leading cause of death worldwide. Breast cancer is difficult to diagnose and treat at an early stage because it grows outward rapidly from deep within the organ and is usually not recognized as a foreign invader by our own body's defense system. Most current anticancer agents do not greatly differentiate between cancerous and normal cells, leading to systemic toxicity and adverse effects. This greatly limits the maximum allowable dose of the drug. In addition, rapid elimination and widespread distribution into targeted organs and tissues requires the administration of a drug in large quantities, which is not economical and often results in undesirable toxicity. Thus, drug targeting has evolved as the most desirable but elusive goal in drug delivery science. It can potentially increase efficacy and reduce toxicity of new and pre-existing drugs by altering their pharmacokinetics and biodistribution and restricting the action of drugs to the treated tissue. Hence, the major challenge is to design drug delivery strategies that deliver the therapeutic agents to the desired intracellular targets based on ability to understand, utilize, modify and exploit membrane trafficking pathways.

Recent advances in nanomaterial technology enable us to control size, shape and surface functionality of nanoconstructs in nanoscale. Because most cancer related biological processes occur at the nano scale, there are many chances to use nanomaterials to diagnose and treat cancers at an early stage. Nanoparticles and liposomes as nanocarriers systems have been used as a physical approach to alter and improve the pharmacokinetic and pharmacodynamic properties of various types of drug molecules. They have been used in vivo to protect the drug entity in the systemic circulation, restrict access of the drug to the chosen sites and to deliver the drug at a controlled and sustained rate to the site of action. In addition, Polymer conjugates, especially those prepared using N- (2-hydroxypropyl) methacrylate (HPMA) have been extensively studied for intracellular and cytoplasmic drug delivery. HPMA conjugated to oligonucleotides via lysosomally degradable spacers were shown to enter the cytoplasm and nucleus of the cells.

Site-specific targeting can be achieved by attaching targeting ligands to surface of nanoconstructs. Various ligands which have been employed include transferrin, folic acid, lectins, RGD petides etc. Many different RGD peptides have been developed. Linear and cyclic RGD peptides, and chemically designed peptidomimetics are currently being tested by researchers. Cyclic RGD peptides are much more potent and more specific than their linear counterparts, and their advantage is their resistance against proteolysis. They have been shown to have selective binding affinity for $\alpha_V\beta_3$ integrin for treatments of human tumor metastasis and tumor-induced angiogenesis. Due to cytoadhesion, cytoinvasion and partial lysosomal accumulation, RGD-mediated drug delivery may provide for improved intracellular availability of conjugated nanocarriers systems.

Docetaxel belonging to the taxane class of anticancer agent is perhaps the most important chemotherapeutic agent against cancer to have emerged over the past several decades. In clinical trials both taxanes are successfully used, mostly against ovarian carcinoma, advanced breast cancer, lung cancer and head/neck cancer. Docetaxel is formulated using polysorbate 80 and ethanol (50:50 v/v). In phase I clinical trials, majority of patients showed acute hypersensitivity reactions with Docetaxel formulated *i.v.* injection. This leads to a need of reformulating Docetaxel with dosage forms to eliminate the toxicity. The objectives of present investigation were development of three types nanoconstructs of docetaxel (PLGA nanoparticles, liposomes and HPMA copolymer drug conjugates), RGD-conjugation onto the nanoconstructs systems, characterization, and evaluation of these nanoconstructs on breast cancer cell lines to understand their role in breast cancer chemotherapy.

The estimation in the nanoparticles, liposomes and *in vitro* release studies for DC was performed by HPLC method. The calibration curve of DC was established in acetonitrile: water gradient system by HPLC at 227nm. The linearity of DC was found to be 0.5-10µg/ml (R^2=0.9985). To determine the amount of drug entrapped nanoparticles were dissolved in acetonitrile. The resulting system was centrifuged to remove the precipitated components and the supernant was diluted with the solvent system and subjected to analysis.

The *in vitro* release study was performed using the tube shaking method. At different time intervals, the samples were removed and centrifuged at 25000 rpm and the settled nanoparticles were dissolved in acetonitrile and analyzed for the drug remaining in the nanoparticles as the same method for entrapment efficiency. The drug released was calculated by taking the difference of the drug taken initially and the drug remaining in the nanoparticles.

The estimation of RGD conjugation was carried out using BCA protein estimation. The calibration curve was established at 12.5-1000 μg/ml (R^2=0.9935). The amount of PVA associated with nanoparticles was determined by a colorimetric method based on the formation of a colored complex between two adjacent hydroxyl groups of PVA and an iodine molecule. A standard plot for known concentrations of PVA was established at 5-250 μg/ml. (R^2=0.9994)

Liposomes were prepared by Supercritical fluid technology using CO_2 as an Antisolvent using SPC/drug/HSPC. Process parameters, such as operating temperature, pressure and flow rate of the SCF were found to have significant influence on preparation of liposome (SCF-LP). Hence, process parameters were optimized and kept unaltered in subsequent experiments. In order to optimize process parameters, a Box Behnken Design (BBD) of RSM was used. Fifteen batches of SCF-LP were prepared by SAS process using a 3-factor, 3-level "Box-Behnken" design (BBD) of Response Surface methodology varying three independent variables (Temperature (A), Pressure (B) and CO_2 flow rate (C) of the formulation. The Design Expert (Version 7.1, State Ease Inc, USA) program was used for design of experiment and analysis of this second-order model and for drawing of three dimensional response surface and contour plots.

The attempt of liposomes formation was carried out by using mixture of lipids containing both unsaturated and saturated lipid in one liposomal system to improve hydration and encapsulation. The unsaturated and saturated lipids were SPC and HSPC respectively along with cholesterol to design conventional liposomes. The ratio of drug to total lipid was taken as 1:15, 1:20 and 1:25 mole%. The liposomes were characterized for particle size, percent entrapment, vesicle morphology and zeta potential. The optimized process parameters were kept constant and the formulation parameters were further optimized by the BBD of Response surface methodology.

It has been observed that the increase in CO2 flow rate results in decrease in particle size and increase in the yield of the SC-LP. The possible explanation for this is the high mixing energy and fine atomization of solvent droplets in the stream of SC-CO2 at high flow rate. Generally, a higher mixing energy leads to smaller particles of spherical morphology. Due to the high flow rate, the incoming solvent droplet converts in to fine form and the supercritical fluid removes the organic solvent and leaves behind the small particles in the vessel. As a result of the rapid removal of organic solvent from each droplet, the solute precipitates faster in the high pressure vessel and it is a factor responsible for high yield. It has been found that, as the pressure increases at high temperature the particle size and yield decreases. While at the pressure increases at moderate temperature the particle size decreases but yield increases. The pressure of the SC-CO_2 in the high pressure vessels depicts its quantity. This means at high pressure, more amount of CO_2 is available in the vessel. The proportion of CO_2 directly affects the process of supersaturation for the particle production. The high amount of CO_2 hastens the supersaturation process and results in the precipitation of small particles with spherical morphology.

The temperature has significant ($p<0.05$) influence on the yield but non-significant ($p>0.05$) influence on particle size. With increase in temperature along with high pressure, yield decreases might be because of the low T_g (49°C) of the mix lipid system. It is known from the literature that the SC-Co$_2$ lowers the T_g of the polymers. We are anticipating the similar effect responsible for low yield of the final product. The process variables with minimum particle size and maximum yield were considered as optimum and kept constant for further processing.

In our initial trials, we found difficulty in hydration during the preparation of liposomes for docetaxel with saturated lipid (HSPC). Hence, we applied a mix lipid system containing unsaturated lipid (SPC) and saturated lipid with cholesterol. In mix lipid system, the saturated phospholipids and cholesterol provide the rigidity to the membrane and hence improve the stability while unsaturated phospholipid improves the hydration through its polar head groups. The drug entrapment was found to be increase from 72.82±2.18% to 81.4±4.6%

with decrease in drug to total lipid ratio from 1:15 to 1:20 mole % in an optimized batch. However, further decrease in drug to total lipid ratio from 1:20 to 1:25mole% did not have any significant effect on %EE. Hence, 1:20 mole % was considered as an optimum drug to total lipid ratio for maximum drug entrapment.

The Different mol % of DSPE- PEG 2000 was incorporated in the bilayer and effect on percent encapsulation efficiency of DC liposomes was studied. It was found that 6 mol % of DSPE-PEG_{2000}-COOH incorporated in liposomes gave optimum entrapment i.e. 79.2±4.4 % among the other molar percentage tried. The percent entrapment was found from 81±4.6 and %, 75.8±2.2%, to their respective molar percent 2 and 8 mole % of DSPE-PEG_{2000}-COOH. Entrapment was decreases to 75.8±2.2% when 8 mol % of the polymer was incorporated in the liposome composition. Fall in the percent entrapment was supported by theory that the hydrophobic chain of DSPE-PEG_{2000}-COOH would align with the hydrophobic chain of lipids in bilayer and therefore competes with the DC to accommodate in bilayer. There was no significant effect on the particle size observed when the ratio of polymer increased up to 8 mol%. The particle size was found in the range of 260 to 274 nm.

Drug loaded PLGA nanoparticles were prepared by emulsion solvent evaporation method. The process parameters *viz.* homogenization pressure and no. of cycles were optimized for maximum %EE and minimum particle size <250nm. To optimize the process parameters for lowest particle size and highest % entrapment efficiency, the primary emulsion was subjected to different number of homogenization cycles and pressures. The results show that when the pressure was kept constant, the particle size and the % entrapment efficiency decreased with the increase in number of homogenization cycles from one to three. Increase in the pressure from 45 to 125MPa also decreased the particle size as well as the entrapment efficiency. With the decrease in particle size, the total surface area of the particles increases resulting in diffusion of drug from the particles. This may be the reason for decreased entrapment with decrease in particle size. Two cycles at 125MPa was found to be the optimized process parameter. Further increase in the number of cycles resulted in lower particle size which was also accompanied by decreased entrapment efficiency.

Based on the results obtained in preliminary experiments, drug concentration, polymer concentration and PVA concentration were found to be the major variables in determining the entrapment efficiency. The optimized process parameters were kept constant and the formulation parameters were further optimized by the BBD of Response surface methodology. The highest %EE achieved was 72.4 ± 4.6 % with particle size of 240 ± 3 nm for DC-NPs. This was at low level of drug (1%), high level of polymer (10%) and at medium level of PVA (1.5%). The drop in the particle size and higher % EE with the increase in PVA concentration is probably due to the differences in the stability of the emulsions formulated with different concentrations of PVA. Further, the viscosity of PVA solution increases with increasing PVA concentrations. This could result in the formation of a stable emulsion with smaller and uniform droplet size, leading to the formation of smaller sized nanoparticles. There was not much reduction in particle size or increase in %EE when the PVA was increased from 1.5 to 2%. Hence, drug: polymer ratio 1: 10 and 1.5% w/v PVA as an emulsifier were taken as optimized parameters for the preparation of NPs for further studies. The drug loaded nanoparticles were also prepared by nanoprecipitation technique. The major process parameter effecting the formation of nanoparticles was the speed of the stirring. Evaluation of the variation of the stirring speed was carried out at slow, moderate and high speed. Moderate speed was optimized as the best suitable for the preparation of uniform nanoparticles dispersion. The rate of addition of organic phase to the aqueous was kept constant at 0.5ml/min throughout the entire experimentation. Based on preliminary investigations drug: polymer ratio, PVA concentration in aqueous phase (%w/v) and the ratio of the organic: aqueous phase were found to influence the major variables of particle size and entrapment efficiency. Hence, drug: polymer ratio (represented as polymer concentration, as the amount of the drug was kept constant), PVA concentration in aqueous phase (%w/v) and the ratio of the organic: aqueous phase (represented in decimal form) were kept as independent variables to find optimized condition to obtain optimum particle size (<250nm) with highest entrapment efficiency (dependent variables).

The particle size and entrapment were strongly influenced by the independent variables. The increase in the amount of PLGA (keeping the drug amount constant) resulted in the increase in the particle size of the nanoparticles. The viscosity of the organic phase in which the PLGA is dissolved appears to affecting the nanoparticles size due to hindrance in rapid dispersion of PLGA solution into the aqueous phase and resulted increase in the droplet and nanoparticles size. Increasing the polymer amount also increased the entrapment efficiency may be due to increase in drug entrapping polymer and due to the decrease in the diffusion of the drug towards the aqueous phase.

Increase in the PVA concentration led to increase in the particle size of the nanoparticles. This increase in the nanoparticles size may be due to increase in the viscosity of the aqueous phase thereby increasing the resistance to the diffusion rate of the organic phase. The miscibility of organic phase (acetone) with aqueous phase results in orientation of PVA at the interface of PLGA solution in acetone present as droplets in the system. Increase in PVA concentration also leads to increase in entrapment efficiency, probably due to reduction in diffusion rate of the organic phase in the aqueous phase.

Increase in the ratio of organic phase: aqueous phase leads to decrease in the particle size and entrapment efficiency. The increase in the organic phase ratio leads increased evaporation time causing slower polymer precipitation, due to the increased microenvironment provided by organic phase after dispersing in the aqueous phase, and thereby formation of small particles. Due to the increased evaporation time and slower polymer precipitation, the tendency of the drug to escape in the aqueous phase before polymer precipitation increases leading to lower drug entrapment efficiency.

The optimized batch was subjected to lyophilization using sucrose, mannitol and trehalose as cryoprotectant at 1:1, 1:2 and 1:3 (nanoconstructs: cryoprotectants). The redispersibility of the lyophilized product and particle size of the nanoconstructs was measured after lyophilization. The redispersibility of nanoparticles with sucrose was poor and was only possible after sonication and show significant increase in particle size. The increase in the particle size could have been due to the cohesive nature of the sucrose. With mannitol, the redispersion was possible only after vigorous shaking and the particle size of the NPs increased on lyophilization. This effect may be due to the low solubility of mannitol in water i.e. 0.18 part of mannitol soluble in 1 parts of water. With trehalose as cryoprotectant, the lyophilized nanoparticles were redispersed easily and the increase in particle size was not significant as indicated by Sf/Si of 1.03 and 1.04 for 1:3 of nanoparticles: trehalose and liposomes: trehalose, respectively. Hence, trehalose at a ratio of 1: 3 (nanoconstructs: trehalose) was used as cryoprotectant for lyophilization of optimized batch of nanoconstructs for further studies.

The Cyclic RGD peptide was conjugated to the surface of the PLGA nanoparticles by using a two step process. In the first step, the nanoparticles were activated using a sulfoNHS/EDC and in the second step the NH_2-PEG-COOH was attached to the activated nanoparticles. The RGD was attached to pegylated nanoparticles by the same process with repetition of conjugation steps.

The surface modification of PLGA-NPs with RGD was achieved in two steps using carbodiimide coupling method. This active ester method yields stable amide bonds. As a prerequisite, the polymer has to contain free carboxyl groups at the surface as represented by the H-type of PLGA which are activated by carbodiimide/N-hydroxysuccinimide. In contrast to the activation of carboxyls with only carbodiimide, the presence of N-hydroxysuccinimide yields N-hydroxysuccinimide esters as stable intermediates which rather acylate amino groups of proteins than to be subject of hydrolysis in aqueous medium. The amounts of activating agents (EDAC/NHS) and RGD were optimized to achieve minimum particle size and maximum RGD density on the surface of NPs.

To check the influence of concentration of activating agents on density of surface RGD, 5 mg of NPs were activated with different concentrations of EDAC/NHS, and the density of surface RGD and particle size of conjugated NPs were measured. It was found that at 0.5/0.3 mmol EDAC/NHS, the surface bound RGD was detectable for conjugated NPs of DC. Increase of EDAC/NHS concentration from 1/0.7 mmole to 2/1.5 mmol increased the RGD density of PLGA-DC-NPs from 14.2 ± 3.7 to 26.4 ± 3.5 µg/mg of nanoparticle surface and further increase in the concentration of EDAC/NHS did not increase the RGD density significantly. The presence of the peptide on the surface, as well as the loss of the fine particles during processing caused the NPs to increase in mean particle size after surface modification. Therefore 2/1.5 mmole EDAC/NHS was taken as the optimized concentration for the activation of PLGA-DC-NPs for the conjugation process.

To maximize conjugation efficiency, different amounts of RGD solution were added to 5 mg of activated PLGA-DC-NPs and the density of conjugated RGD was measured. For

PLGA-DC-NPs as the amount of RGD was increased from 0.5 to 4 mg, the density of conjugated RGD /NPs increased from 6.2 ± 1.7 µg/mg to 30.2 ± 4.5 µg/mg. However, the % conjugation efficiency was found to be insignificant with increased amounts (4mg) of RGD. Therefore, 2mg was taken as the optimized amount of RGD to be used for conjugation of 5 mg of PLGA-DC-NPs.

Mean particle size and zeta potential of PLGA-DC-NP and PLGA-DC-RGD-NP were found to be 210.3 ± 2.7nm and -38.4 ± 2.6mV and 230.7 ± 2.3nm and -10.2 ± 2.8mV respectively. Increase in the particle size after RGD conjugation was due to RGD conjugated. The %EE for PLGA-DC-NP and PLGA-DC-RGD-NP was found to be 71.6 ± 2.4 % and 58.4 ± 1.6 respectively. The reduced drug entrapment efficiency for PLGA-DC-RGD-NP may be due to dissociation of the drug on the surface of PLGA-DC-NP during the RGD conjugation process.

Similarly, the particle size and zeta potential for LP-DC, LP-DC-PEG and LP-DC-RGD were analyzed. Mean particle size and zeta potential of LP-DC & LP-DC-PEG were found to be 260.4 ± 4.6nm& 269.2 ± 2.8nm and -28.7 ± 1.3 & -27.2±1.8mV respectively. While the LP-DC-PEG-RGD demonstrated 278.6±3.4nm particle size and -11.6±0.4mV zeta potential. The %EE for LP-DC, LP-DC-PEG and LP-DC-PEG-RGD was determined to be 72.8 ± 2.2 %, 67.9 ± 3.1% and 64.5±1.5%, respectively.

The release studies of docetaxel from the optimized nanoparticles batch were conducted in phosphate buffer pH 7.4 + 0.1%w/v polysorbate-80. For PLGA-DC-NP there was an initial burst release of about 19% in 12hrs and then there was a lag phase and about 80% release resulted in 21 days. The unconjugated nanoparticles showed a high initial burst which can be attributed to the immediate dissociation and dissolution of drug adhered on the surface and located near the surface of the NPs. The burst effect was absent in PLGA-DC-RGD-NP and the release in 21 days was found to be about 60%.

For docetaxel encapsulated liposomes, it was found that both formulations produced an initial burst release in which docetaxel release was more than 10 % and 8 % for pegylated and non-pegylated liposomes, respectively, within the initial sampling time (30min). The burst release in both forms of liposomes is related to release of surface adsorbed drug. After the initial burst release, a constant drug release was found and maximum of 75% and 60%

drug was released in 48hr of time period with pegylated and non pegylated liposomes respectively. Faster release in pegylated liposomes may be due to the fast hydration process of PEG molecules on the surface of the particles.

Transmission Electron Microscopy and Scanning Electron Microscopy images of the unconjugated and conjugated NPs and liposomes showed spherical configuration with smooth surfaces. DSC thermogram of plain Docetaxel depicts a sharp melting peak from 169-171°C, indicating the crystalline nature of the drug. The drug in the amorphous form is entrapped in the nanoparticles. For PLGA-DC-NP the peak of docetaxel is absent indicating the conversion of DC into amorphous state during the nanoparticles formulation and thereby entrapped in the PLGA polymer. Similarly, for LP-DC, the peak of docetaxel is absent indicating the conversion of DC into amorphous state during the liposome formulation and thereby entrapped in the liposomes. XRD patterns of the PLGA-DC-RGD-NPs and LP-DC-RGD depict that the formulations were in amorphous forms.

The stability studies were carried out in accordance with the ICH guidelines for drug substances intended to be stored in a refrigerator. The stability of the nanoparticles and liposomes were assessed for physical observation, particle size, zeta potential and the drug content (with respect to the initial) at 5°C ± 3°C for 6M and 25°C ± 2°C/60% RH ± 5% RH for 6 months.

It was observed that unconjugated and conjugated nanoparticles of docetaxel there was no significant change ($P>0.05$) observed in particle size, zeta potential and drug content at 5°C ± 3°C for 6M. The storage of the unconjugated and conjugated nanoparticles of docetaxel at 25°C ± 2°C/60% ± 5% RH, led to increase in the particle size. The increase in the particle size was not significant during the first month, however became significant and more prominent after 2, 3 and 6 months. During our analysis of samples, the polydispersity index of the nanoparticles stored at 25°C ± 2°C/60% ± 5% RH was found to increase as compared to the initial. The increase in the particle size may be due to the absorption of the moisture by the nanoparticles resulting in the coalescence of the small nanoparticles forming particles larger in size.

The nanoparticles were also observed for physical appearance. After 3 and 6 months the physical appearance was also changed, with loss of the free flowing property followed by the difficulty in redispersibility. Also, the RGD conjugated nanoparticles demonstrated difference in the color than the initial powder. At 6 months the color of the powder was light pink. This could be indicative of the degradation of the surface RGD.

At 25°C ± 2°C/60% ± 5% RH, the zeta potential of the nanoparticles shifted towards the zero for both unconjugated and conjugated nanoparticles. This may be due to the acidic conditions produced due to the degradation of PLGA into lactic and glycolic acid. The lowered zeta potential values also might have contributed toward the aggregation of particles. The drug content of the unconjugated and conjugated nanoparticles was not altered up to 6M at 5°C ± 3°C. However, the drug content was reduced after 6M storage at 25°C ± 2°C/60% RH ± 5% RH. This impact could be due to the moisture absorbed by the nanoparticles upon storage at 25°C ± 2°C/60% RH ± 5% RH, possibly resulting in the degradation of the drug. The initial drug entrapment was found to be 72.6±2.4% and 69.6±3.4% and initial particle size 260.6±2.4 nm, 260.6±2.4 nm for Non-PEGylated and PEGylated liposomes respectively. Reduction in the entrapment after 3 months, were observed 69.2±2.8 (2-8°C) and 61.2±3.8 mg (25°C) while particle size was 269.2±4.4 nm (2-8°C) and 288.2±7.6 nm (25°C) for Non-PEGylated. In case of PEGylated liposomes, minor reduction in the drug entrapment was seen (68.2±2.1 and 61.2±3.8) at 2-8°C and 25°C respectively and increase in the particles size was in the range of 8-12 nm from the initial.

From the above study, we can demonstrate that the unconjugated and RGD-conjugated PLGA nanoparticles and liposomes of docetaxel when stored at 25°C ± 2°C/60% RH ± 5% RH for 6M show instability reflected by change in physical appearance, increase in the particle size, zeta potential and reduction in the drug content. Hence, we can conclusively specify that both unconjugated and conjugated nanoparticles and liposomes of docetaxel were stable and can be stored 5°C ± 3°C for 6M retaining its original formulation characteristics.

In vitro cell culture studies were performed on BT-20 and MDA-MB-231cells to assess the intracellular nanoparticles and liposomes uptake, to study the antiproliferative action, to assess the DNA content and to evaluate the mode of cell death by nanoparticles and liposomes with compare to the drug solution. BT-20 and MDA-MB-231 cells were cultured and maintained as monolayer, growing as adherent monolayer in DMEM. DMEM was supplemented with 10% fetal bovine serum at 37°C in the atmosphere of 5% CO_2 and 95% relative humidity.

Intracellular uptake of the nanoparticles and liposomes into the cell was studied by incorporating 6-coumarin (fluorescent dye) into the nanoparticles (PLGA-NP) & liposomes (LP) and further conjugated with RGD (RGD-PLGA-NP & RGD-LP). Quantative intracellular uptake of the nanocarriers was performed to assess the influence of time and concentration. The uptake of the nanoparticles was directly proportional to the concentration of the nanoparticles in the medium. It was observed that the cellular uptake of the nanoparticles increased with increase in the concentration. However, the cellular uptake efficiency was found to be highest at the lowest concentration and found to decrease with increase in concentration. The decrease in the uptake efficiency indicates that the cells might have reached the saturating capacity for uptake. RGD-conjugated nanoconstructs at all concentrations demonstrate 1.6-2.1 folds increased uptake over unconjugated nanoconstructs uptake. The superior uptake of the RGD conjugated nanoparticles could be due to specific active endocytosis process mediated through the RGD adhesion to the integrins.

The results of quantitative uptake studies indicate the uptake of the nanoparticles into the cell. The untreated cells did not demonstrate any fluorescence. The nanoconstructs cell uptake efficiency was found to increase with time from 0.25-4hrs for both the unconjugated and RGD conjugated nanoconstructs. At all time points, the uptake efficiency of RGD conjugated systems were approximately 1.6~2.1 folds higher than the unconjugated systems. At 5hrs there was not much increase in the uptake efficiency suggesting the saturation of uptake with time. Hence, the influence of the concentration was performed by keeping the incubation time at 4hrs for all concentrations.

The uptake of the nanocarriers in the cells was qualitatively confirmed by visualizing under fluorescent microscope. The fluorescent microscopic images showed green fluorescence in the cell cytoplasm and around the nucleus which reflects the internalization of the nanocarriers into the cell. Based on this observation, it is reasonable to believe that the nanoparticles may carry the active drug across the cell membrane into the cytoplasm. The RGD conjugated nanocarriers at all the time points demonstrated higher fluorescence intensity than the unconjugated nanocarriers confirming the results of the quantitative uptake studies. Also the RGD conjugated nanocarriers show higher number of the cells showing fluorescence than the unconjugated nanoparticles.

The cytotoxicity studies were performed using CCK-8 assay. Cytotoxicity studies were performed at different nanomolar concentration range for free docetaxel and docetaxel encapsulated targeted and nontargeted nanoconstructs. The cytotoxicities of unconjugated and RGD conjugated nanoconstructs were significantly ($p<0.05$) higher than drug solution. The cytotoxicity was found to be dose and time dependent.

The cytotoxicity indicated by IC_{50} values suggests that RGD conjugated nanoparticles at 72hrs are 2.1 and 10 time more cytotoxic than unconjugated nanoparticles and drug solution for BT-20 cell lines. Similarly, for MDA-MB-231 cells, the RGD conjugated nanoparticles are 2 and 4 time more cytotoxic than unconjugated nanoparticles and drug solution.

The RGD conjugated docetaxel nanoparticles produced significantly higher toxicities at all time points, i.e 24, 48, 72hrs, than the drug solution and unconjugated nanoparticles. After 24hrs, RGD conjugated nanoparticles at the higher concentrations showed superior toxicity differences compared to drug solution and unconjugated nanoparticles. An important observation was that with increase in incubation time at 72hrs, the lowest concentration of RGD conjugated nanoparticles showed greater toxicity than drug solution and unconjugated nanoparticles. However, the higher concentrations didn't show much toxicity difference than the drug solution and unconjugated nanoparticles.

The cytotoxicity indicated by IC_{50} values suggests that RGD conjugated liposomes at 72hrs are 1.875 and 8.3 time more cytotoxic than unconjugated liposomes and drug solution for BT-20 cell lines. Similarly, for MDA-MB-231 cells, the RGD conjugated liposomes are 1.82 and 4.7 time more cytotoxic than unconjugated liposomes and drug solution.

Cell cycle analysis was done to determine the growth phase in which the cells were accumulating due to inhibition of cell cycle progression. Docetaxel inhibits cell growth and proliferation primarily through its effect on the cell cycle and induction of apoptosis and necrosis.

In case of free drug, the arrest in G2 phase was observed at lower concentration of 1nM and 2 nM but due to the high amount of debris, the exact percentage of each phase was difficult to calculate by Modfit software. At 24hrs, the cell cycle arrest in G2 phase was increasing significantly ($p<0.05$) as increase in concentration from 10nM to 30nM for free drug. However, the difference was insignificant ($p>0.05$) at 48hrs between intra concentrations of free drug at 48hrs. It was observed at 48hrs, that with 10nM of free drug solution, the percentage G2 phase arrest was increased significantly compared to 24hrs effect. But the difference was insignificant with 30nM and 50nM of free drug. As shown in table 7.11 the RGD conjugated nanoparticles at the drug equivalent concentration of 5nM showed 51% G2 phase arrest as compared to 30% G2 phase arrest with unconjugated nanoparticles at the same concentration at 24hrs. The block in G2 phase was found to be time and concentration dependent. At 48hrs, there is no significant difference between the effects of conjugated and unconjugated nanoparticles at 10nM concentration. Similarly, RGD conjugated drug encapsulated liposomal system was found to have significantly high arrest of cell cycle as compared to unconjugated system at same concentrations. The cell cycle arrest was found to be concentration and time dependent.

Cell cycle analysis demonstrated that all free DC, PLGA-DC and PLGA-DC-RGD arrested BT-20 cells in the G-2 phase of the cell cycle. However, in cells treated with PLGA-DC and PLGA-DC-RGD, the appearance of populations shown to be in G-2 was found to be more by at least 2 fold as compared to those treated with free DC. Further, the accumulation of cells in G-2 was accompanied by a 7-8 fold decrease in the number of cells in S phase compared to control cells, an indication of DNA replication inhibition. Blank PLGA and RGD peptide alone had no effect on cell cycle progression when applied using the same range of concentrations as PLGA-DC and PLGA-DC-RGD.

The apoptosis and necrosis effect was found to be concentration and time dependent for both types of drug delivery systems. In case of nanoparticles, the RGD conjugated nanoparticles have more apoptotic cell fragments than the unconjugated nanoparticles and drug solution at the same drug equivalent concentrations. At 24 hrs, the treatment of 5nM of drug solution with cells resulted in 13.6% & 3.4 % necrotic & apoptotic cell fragments respectively. While at similar drug equivalent concentration, the PLGA-DC-RGD and PLGA-DC nanoparticles showed 6.4% & 28.3% and 5.1% & 25.6% necrotic & apoptotic cell fragments respectively. At 72hrs, the percent apoptotic cell fragments were significantly high for targeted nanoparticles as compared to untargeted nanoparticles and drug solution at 5nM concentration. While at 72hrs, the 5nM drug solution had significant high necrotic cell fragments as compared to targeted and untargeted Nanoparticulate systems. The free drug has found to have two mode of action at two different concentrations. At 5nM concentration it produces significantly high necrosis and low apoptosis. While at 10nM concentration the observed effect was reversed i.e. high apoptosis and low necrosis. The necrosis effect was significantly low in case of targeted and untargeted nanoparticles at both concentrations. At 10nM drug eq. concentration, the PLGA-DC-RGD nanoparticles have shown to be significantly high percentage of apoptosis with compared to same concentration of drug solution at all time points i.e. 24hrs, 48hrs and 72hrs. However the difference is insignificant with compared to PLGA-DC nanoparticles. Similar kinds of effects were observed with liposomal systems also.

9.2. Conclusions

To conclude, docetaxel encapsulated PLGA loaded nanoparticles and liposomes, and docetaxel conjugated HPMA copolymer were successfully prepared using solvent evaporation, Supercritical CO_2 as anti-solvent method and free radical polymerization techniques respectively. Cyclic RGD peptide was attached to these nanoconstructs to impart ability to target breast cancer. The characterization of nanoparticles and liposomes demonstrated small particle size (< 300nm) suitable for intravenous administration, optimum drug encapsulation and prolonged drug release. The intracellular uptake of nanoparticles and liposomes loaded with fluorescent dye 6-coumarin showed significantly higher cell uptake after RGD conjugation of nanoparticles due to the receptor mediated uptake through the RGD receptors located on the BT-20 and MDA-MB-231 breast cancer cells. The HPMA-docetaxel copolymer conjugates were found to have high molecular weight (>30KDa), optimum drug content .Hydrolysis of conjugates by lysosomal enzyme to release drug for pharmacological response was found to be above 50% of conjugated drug when assessed *in-vitro* by Cathepsin B enzyme hydrolysis.

The docetaxel encapsulated liposomes were found to be more effective than PLGA nanoparticles, HPMA copolymer conjugates and free drug solutions at equivalent drug concentrations when assessed for cytotoxicity, DNA content and mode of cell death analysis.

The difference may be attributed to the quick drug release inside the cytoplasm from the liposomes due to the rapid hydrolysis of pegylated lipid membranes. Drug release from PLGA nanoparticles was slow due to the more hydrophobic nature of PLGA and slow biodegradability of the surface ester bonds and hence, had moderate chemotherapeutic efficacy for prolonged period. The docetaxel conjugates with HPMA copolymer with tetrapeptidyl linker (Gly-Phe-Leu-Gly), cleave by endolysosomal proteases after endocytic uptake by the cells and are stable in circulation. The cleavage of the linkage delays the drug release inside the cell and hence, chemotherapeutic efficacy of the conjugates. But, chemotherapeutic response of the conjugates was prolonged to the maximum extent compared to other nanoconstructs prepared in this investigation. Chemotherapeutic efficacy of RGD conjugation to any of nanoconstructs prepared in this investigation was found to be more than those nanoconstructs without RGD conjugation. All nanoconstructs formulations were found to be stable for six months when stored at refrigerated condition (2-8°C). The in vitro serum drug release data suggest that the nanoparticles release least (6.5%) drug in 24hrs followed by liposomes (35%) HPMA copolymer conjugates (above 50%).

The RGD attachment via a Glycyl- glyceine non cleavable linkage makes drug HPMA conjugates fairly stable in blood circulation and surface density of RGD is also maximum compared to drug nanoparticles and liposomes providing most target specific drug delivery. Moreover the drug release been slower, it provides prolonged chemotherapeutic response and also helps in prevention of development of drug resistance. These benefits made RGD attached docetaxel HPMA conjugates most attractive among the nanoconstructs studied in this investigation. The advantages are also in terms of ease of chemical synthesis of HPMA copolymer conjugates in high quantity and least expensive set of equipment requirement favoring scale up of developed technology as compared to liposomes or nanoparticles. However, more extensive animal experimentation in terms of chemotherapeutic efficacy and side effects are necessary to take up findings of this investigation to clinical evaluations.

CPSIA information can be obtained
at www.ICGtesting.com
Printed in the USA
BVHW052241160423
662367BV00001B/97

9 781805 251996